Pathways of Care in Vascular Surgery

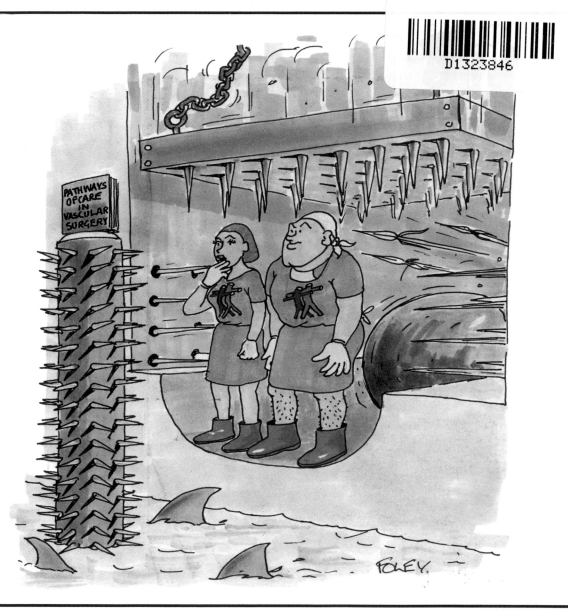

Edited by
Jonathan D Beard &
Shelagh Murray

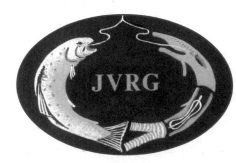

Publisher

tfm Publishing Limited
Castle Hill Barns
Harley
Shrewsbury
SY5 6LX
UK

Tel: +44 (0)1952 510061
Fax: +44 (0)1952 510192
E-mail: nikki@tfmpublishing.co.uk
Web site: www.tfmpublishing.co.uk

Design and layout: Nikki Bramhill
Cartoons: Barry Foley

First Edition   June 2002

ISBN 1 903378 09 5

Printed by Ebenezer Baylis & Son Ltd.
The Trinity Press
London Road
Worcester
WR5 2JH
UK

Tel: +44 (0)1905 357979
Fax: +44 (0)1905 354919

Contents

Contributors

Editors

JD Beard MB BS BSc ChM FRCS, Consultant Vascular Surgeon, Sheffield Vascular Institute, The Northern General Hospital, Sheffield.

S Murray RGN BSc (Hons), Senior Clinical Nurse, Department of Vascular Surgery, St. George's Hospital, London.

Sub-Editors

P Dobson BSc MBChB FRCA, Consultant Anaesthetist, Sheffield Vascular Institute, The Northern General Hospital, Sheffield.

MJ Gough ChM FRCS, Consultant Vascular Surgeon, Vascular Surgical Unit, The General Infirmary at Leeds, Leeds.

S Johnson BSc (Hons) RGN PGCEA RNT, Director, Venture Training & Consulting Ltd, Chichester, & Editor, Journal of Integrated Care Pathways (published by the Royal Society of Medicine Press, London).

C McGrath MSc BSc (Hons) RGN, JVRG Co-ordinator & Senior Research Nurse, Vascular Studies Unit, Bristol Royal Infirmary, Bristol.

JA Michaels MChir FRCS, Consultant Vascular Surgeon, Sheffield Vascular Institute, The Northern General Hospital, Sheffield.

P Morris-Vincent BSc (Hons) RGN, Nurse Specialist, The Royal Free Hospital, London.

BMF Ridler MB ChB, Vascular Research Associate, Royal Devon and Exeter Hospital, Exeter.

A Watkinson BSc MSc (Oxon) MBBS FRCS (Eng) FRCR, Consultant Radiologist, The Royal Free Hospital, London.

Web site Co-ordinator

SJA Baker BSc (Hons) Dip N RGN, Deputy Theatre Manager/Vascular Surgical Assistant, The Vascular Surgical Unit, Royal Bournemouth Hospital, Bournemouth.

J Andrew MSc RGN Cert Ed, Community Dialysis Sister, Renal Unit, Morriston Hospital, Swansea.

M Aukett BSc RN, Vascular Nurse Practitioner, Department of Vascular Surgery, Guy's & St. Thomas' Hospital, London.

DM Baker BSc PhD FRCS, Consultant Vascular Surgeon, Department of Surgery, The Royal Free Hospital, London.

DK Beattie MD FRCS (Gen Surg) FRCSI, Specialist Registrar, Imperial College School of Medicine, Charing Cross Hospital, London.

T Beresford MB BS FRCS, Research Fellow in Vascular Surgery, Department of Vascular Surgery, Charing Cross Hospital, London.

PHB Blair MD FRCS, Consultant Vascular Surgeon, Regional Vascular Unit, Royal Victoria Hospital, Belfast, Northern Ireland.

A Bradbury BSc MD FRCS, Professor of Vascular Surgery, University of Birmingham and Birmingham Heartlands Hospital, Birmingham.

AS Brown MB BS FRCS (Ed), Specialist Registrar in Vascular Surgery, Northern Vascular Centre, Freeman Hospital, Newcastle-upon-Tyne.

WB Campbell MS FRCP FRCS, Professor and Consultant Surgeon, Department of Surgery, Royal Devon and Exeter Hospital, Exeter.

H Chant BSc (Hons) MB BS FRCS, Specialist Registrar, Vascular Surgery, Derriford Hospital, Plymouth.

MJ Clarke MD FRCS (Ed) FRCS (Vasc), Consultant Vascular Surgeon, Northern Vascular Centre, Freeman Hospital, Newcastle-upon-Tyne.

T Cleveland FRCS FRCR, Consultant Vascular Radiologist, Sheffield Vascular Institute, The Northern General Hospital, Sheffield.

AH Davies MA DM FRCS, Reader in Surgery and Consultant Surgeon, Imperial College School of Medicine, Charing Cross Hospital, London.

K de Brett BSc (Hons) RGN, Pain Nurse, Department of Anaesthetics, Royal Devon and Exeter Hospital, Exeter.

V Ducker BSc RN, Staff Nurse, Exeter Vascular Service, Royal Devon and Exeter Hospital, Exeter.

S Dugdill RGN BSc MA, Vascular Nurse Practitioner, Northern Vascular Centre, Freeman Hospital, Newcastle-upon-Tyne.

JJ Earnshaw DM FRCS, Consultant Vascular Surgeon, Department of Vascular Surgery, Gloucestershire Royal Hospital, Gloucester.

N Edwards MB BS FRCA, Consultant in Pain Management, Chronic Pain Clinic, The Northern General Hospital, Sheffield.

M Ellis AVT, Chief Vascular Technologist, Imperial College School of Medicine, Charing Cross Hospital, London.

CJ Ferguson MB ChB FRCS MCh, Consultant Surgeon, Department of Surgery, Morriston Hospital, Swansea.

LJ Fligelstone MB BCh FRCS (Eng) FRCS (Gen), Consultant Surgeon, Department of Surgery, Morriston Hospital, Swansea.

P Gaines MRCP FRCR, Consultant Vascular Radiologist, Sheffield Vascular Institute, The Northern General Hospital, Sheffield.

RB Galland MD FRCS, Consultant Vascular Surgeon, Department of Surgery, Royal Berkshire Hospital, Reading.

C Gibbons MA DPhil MCh FRCS, Consultant Vascular and General Surgeon, Department of Vascular Surgery, Morriston Hospital, Swansea.

GL Gilling-Smith MS FRCS, Consultant Vascular Surgeon, Regional Vascular Unit, Royal Liverpool University Hospital, Liverpool.

S Gough MD FRCP, Reader in Medicine, University of Birmingham and Birmingham Heartlands Hospital, Birmingham.

GD Griffiths MD FRCS, Consultant Vascular Surgeon, Department of Vascular Surgery, Ninewells Hospital, Dundee.

G Hamilton FRCS, Consultant Vascular Surgeon, University Department of Surgery, The Royal Free Hospital & University College Medical School, London.
BP Heather MS FRCS, Consultant Vascular Surgeon, Department of Vascular Surgery, Gloucestershire Royal Hospital, Gloucester.
B Higgs MB BS MSc FRCA, Consultant Vascular Anaesthetist, The Royal Free Hospital, London.
M Horner RGN Cert. Ed., Vascular Nurse Specialist, Department of Vascular Surgery, Southampton General Hospital, Southampton.
SP Hutchinson BSc MBChB MRCP FRCA, Consultant in Anaesthesia and Intensive Care, Department of Critical Care, Sheffield Teaching Hospitals Trust, Sheffield.
C Jackson MSc Exercise and Health Science, Smoking Cessation Co-ordinator, North and East Devon Health Authority, Exeter.
C Johnstone RGN CMS BSc (Hons) MSc, Lecturer in Nursing, University of Dundee, Dundee.
C Judge RGN, Vascular Research Sister, Department of Surgery, The Royal Free Hospital, London.
SP Kelley MB ChB, Senior House Officer, Vascular Surgical Unit, The General Infirmary at Leeds, Leeds.
K Khaw MA MRCP FRCR, Consultant Radiologist, Department of Radiology, St George's Hospital, London.
PM Lamont MA MD FRCS, Consultant Vascular Surgeon, Vascular Surgery Unit, Bristol Royal Infirmary, Bristol.
NJM London MB ChB MD FRCS FRCP (Edin), Professor of Surgery and Honorary Consultant Vascular Surgeon, Leicester University and University Hospitals of Leicester Trust, Leicester.
S Macdonald FRCR, Endovascular Fellow, Sheffield Vascular Institute, The Northern General Hospital, Sheffield.
P MacIntyre FRCA, Consultant Anaesthetist, Department of Anaesthetics, Royal Devon and Exeter Hospital, Exeter.
JG McClements RGN, Vascular Ward Sister, Regional Vascular Unit, Royal Victoria Hospital, Belfast, Northern Ireland.
R Morgan FRCR, Consultant Vascular Radiologist, St George's Hospital, London.
SA Murray BSc (Hons) Dip HSM RGN, Clinical Research Nurse, Regional Vascular Unit, Royal Victoria Hospital, Belfast, Northern Ireland.
F Myint FRCS, Consultant Vascular Surgeon, University Department of Surgery, The Royal Free Hospital & University College Medical School, London.
AR Naylor MD FRCS, Consultant Vascular Surgeon and Honorary Reader in Surgery, The Department of Surgery, Faculty of Medicine and Biological Sciences, Leicester Royal Infirmary, Leicester.
C Nocton RGN, Vascular Nurse Specialist and Cardiology Project Manager, Swindon and Marlborough NHS Trust, Swindon.
S Palfreyman BSc (Hons) RGN MSc, Research Nurse, Sheffield Vascular Institute, The Northern General Hospital, Sheffield.
D Parkin MSc RGN, Consultant Nurse, Department of Vascular Surgery, Gloucestershire Royal Hospital, Gloucester.
JA Potterton RGN BSc (Hons), Vascular Nurse, Department of Surgery, Royal Berkshire Hospital, Reading.
JF Reidy FRCR FRCP, Consultant Radiologist, Department of Radiology, Guy's & St. Thomas' Hospital, London.
JE Scoble MA MD FRCP, Consultant Nephrologist, Department of Nephrology, Guy's & St. Thomas' Hospital, London.
E Shaw SRN, Aneurysm Screening Co-ordinator, Department of Vascular Surgery, Gloucestershire Royal Hospital, Gloucester.
C Shearman BSc (Hons) MS FRCS, Professor of Vascular Surgery, Department of Vascular Surgery, Southampton General Hospital, Southampton.
FCT Smith BSc MD FRCS FRCSEd FRCS (Glas), Consultant Senior Lecturer in Vascular Surgery, Vascular Surgery Unit, Bristol Royal Infirmary, Bristol.
PR Taylor MA MChir FRCS, Consultant Vascular Surgeon, Department of Vascular Surgery, Guy's & St. Thomas' Hospital, London.
T Theophilus RGN Dip. Health/Fitness, Specialist in Therapeutic Exercise, The Royal Free Hospital, London.
M Thomas MS FRCS, Consultant Vascular Surgeon, Chairman Surrey Vascular Group, St. Peters Hospital, Chertsey, Surrey.
JF Thompson MS FRCSEd FRCS, Consultant Surgeon, Exeter Vascular Service, Royal Devon and Exeter Hospital, Exeter.
A Tiwari MRCS, Clinical Research Fellow, University Department of Surgery, The Royal Free Hospital & University College Medical School, London.
H Trender RGN RM, Vascular Nurse Specialist, Sheffield Vascular Institute, The Northern General Hospital, Sheffield.
J Tsui MA MB BChir MRCS, Vascular Research Registrar, The Royal Free Hospital, London.
R Vallabhaneni FRCS (Gen Surg), Endovascular Fellow, Regional Vascular Unit, Royal Liverpool University Hospital, Liverpool.
V Vijayan MRCS, Vascular Research Fellow, Vascular Surgery Unit, Bristol Royal Infirmary, Bristol.
A Wallbridge RGN DipCBT DipAcc, Clinical Nurse Specialist, Chronic Pain Clinic, The Northern General Hospital, Sheffield.
AR Warin MD FRCP, Consultant Dermatologist, Royal Devon and Exeter Hospital, Exeter.
D White MSc RGN, Executive Nurse, Exeter Primary Care Trust, Exeter.
B Whitman BA (Hons), Research Co-ordinator, Department of Vascular Surgery, Gloucestershire Royal Hospital, Gloucester.
A Williams RN MSc, Vascular Nurse Specialist, Department of Vascular Surgery, Charing Cross Hospital, London.
L Wilson RGN, Vascular Research Sister, Northern Vascular Centre, Freeman Hospital, Newcastle-upon-Tyne.
MG Wyatt MSc MD FRCS, Consultant Vascular Surgeon, Northern Vascular Centre, Freeman Hospital, Newcastle-upon-Tyne.

Foreword

Following the success of its last symposium and book entitled *The Evidence for Vascular Surgery*, the Joint Vascular Research Group (JVRG) brings you Pathways of Care in Vascular Surgery. This book describes recent developments and best practice in vascular surgery, with an emphasis on multi-disciplinary care pathways. It is based upon a symposium held in Sheffield in June 2002, which aimed to improve the provision and equality of care for patients with peripheral arterial and venous disease. Many members of the JVRG have contributed to this book, including vascular surgeons, anaesthetists, radiologists, nurses and vascular technologists.

The book consists of five sections covering the main areas of management of patients with peripheral vascular disease: out-patients and medical management; vascular imaging and endovascular intervention; vascular surgery; anaesthesia and theatres; and organisational aspects of care. We have focused on the most important aspects of care rather than the comprehensive approach of larger (and more expensive) textbooks. Each chapter describes a care pathway based on pragmatism and the evidence, where available. Each chapter lists one or more books for further reading rather than exhaustive references. The following books complement this one:

◆   The Evidence for Vascular Surgery. Earnshaw JJ and Murie JA (eds). tfm Publishing Limited, 1999.

◆   Vascular and Endovascular Surgery, 2nd Edition. Beard JD and Gaines PA (eds). WB Saunders, 2001.

◆   Vascular Disease: Nursing and Management. Murray S (ed). Whurr Publishers, 2001

We have used a simplified classification of grading evidence and recommendations for use with clinical guidelines, recently developed by Jonathan Michaels. This is referenced in the text by the appropriate bold numeral or letter in brackets. The classification is outlined below:

Grading of Evidence

I   Beyond reasonable doubt

Evidence from high quality randomised controlled trials, systematic reviews, decision analyses, cost-effectiveness analyses or large observational data-sets which is directly applicable to the population of concern and has clear results.

II   On the balance of probabilities

Evidence of "best practice" from a high quality review of the literature, which fails to reach the highest standard of proof due to heterogenicity, questionable trial methodology or lack of evidence in the population to which the guidelines apply.

III Unproven

Contradictory evidence or insufficient evidence upon which to base a decision.

Grading of Recommendations

A A strong recommendation, which should be followed unless there are compelling reasons not to do so.

B Recommendation based on evidence of effectiveness that may need interpretation in the light of other factors (e.g. patient preferences, local facilities, local audit results or available resources).

C Recommendation where there is inadequate evidence on effectiveness but pragmatic or financial reasons to institute an agreed policy.

One reason for writing this book was to pool the valuable expertise that the members of the JVRG possess with regard to care pathways. Integrated care pathways and their related protocols take many hours to write and further work to validate. It was not possible to include all the associated paperwork, protocols and forms in this book. These can be found on the JVRG website at **www.jvrg.org** and are referenced in the relevant chapters. We hope that this website will become a dynamic resource for the development of care pathways in the future. Please download those that seem of use to you, adapt them as required and return them to us with any improvements.

This book represents an exciting move towards multi-disciplinary care in peripheral arterial and venous disease. We hope it stimulates you to develop your own pathways of care without needing to reinvent the wheel!

Jonathan D Beard MB BS BSc ChM FRCS
Consultant Vascular Surgeon
Sheffield Vascular Institute
Northern General Hospital

Shelagh Murray RGN, BSc (Hons)
Senior Clinical Nurse
Department of Vascular Surgery
St George's Hospital, London

Chapter 1

Nurse-led claudication clinics

Simon Palfreyman Research Nurse

Hazel Trender Vascular Nurse Specialist

SHEFFIELD VASCULAR INSTITUTE, THE NORTHERN GENERAL HOSPITAL, SHEFFIELD, UK

Introduction

The effective management of patients referred to the vascular out-patient clinic with possible intermittent claudication has implications for both the patient and health service providers. The patients who are presenting with a referral for intermittent claudication (IC) are likely to be those people whose symptoms are having some impact on their life-style. In addition to their physical symptoms these patients can have significant emotional requirements, with feelings of powerlessness and frustration [1]. The patients therefore have complex symptoms and emotional requirements that can have significant resource implications.

The patients may need multiple hospital appointments for investigations and subsequent management. This can have an impact on the out-patient service provided by medical staff as adequate time has to be allocated for this process. There is also a need to ensure that IC is correctly diagnosed, risk factors identified and modified, patients selected that may benefit from intervention and to detect those that might be at risk of limb loss due to impending critical limb ischaemia.

One method of organising the out-patient service, and making the most effective use of time and resources, is to use specialist vascular nurses to provide a nurse-led out-patient claudication clinic. The Government has advocated such nurse-led clinics in the NHS Plan [2] as a way of extending the scope of nursing practice and meeting NHS targets. Nurse-led clinics have become established in pre-operative assessment [3, 4], oncology [5], respiratory medicine [6,7], leg ulcer care [8, 9], and a number of other specialities. The clinics seem to be well received by patients [10] and to have some impact on patient outcomes [5,7].

Intermittent claudication

Intermittent claudication is a consequence of atherosclerotic peripheral arterial disease (PAD) and is present in around 19% of the population [11,12]. It has been defined as cramping leg muscle pain caused by

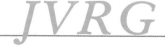

Figure 1 A pathway of care for a nurse-led claudication clinic.

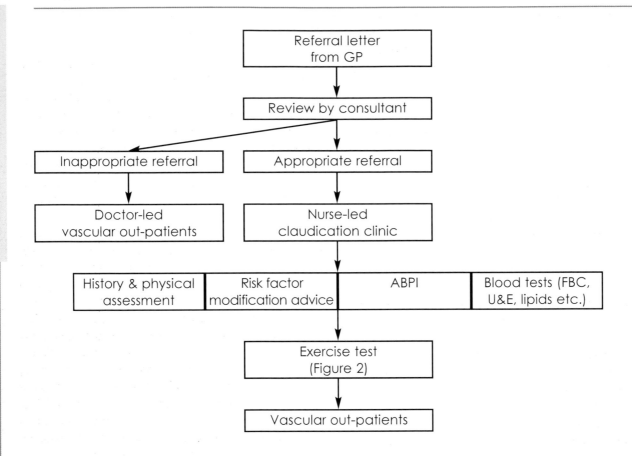

exercise and rapidly relieved by rest [13]. The prevalence of patients experiencing symptoms of IC in the general population is between 2.2 and 4.5% [11,14]. The prevalence increases with age and 6% over the age of 85 report symptoms of IC [11]. The most common cause of claudication is narrowing or occlusion of the iliac and femoral arteries [15] (I).

Intermittent claudication is a subjective experience with patient reporting of their walking distance perceived as unreliable by medical staff [16]. It can also be difficult to measure in a reliable fashion using objective measures. Treadmill exercise tests may not have any relationship to the patient's normal walking pace or total distance they are able to walk pain-free [17].

Although IC is a chronic condition it can be relatively benign; the risk of symptom progression has been estimated at between 10 and 25% [13,15]. Furthermore, patients can also spontaneously improve in terms of their symptoms and walking distance [15]. The main aims of treatment are to prevent symptom progression, improve symptoms and to decrease morbidity and mortality. The basis of treatment has been summed-up in the phrase "stop smoking and start walking" [18].

Intermittent claudication is an indicator of systemic atherosclerosis [19] (I). Claudicants have an increased risk of mortality of between 2 and 4% compared to the general population and patients with asymptomatic PAD [13]. The increased mortality for this group of patients is usually from ischaemic heart disease or cerebrovascular disease. The risk of limb loss due to PAD, and the associated need for revascularisation is much lower than the risk of having a MI or stroke [20].

Nurse-led clinics

Nurse-led clinics are as a result of a number of factors including the reduction in junior doctors' hours and response to local service needs. The trend is likely to be for an increase in the scope and extent of such clinics as they are perceived by the Government as a way of reducing out-patient waiting times [21]. In addition, nurse-led clinics are broadly welcomed by the nursing profession and are seen as a way of increasing job satisfaction and having a positive impact on patient care [22].

The evidence for the effectiveness of nurse-led services is very mixed with few rigorous evaluations [23] - this is especially true from an economic perspective. There is some evidence to suggest that nurse-led clinics can have an impact on risk factor modification in terms of diet, physical activity and compliance with drug treatment [24] **(I)**. Other benefits that have been cited include holistic assessment, decreased waiting times, screening, ensuring consistency, health promotion and health education [5]. One large randomised controlled trial did find that nurse-led services were at least equivalent to house officers in terms of cost and quality and that nurses order fewer inappropriate tests [25] **(I)**. Nurses are also no more likely to make mistakes in their new roles compared with doctors but clear structures are needed when establishing these services for risk assessment and clinical governance [26].

Any nurse-led services should be focused on improving patient care and not just a way for nurses to take on some of the roles previously undertaken by medical staff [26]. For such clinics to be effective there has to be clearly defined roles for both the medical and nursing staff if there is to be no negative impact on patient care [27]. However, the provision of such clinics, in common with other clinical nurse specialist roles, has been haphazard and there have been no corresponding developments in terms of job descriptions, educational requirements or training [28].

Nurse-led vascular clinics

Nurse-led vascular clinics, in common with initiatives in other such areas, are a response to the need to meet Government targets on waiting times. However, any expansion of the role of nursing staff must be based on the principle of being of benefit to patients and not purely as a way of offloading tasks from medical staff to nurses. Therefore, such clinics must be evaluated for their cost-effectiveness and impact on patient outcomes.

There has been only one published evaluation of a nurse-led clinic for patients with intermittent claudication [29]. This was a questionnaire based patient satisfaction survey of 41 patients attending the clinic. The study revealed high levels of satisfaction with the service provided and no negative feelings of the patients to being seen by a nurse rather than a doctor. However, there is a need for a more rigorous study involving proper costings and assessment of outcomes.

Nurse-led clinics provide most benefit where there are clearly defined care pathways and guidelines [30] **(I)**. One of the main reasons for this is that nurses are more able to adhere to guidelines, find them reassuring and can provide care equivalent to standard medical care. This can be compared with doctors who tend to dislike the restrictions care pathways place on their autonomy and authority [31]. The advantages of having clearly defined care pathways include decreasing costs, improving communication, allowing audit against agreed standards, and ability to include clinical governance systems [32,33,34]. However, there have been no randomised controlled trials conducted to evaluate the impact of care pathways [34]. The disadvantages include the need for a champion, inflexibility and need for constant review [34]

Clinic configuration

There are three possible configurations of nurse-led clinics for intermittent claudication:

- ◆ Primary assessment. Patients are seen by the nurse prior to them attending to see the medical staff.

- ◆ Follow-up. Patients are seen by the medical staff and then referred to the nursing staff for follow-up.

- ◆ Primary assessment plus follow-up. Patients are seen by the nurse for assessment and follow-up.

In Sheffield we have adopted the primary assessment model where the nurse sees the patient first (Figure 1).

Figure 2 Investigation of suspected intermittent claudication.

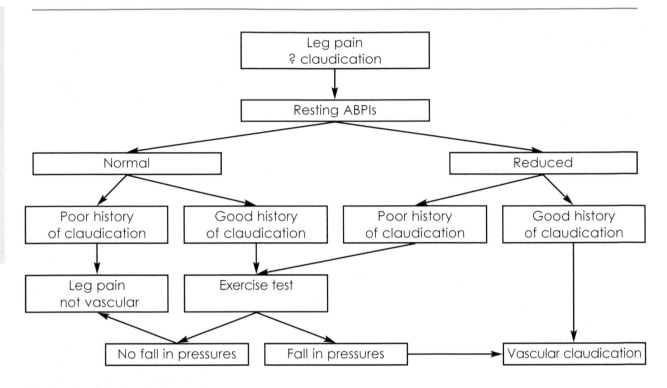

Primary assessment clinic

The main ethos of setting the clinics up in this fashion is for the nurses to take a structured history and physical assessment, order blood tests and other investigations, plus provide life-style modification and smoking cessation advice. The patients are then brought back to the vascular out-patients for review by the medical staff who have all the information on which to base a clinical decision.

Patient identification

The identification of patients with intermittent claudication referred to vascular clinics by GPs can be difficult. Review of the referral letters by a consultant vascular surgeon can minimise the number of patients referred to the nurse-led clinic with other conditions.

History taking and physical examination

History taking and physical examination have been identified as one of the most time consuming tasks undertaken by junior medical staff [35]. The value of nursing staff undertaking these tasks are that it frees up medical staff to see other patients and undertake other tasks. A comparison of nurses and junior medical staff performing physical assessments showed that nurse specialists were as effective as the medical staff in conducting physical assessments [25] **(I)**. The study also found that from an economic perspective the use of appropriately trained nurses was cost neutral.

Physical assessment using specific forms and guidelines to assist the assessor are helpful in ensuring that a complete examination is undertaken (see website). The assessment of patients should

Chapter 1

include examination of foot pulses, popliteal and femoral pulses, blood pressure, ankle-brachial pressure index (ABPI), past medical history, self-reported claudication distance, and risk factor assessment (including smoking). The following blood tests are requested: FBC, ESR, U&E, Lipids, Glucose, LFTs and HbA1c if diabetic.

Smoking cessation

Medical staff can often miss opportunities to promote smoking cessation in their patients [36]. Nurses can provide valuable information to the patients on how to stop smoking in nurse-led clinics [37] (I). Providing training in smoking cessation techniques increases the frequency of patients stopping smoking but has not been proved conclusively to have any effect on patient outcome [38] (I). The problem with smoking cessation advice appears to be that patients either ignore it or are unable to stop smoking. The chapter on smoking cessation explores this topic in more detail.

Exercise

Advice to the patient to take more exercise does not appear to have much effect [39]. Exercise programmes have been shown to increase the pain free distance claudicants can walk [40] (I) but there have been doubts expressed regarding the over estimation of their treatment effect [15]. The value of structured exercise programmes to the population of claudicants as a whole is likely to be limited to those who are able to follow the programmes and there has been no evaluation of long-term compliance (see chapter on exercise programmes).

Cholesterol

Drug therapy to lower cholesterol has been shown to be of benefit in preventing deterioration of patients with lower limb atherscleorosis [41] (I). Dietary advice given by dieticians or nurses rather than medical staff has been shown to reduce cholesterol [42] (II). However, this was based on a systematic review that included relatively poor evidence and a low number of trials (see chapter on risk factor modification).

Patient education

Patient education within the nurse-led clinic should be centred on risk factor modification. The nurse should draw up goals with the patient for any changes in life-style that the patient may need to implement. These goals need to be specific to each patient, measurable and realistic [43]. We have found information leaflets to be extremely useful in this respect (see website).

Further investigation

There are many causes of leg pain that can occur in the presence of asymptomatic PAD. Therefore, the presence of pulses does not necessarily imply a causal link. Furthermore, the presence of pulses at rest does not exclude symptomatic PAD. A good history together with an ABPI < 0.9 confirms the diagnosis without the need for further tests.

Exercise testing provides an objective measurement of walking distance, and highlights other exercise-limiting conditions such as arthritis and breathlessness. However, exercise testing takes time, and many elderly patients find it difficult to walk on a treadmill. Only those with a good history of claudication and normal resting ABPIs require an exercise test (Figure 2).

An audit of a primary assessment clinic

A recent audit of the vascular nurse specialist claudication clinic in Sheffield showed the benefits such a service can provide. The clinic was established because the waiting times for a routine vascular out-patient appointment exceeded 5 months. A routine audit of the medical records found that risk factors had often not been recorded and blood tests not requested despite a specific proforma. A subsequent audit of the medical records of 56 patients in the first year of the primary assessment clinic revealed 100% recording of risk factors and blood tests. Only 29% patients had had their cholesterol checked by their GP and only 41% had been prescribed low-dose aspirin despite primary health care guidelines.

The audit also highlighted the problems of giving verbal and leaflet advice to patients to encourage smoking cessation. Only one smoker had stopped smoking at follow-up in the vascular out-patients. The overwhelming outcome for 82% of the patients subsequently seen by the medical staff in the vascular clinic was "discharge with no further appointment". This suggests that the clinic could be converted into a nurse only clinic - dependent upon sufficient clinical governance and resources.

Medical referral to nurse-led clinics

These types of clinics are usually centred on risk factor modification for those patients who would not benefit from any surgical intervention. The patients are referred to the medical staff by GPs or other agencies, assessed by the medical staff and then their follow-up is undertaken by nursing staff. The main advantage is that the patients can be followed-up by nursing staff and encouraged to make any life-style modifications that may be necessary to improve their claudication. This means that appointment slots can be freed in the medical out-patient clinics for other patients. The disadvantage of this type of clinic is that the patient may need to attend several appointments, for investigations and tests, before the medical staff can complete their assessment and decide on what action is necessary.

Assessment and follow-up

A future direction for nurse-led claudication clinics could be for GP referrals to be directed straight to the nurse. Only those patients who deviate from the normal presentation of claudication, or those where the diagnosis in doubt, are then seen by the medical staff. Such clinics would need clear care pathways and treatment protocols to ensure confidence of the nurses supervising the clinics and also of the medical staff. The clinics would include all aspects of assessment and follow-up for this group of patients. However, the evidence for cost-effectiveness of such clinics is not yet available.

Summary

♦ The evidence for cost-effectiveness of nurse-led claudication clinics is not yet available.

♦ The initial assessment and ordering of investigations prior to medical staff seeing the patient can provide additional out-patient slots and ensure more effective management of patients with claudication (II).

♦ Nurse-led clinics can provide a means of giving patient life-style advice and monitoring their compliance with such advice (III).

♦ Patients with intermittent claudication can be reviewed and managed effectively by nurse-led clinics (II).

♦ Nurse-led clinics should be based on clear, agreed care pathways (B).

♦ Life-style modification advice on exercise, stopping smoking and losing weight should be given by appropriately trained nurses and the patient's compliance with these monitored (B).

Further reading

1   Herbert LM. *Caring for the Vascular Patient.* Churchill Livingstone, London, 1997.

2   Fahey VA. *Vascular Nursing* (3rd Ed). WB Saunders, Philadelphia, 1999.

3   Humphries D, Ed. *The Clinical Nurse Specialist.* Palgrave MacMillan, UK, 1994.

References (grade I evidence and grade A recommendations in bold)

1   Gibson JME, Kenrick M. Pain and powerlessness: the experience of living with peripheral vascular disease. *Journal of Advanced Nursing* 1998; 27(4): 737-45.

2   Department of Health. The NHS Plan. A plan for investment. A plan for reform. DOH, London, 2000.

3   Rushforth H, Bliss A, Burge D, Glasper EA. A pilot randomised controlled trial of medical versus nurse clerking for minor surgery. *Archives of Disease in Childhood* 2000; 83: 223-6.

4   Barnes P. The nurse clinician in surgical services. *Prof Nurse* 2000; 15: 240-3.

5   Loftus LA, Weston V. The development of nurse-led clinics in cancer care. *Journal of Clinical Nursing* 2001; 10(2): 215-20.

6   Gibbons D, Hamilton J, Maw G, Telford J. Developing a nurse-led service for COPD patients. *Prof Nurse* 2001; 16(4): 1035-7.

7   Porter-Jones G, Francis S, Benfield G. Running a nurse-led nebulizer clinic in a district general hospital. *British Journal of Nursing* 1999; 8: 1079-84.

8   Rotchell L. Introducing and auditing a nurse-led leg ulcer service. *Prof Nurse* 1999; 14: 545-50.

9   Bedo J. A nurse-led service for leg ulcer care. *Community Nurse* 1999; 5: 25.

10   Shaw C, Williams KS, Assassa RP. Patients' views of a new nurse-led continence service. *Journal of Clinical Nursing* 2000; 9: 574-82.

11   Meijer WT *et al*. Peripheral arterial disease in the elderly: The Rotterdam study. *Arteriosclerosis, Thrombosis and Vascular Biology* 1998; 18: 185-92.

12   Hooi JD, Stoffers HE, Knottnerus JA, van Ree JW. The prognosis of non-critical limb ischaemia: a systematic review of population-based evidence. *British Journal of General Practice* 1999; 49: 49-55.

13   Newman AB. Peripheral arterial disease: insights from population studies of older adults. *J Am Geriatr Soc* 2000; 48: 1157-62.

14   Fowkes FG *et al*. Edinburgh Artery Study: prevalence of asymptomatic and symptomatic peripheral arterial disease in the general population. *Int J Epidemiol* 1991; 20: 384-92.

15   Girolami B *et al*. Treatment of intermittent claudication with physical training, smoking cessation, pentoxifylline, or nafronyl: a meta-analysis. *Archives of Internal Medicine* 1999; 159: 337-45.

16   Perakyla T, Lepantalo M. Accuracy of patients own estimate of intermittent claudication. *International Journal of Angiology* 1998; 7: 62-4.

17   Watson CJE, Phillips D, Hands L, Collin J. Claudication distance is poorly estimated and inappropriately measured. *Br J Surg* 1997; 84: 1107-9.

18   Housley E. Treating claudication in five words. *BMJ* 1988; 296: 1483-4.

19   Hiatt WR. Drug therapy. Medical treatment of peripheral arterial disease and claudication. *N Engl J Med* 2001; 344: 1608-21.

20   Weitz J, Byrne J, Clagett P. Diagnosis and treatment of chronic arterial insufficiency of the lower extremities: A critical review. *Circulation* 1996; 94: 3026-49.

21   National Audit Office. Inpatient and out-patient waiting in the NHS. HC 221. HMSO, London, 2002.

22   Royal College of Nursing. Developing a national plan for the new NHS. Nursing's views on NHS modernisation in England. RCN, London, 2001.

23   Rushforth H, Glasper EA. Implications of nursing role expansion for professional practice. *British Journal of Nursing* 1999; 8: 1507-13.

24   Campbell NC *et al*. Secondary prevention in coronary heart disease: a randomised trial of nurse led clinics in primary care. *Heart* 1998; 80: 447-52.

25   Kinley H *et al*. Extended scope of nursing practice: a multicentre randomised controlled trial of appropriately trained nurses and pre-registration house officers in pre-operative assessment in elective general surgery. *Health Technology Assessment* 2001; 5: 1-87.

26   Dowling S *et al*. Nurses taking on junior doctors' work: a confusion of accountability. *BMJ* 1996; 312: 1211-14.

27   Sweet SJ, Norman IJ. The nurse-doctor relationship: a selective literature review. *J Adv Nurs* 1995; 22: 165-70.

28   Bamford O, Gibson F. The clinical nurse specialist: perceptions of practising CNSs of their role and development needs. *Journal of Clinical Nursing* 2000; 9: 282-92.

29   Murray S. A nurse-led clinic for patients with peripheral vascular disease. *British Journal of Nursing* 1997; 6: 726-8.

30   Gooch S. Review: nursing care driven by guidelines improves some process measures and patient outcomes (Cochrane Review, latest version 24 Nov 1998). Cochrane Library 2002; Oxford.

31   Manias E, Street A. Legitimation of nurses' knowledge through policies and protocols in clinical practice. *J Adv Nurs* 2000; 32: 1467-75.

32   Ellis BW, Johnson S. The care pathway: a tool to enhance clinical governance. *Br J Clin Governance* 1999; 4: 61-71.

33   Barker SG *et al*. Integrated care pathways for vascular surgery. *Eur J Vasc Endovasc Surg* 1999; 18: 207-15.

34   Campbell H *et al*. Integrated care pathways. *BMJ* 1998; 316: 133-7.

35   Rushforth H, Warner J, Burge D, Glasper EA. Specialist nursing. Nursing physical assessment skills: implications for UK practice. *British Journal of Nursing* 1998; 7: 965-70.

36   Doescher MP, Saver BG. Physicians' advice to quit smoking. The glass remains half empty. *Journal of Family Practice* 2000; 49: 543-7.

37   West R, McNeill A, Raw M. Smoking cessation guidelines for health professionals: an update. Health Education Authority. *Thorax* 2000; 55: 987-99.

38   Silagy C, Lancaster T, Gray S, Fowler G. Effectiveness of training health professionals to provide smoking cessation interventions: systematic review of randomised controlled trials. *Quality in Health Care* 1994; 3: 193-8.

39   Currie IC, Wilson YG, Baird RN, Lamont PM. Treatment of intermittent claudication: the impact on quality of life. *Eur J Vasc Endovasc Surg* 1996; 10: 356-61.

40   **Gardner AW, Poehlman ET. Exercise rehabilitation programmes for the treatment of claudication pain. A metaanalysis.** *JAMA* **1995; 274: 975-80.**

41   **Leng G, Price J, Jepson R. Lipid-lowering for lower limb atherosclerosis.** *Cochrane Database of Systematic Reviews* **2001; Issue 4, 2001.**

42   Thompson R, Summerbell C, Hooper. Dietary advice given by a dietitian versus other health professional or self-help resources to reduce blood cholesterol. *Cochrane Database of Systematic Reviews* 2001; Issue 4, 2001.

43   Goodall S. Risk factor assessment for patients with peripheral arterial disease. *Prof Nurse* 2001 17(1):27-30.

Chapter 2

Risk factor modification

Simon P Kelley Senior House Officer

Michael J Gough Consultant Vascular Surgeon

Vascular Surgical Unit, The General Infirmary at Leeds, Leeds, UK

Introduction

Atherosclerotic peripheral arterial occlusive disease (PAOD) affects 5-10% of the population aged > 55 years and is a systemic disease. Thus PAOD patients have a similar relative risk of death from myocardial infarction, stroke, and other vascular causes as patients with symptomatic coronary or cerebrovascular disease. These risks are closely linked to the severity of disease, increasing, as the ankle-brachial pressure index becomes lower.

Although the major risk factors for the development and progression of PAOD are well known (smoking, hyperlipidaemia, hypertension, diabetes) modification of these, particularly the management of hyperlipidaemia and the prescription of antiplatelet drugs, is less assiduously pursued than in patients with coronary artery disease [1,2].

In patients with PAOD the aims of treatment are:

- To alleviate disability.

- To prevent disease progression leading to major amputation.

- To reduce the secondary morbidity and mortality from cardiac and cerebrovascular events.

Since 75% of PAOD patients are treated conservatively this chapter focuses upon the modification of risk factors that may have an impact upon progression of atherosclerotic disease in both peripheral vessels and other vascular territories. In this respect, previous work has shown that modification of tobacco use, and control of both hypertension and hypercholesterolaemia is cost-effective (cost/year of life saved) and improves clinical outcomes [3] **(II)**.

Risk factors

Age and sex

Deposition of fatty streaks in major vessels, a precursor of atherosclerosis, commences during childhood and the impact and prevalence of PAOD increases with age. Although more than 90% of patients have at least one risk factor for the development of symptomatic PAOD a minority present

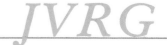

late in life with claudication or other manifestations of PAOD in whom no obvious risk factors are present. Thus atherosclerosis appears to be part of the normal ageing process and in some patients modification of risk factors may have little impact on their future progress.

Symptomatic PAOD is more common and occurs earlier in males, the incidence being twice as high in men below the age of 60 years. Female sex hormones have been proposed as the basis for this difference. After the menopause this effect is reduced and symptomatic disease in women becomes more common. This hypothesis is supported by observational studies suggesting a 50% reduction in cardiac morbidity and mortality in women receiving hormone replacement therapy (HRT). Potential mechanisms for this benefit include alterations in lipid profile (lower LDL and total cholesterol levels), a reduction in serum markers of coagulation, improved insulin sensitivity, a reduction in central body fat, improved endothelium-dependent vasodilatation and a global improvement in systolic cardiac function [4]. However, women taking HRT appear to have fewer risk factors for coronary artery disease and it is unclear whether HRT has a direct effect on the prevalence of coronary artery disease [5] **(II)**. Furthermore HRT therapy in women with established coronary artery disease confers no secondary prevention benefit [6] **(I)** and does not reduce subsequent peripheral arterial events [7] **(I)**.

In contrast, population studies show a decreased risk of developing peripheral vascular disease in women receiving HRT [8] **(I)**. Thus it would appear that the principle benefit of HRT is in the primary prevention of atherosclerotic disease rather than in providing a secondary benefit for patients with established vascular disease, and there is no sound basis for recommending its prescription in female vascular patients.

Smoking

Cigarette smoking is potentially the most preventable cause of cardiovascular morbidity and mortality. Despite the well established association between the two, approximately 70% of patients with atherosclerosis continue to smoke.

Tobacco smoke promotes many potentially atherogenic effects although it remains unclear which of > 4000 active chemicals are most harmful. Both nicotine, via the release of catecholamines, and carbon monoxide (hypoxia) have a major role in the cardiovascular effects of smoking by adversely affecting the myocardial oxygen supply/demand ratio. Other harmful effects of smoking are related to the activity of agents that promote endothelial injury and atherogenesis **(I)**. These include alterations in the lipid profile (reduced HDL and increased LDL, total cholesterol and triglyceride levels) and in haemostatic or haemorrheologic factors (vasoconstriction, platelet activation, increased plasma fibrinogen levels, fibrin degradation products, platelet aggregation, ß-thromboglobulin and blood viscosity). Furthermore rises in circulating tissue plasminogen activator and vWF antigen levels reflect endothelial disruption. Despite this the precise mechanism by which smoking promotes PAOD remains unclear. Nevertheless the circumstantial evidence clearly suggests that it has a major role **(I)**.

Finally, heavy cigarette smoking (> 15 cigarettes/day) appears to counteract the local anti-thrombotic potency of aspirin, which may further increase the risk of arterial occlusion [9] **(II)**.

Free radical-induced oxidation of atherogenic lipoproteins is also promoted by smoking and is associated with a reduction in circulating anti-oxidant levels. Thus vitamin C, ß-carotene, vitamin E and selenium levels are reduced in smokers. Although there is some evidence that smoking directly reduces vitamin C levels it is probable that reduced dietary intake is a more important factor than anti-oxidant consumption. Although these can be replenished by dietary supplementation, and vitamin C replacement appears to reduce oxidative injury [10], there is conflicting evidence that this is of clinical benefit. Thus the Rotterdam Study suggested that high ß-carotene intake reduced the risk of cardiac events in previously asymptomatic subjects and that increases in vitamin C and vitamin E intake improved peripheral vascular disease in women and men respectively [11]. Conversely a randomised trial of dietary supplementation with ß-carotene, ∝-tocopherol, both, or placebo, in patients with known coronary artery disease showed no reduction in future cardiac events

Table 1 Additional benefit over placebo of interventions for smoking cessation.

Treatment	Patient Group	Benefit	95% CI
Simple physician advice	GP/outpatient clinic	2%	1-3%
Specialist behavioural support	Smokers seeking help	7%	3-10%
Specialist behavioural support	Smokers in hospital	4%	0-8%
Written self-help guides	Smokers seeking help	1%	0-2%
Nicotine Replacement Therapy			
gum + limited support	Moderate/heavy smokers	5%	4-6%
gum + intensive support	Moderate/heavy smokers	8%	6-10%
patch + limited support	Moderate/heavy smokers	5%	4-7%
patch + intensive support	Moderate/heavy smokers	6%	5-8%
nasal spray + intensive support	Moderate/heavy smokers	12%	7-17%
inhalator + intensive support	Moderate/heavy smokers	8%	4-12%
sublingual tab + intensive support	Moderate/heavy smokers	8%	1-14%
Other regimes			
Buproprion + intensive support	Moderate/heavy smokers	9%	5-14%
Intensive support + NRT or buproprion	Moderate/heavy smokers who seek help from specialist clinic	13-19%	

CI= Confidence interval

during active treatment and even a possible increase in fatal cardiac events in those receiving ß-carotene or both [12]. Thus there is no sound basis upon which to advise dietary anti-oxidant supplementation for patients with peripheral vascular disease **(III)**.

Finally smoking elicits a significantly higher catecholamine response in hypertensive patients and may reduce the efficacy of anti-hypertensive therapy, particularly with hepatically metabolised ß-blockers such as propranolol.

In summary, smoking is not only an independent risk factor for PAOD but it also enhances the effect of other recognised risk factors **(I)**.

Smoking cessation

An overview of the role of smoking cessation management is considered in another chapter. However it is briefly considered here, as there is evidence that it reduces the risk of developing critical leg ischaemia and the frequency of myocardial infarction and death from other vascular causes in patients with symptomatic PAOD. After 5-10 years abstinence future cardiovascular risk approaches that of non-smokers. Further, a symptomatic improvement in claudication may occur within 3-6 months of cessation due to reversal of haemorrheologic changes and hypoxaemia. Concomitant exercise training may enhance this effect. If symptoms do not improve the risk of starting to smoke again is increased.

Smoking cessation programmes should provide effective education and appropriate aids for PAOD patients to negate the effects of nicotine withdrawal (craving, irritability, anxiety, poor concentration, restlessness, weight gain).

A recent review has collated data from a number of sources, including the Cochrane database, on the efficacy of smoking cessation techniques[13]. This is summarised in Table 1 **(I)**.

Thus a combined approach to smoking cessation involving both pharmacotherapy and psychological support in a dedicated clinic will be most successful **(A)**. Other "life-style changes" such as increased exercise and diet modification can also be encouraged in such a clinic if resources allow.

Hyperlipidaemia

Hyperlipidaemia, as an independent risk factor for PAOD is characterised by:

♦ ↑ total cholesterol, primarily LDL cholesterol.

♦ ↓ in protective HDL cholesterol.

♦ high total: HDL cholesterol ratio (Sheffield table [14]).

♦ ↑ VLDL cholesterol.

♦ ↑ triglycerides (reflecting high non-HDL cholesterol levels).

A systematic review of randomised controlled trials of lipid lowering therapy (diet, cholestyramine, probucol, nicotinic acid) in 698 patients with lower limb atherosclerosis showed that disease progression was reduced together with a non-significant reduction in mortality (0.7% v 2.9%) [15] **(I)**. Several studies also indicate that such therapy stabilises or even promotes femoral and carotid plaque regression, the latter being associated with a reduction in lipid content and inflammation with an increase in tissue inhibitor of metalloproteinase 1 (TIMP-1) and collagen content [16].

Further, five large placebo-controlled randomised trials have shown that statin therapy reduces total mortality and major coronary events by lowering LDL cholesterol levels in patients with coronary artery disease [17] **(I)** whilst in PAOD patients it specifically improves endothelial function, reducing markers of atherosclerotic risk such as serum P-selectin levels [18,19] **(II)**. Finally, in the Scandinavian Simvastatin Survival Study the relative risk of new or worsening claudication in patients receiving simvastatin was 0.6 compared to those given placebo [20] **(I)**. Thus patients with PAOD will benefit from lipid lowering therapy, particularly if they have co-existing coronary artery or cerebrovascular disease.

The aims of treatment for hyperlipidaemias should be to:

♦ ↓ LDL cholesterol to < 2.6mmol/l.

♦ ↓ triglycerides to < 1.7mmol/l.

♦ ↓ total cholesterol to < 5.0 mmol/l.

Since even rigorous dietary manipulation is unlikely to achieve a >10% reduction in these parameters active therapy with a statin is usually advised **(A)**, particularly in view of the potential effects on plaque regression.

Niacin might also be prescribed as this independently increases serum HDL cholesterol levels and lowers serum triglyceride concentrations [21] **(I)**, **(B)**. The effect of niacin on the lipid profile is complex with a reduction in LDL-cholesterol occurring at higher doses (>1500mg/day) whereas an increase in HDL-cholesterol occurs at a lower dose (1500mg/day). This may be important since the main drawback of niacin therapy is its side effect profile (flushing, palpitations, impaired diabetic control). Its use should therefore be limited to patients with severe hyperlipidaemia in whom the side effects can be closely monitored.

Hyperlipidaemia and an unsatisfactory diet are often associated with obesity. Whilst this is not an independent risk factor for PAOD it is likely to be associated with a sedentary life-style and worsening claudication. A strict "low cholesterol" diet should result in weight reduction and improved exercise tolerance.

Chapter 2

Irrespective of cholesterol levels the Heart Protection Study [22] (unpublished) suggests that all patients with symptomatic atherosclerosis should be treated with a statin to reduce vascular mortality.

Diet

The low incidence of atherosclerotic disease in Mediterranean countries and in Greenlandic Eskimos is well recognised and is believed to be related to dietary factors (II). The Mediterranean diet is rich in olive oil, the main constituent of which, oleic acid, directly interferes with the inflammatory response that characterises early atherogenesis. Oleic acid is incorporated into total cell lipids in preference to saturated fatty acids and reduces the expression of adhesion molecules in the endothelium, thereby reducing monocyte recruitment in the intimal layer of arteries. This appears to have a role in preventing atherosclerosis [23].

The Eskimo diet is known to be rich in eicosapentanoic acid, which has a significant effect on platelet reactivity and reducing plasma lipid concentrations, particularly of triglycerides. This may explain why a diet rich in fish oils reduces the risk of atherosclerotic disease in this population [24].

Despite the apparently beneficial effect of these diets there are no prospective studies that examine their benefit in the secondary prevention of vascular complications in patients with established atherosclerosis although fish oils are used in the management of patients with hypertriglyceridaemia. Similarly although it is recommended that a Western diet includes five portions of fruit or vegetables/day, which increases antioxidant intake and may reduce lipoprotein lipid peroxidation and cellular accumulation of cholesterol, its value has not been fully assessed.

Diabetes mellitus

Tight control of blood glucose in diabetic patients reduces the risk of microvascular and cardiac complications. However neither the Diabetes Control and Complication Trial [25] nor the United Kingdom Prospective Diabetes Study [26] (a total of > 5000 patients) reported a significant reduction in the complication rates from PAOD (I). Nevertheless careful control of blood sugar levels are clearly desirable, particularly in patients who may have other risk factors (C).

Hypertension

Blood pressure increases with age and thus it is difficult to provide clear guidelines as to when active treatment is required. However hypertension is associated with an increased risk of stroke, MI, heart failure, renal impairment and peripheral vascular disease, this being 2-3 times that of a normotensive population [27,28] (I). Thus a blood pressure of >140/90 mm Hg is the threshold level above which treatment should be considered, giving a prevalence of hypertension in most developed countries of approximately 20%. Further, older patients with hypertension have a higher absolute benefit from treatment since they have a greater risk of vascular events.

Hypertension causes continuous endothelial trauma and promotes early atherogenesis. In patients with advanced atherosclerosis, plaque growth may also be enhanced. Despite this there is no convincing evidence that anti-hypertensive treatment reduces PAOD progression or the risk of developing claudication. Even so, adequate control of blood pressure reduces the risk of other cardiovascular complications and hypertensive patients with PAOD should be treated according to general guidelines.

Initially management should be aimed at life-style changes to achieve ideal body weight, smoking cessation, a diet low in cholesterol, saturated fat and salt, and a regular exercise programme. This will improve blood pressure control, insulin sensitivity, claudication distance and long-term survival [29] (II). Many patients find this difficult to comply with and pharmacotherapy is usually required.

It may be relatively uncommon for vascular surgeons to institute anti-hypertensive therapy, preferring to leave this to the patient's general practitioner or a physician colleague. Diuretics, calcium channel antagonists, ß-adrenergic antagonists (ß-blockers) and angiotensin-converting enzyme inhibitors are most commonly prescribed and may be used in combination if required.

Although ß-blockers are the most widely prescribed drugs it has been suggested that they may lead to a reduction in exercise tolerance by reducing lower limb blood flow in PAOD patients. However recent reviews indicate that this is not the case except when administered in combination with a calcium-channel antagonist or in patients with advanced PAOD [30,31] **(II)**.

Ramipril (angiotensin-converting enzyme inhibitor) reduces the mortality from all cardiovascular causes in PAOD patients [32] **(I)** and it seems logical that this should be the drug of choice except in patients with mild hypertension controlled by a thiazide diuretic, particularly if aged < 50 years **(A)**. However angiotensin-converting enzyme inhibitors may cause deterioration in renal function in patients with renal artery stenosis and this should be monitored in PAOD patients. If deterioration occurs a calcium channel antagonist or a ß-blocker is preferred **(B)**.

Hyperhomocysteinaemia

A number of studies have shown that elevated total homocysteine levels often occur in patients with atherosclerosis [33] and several cross-sectional case control and cohort studies have linked this with both asymptomatic and symptomatic cardiovascular disease [34]. This may be the result of errors of metabolism (e.g. methylenetetrahydrofolate reductase deficiency), altered vitamin B_{12} metabolism or dietary folate deficiency all of which are involved in homocysteine metabolism. Heavy coffee consumption is also associated with elevated homocysteine levels.

Hyperhomocysteinaemia appears to act independently of other risk factors and its possible mechanisms of action are:

- LDL cholesterol oxidation, endothelial damage, plaque formation.

- Inhibition of vasodilatation by endothelial-derived nitric oxide.

- Promotion of vascular smooth muscle hyperplasia.

Serum homocysteine levels should be checked in patients with PAOD, particularly when presenting at a relatively young age (e.g. < 60). If elevated, a daily supplement of 0.5-5 mg folic acid and 0.5 mg vitamin B_{12} will usually reduce homocysteine levels by about a quarter to a third.

Although reducing homocysteine levels should help prevent PAOD there have been no long-term prospective studies to confirm a reduction in cardiovascular-related morbidity and mortality in these patients. Until such data is available increasing folic acid and vitamin B_{12} intake could have a considerable effect on the prevention of atherosclerotic vascular disease **(C)**.

Chlamydiae pneumoniae

Chlamydiae pneumoniae has been detected in atherosclerotic plaques at various sites including the lower limbs. The organisms produce large amounts of heat shock protein 60 (HSP-60) and localise within plaque macrophages where they induce TNF-a (pro-inflammatory cytokine) and metalloproteinase production thus providing potential mechanisms by which chlamydial infection may promote atherogenesis.

Whilst this organism could have an important role in the pathogenesis of PAOD it may be an incidental finding and further work is required to establish its relevance **(III)**. If its role is proven then therapy with doxycycline may prevent progression of disease and have a role in secondary prevention. This concept is hypothetical.

Additional approaches to risk factor modification

Antiplatelet therapy

A systematic review of antiplatelet therapy in patients with pre-existing cardiovascular disease has shown that these agents reduce the future risk of non-fatal MI, ischaemic stroke, and death from all vascular causes from 11.9% in controls to 9.5% in the treatment group. Since trials of aspirin were most commonly included in the analysis this was recommended for secondary disease prevention in all patients with cardiovascular disease [35] (I).

Despite the overall findings PAOD patients only showed a non-significant reduction in MI, stroke or vascular death although a significant improvement in graft (vein or synthetic) or angioplasty patency was reported. Further, in a primary prevention trial (Physicians' Health Study) aspirin reduced the need for future vascular surgery [36] (I).

The most efficacious dose of aspirin has been debated. As a cyclo-oxygenase inhibitor its antiplatelet effect is due to a reduction in thromboxane activity in platelets and endothelial cells. By the same mechanism, aspirin also reduces endothelial prostacyclin synthesis and theoretically this could have a detrimental effect within diseased vessels. However there is no evidence that the clinical effect of the drug is dose dependent with both low dose (75-325 mg per day) and high dose aspirin (600-1500 mg per day) seem equally effective.

The impact of aspirin alone or in combination with other antiplatelet agents (dipyridamole, ticlopidine) on graft patency has also been assessed and no difference found (I). However a recent trial of aspirin and clopidogrel in patients with acute coronary syndromes has shown that the combination is more effective in preventing death from cardiovascular causes [37] (I). Further, the second European Stroke Prevention Study (ASA/ESPS-2) demonstrated that treatment with a fixed combination of aspirin and extended release dipyridamole was more effective than aspirin alone for the prevention of recurrent stroke [38] (I).

Clopidogrel, which inhibits ADP-dependent platelet aggregation has been extensively investigated in the CAPRIE trial [39] and was more effective than aspirin in reducing the secondary risk of ischaemic stroke, MI, or vascular death in PAOD patients. Further, the therapeutic effect of clopidogrel was greater in PAOD patients than in those with primary cardiac or cerebrovascular symptoms and the safety profile was at least as good as medium dose aspirin.

The choice between aspirin and clopidogrel is difficult. On the basis of a single RCT only the latter is of proven benefit for secondary prevention in PAOD patients. However the evidence in favour of aspirin in many trials involving > 100,000 patients, although just failing to reach statistical significance, has been consistent with additional significant improvements in graft/angioplasty patency where this was applicable. Aspirin is also very cheap and thus it may be reasonable to reserve clopidogrel for patients who are:

◆ Intolerant to aspirin.

◆ Who have a further vascular event despite aspirin therapy.

◆ Considered at particularly high risk (e.g. age < 50, disease in multiple vascular beds).

Trials of combination therapy in PAOD patients are required.

In summary, patients with PAOD are at high risk for cardiovascular disease and death. Although the data are not conclusive, aspirin should be considered the antiplatelet drug of choice for secondary prevention in this group (A). Clopidogrel is now an established treatment option for secondary prevention in PAOD patients although on an economical basis it should be prescribed according to the guidelines indicated above (B).

Summary

◆ HRT has a role in the primary prevention of atherosclerotic disease rather than in providing a secondary benefit for patients with established vascular disease (II).

◆ Smoking is not only an independent risk factor for PAOD but it also enhances the effect of other recognised risk factors. The most effective smoking cessation programmes include intensive counselling and either nicotine replacement therapy or buproprion (A).

Risk factor modification

◆ Hyperlipidaemias (↑total cholesterol, LDL cholesterol, and triglycerides, together with ↓HDL cholesterol) are a major risk factor for PAOD. Aggressive treatment for hyperlipidaemias confers a significant secondary cardiovascular benefit and may result in plaque regression **(I)**.

◆ Tight control of diabetes mellitus reduces the risk of microvascular and cardiac complications but does not appear to influence PAOD-related events **(I)**.

◆ Hypertension is associated with a 2-3 fold increase in the risk of cerebral, cardiac and vascular events. Treatment of hypertension reduces the risk of future cerebral and cardiac events although there is no firm evidence that such a benefit is conferred upon the peripheral circulation. Ramipril reduces the risk of future cardiovascular events in patients with PAOD and should be the antihypertensive of choice except for patients controlled by a thiazide diuretic or those who have renal artery stenosis (risk of deteriorating renal function) **(I)**.

◆ Hyperhomocysteinaemia appears to be an independent risk factor for PAOD. There is currently no proof that treatment reduces the risk of future cardiovascular events **(C)**.

◆ The role of chlamydial infection in atherogenesis and the benefit from its treatment is not proven **(III)**.

◆ Antiplatelet therapy has a proven role in secondary prevention for patients with pre-existing cardiovascular disease and aspirin increases patency after vascular reconstruction or angioplasty **(A)**. Although clopidogrel appears more effective than aspirin in PAOD patients it is usually prescribed selectively **(B)**.

These recommendations are summarised in Figures 1 and 2.

Figure 1 Management of principle risk factors in patients with PAOD.

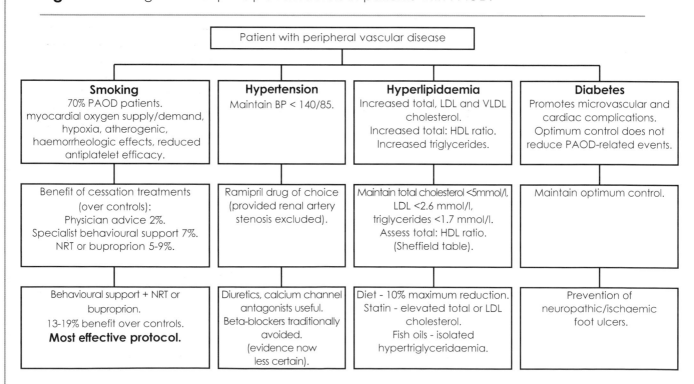

Figure 2 Secondary risk factors and antiplatelet therapy for PAOD.

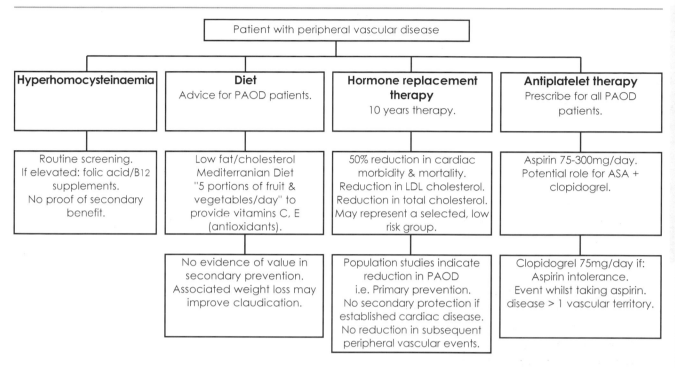

Chapter 2

Further reading

1 Weatherall DJ, Ledingham JGG, Warrell DA, Eds. *Oxford Textbook of Medicine*, 3rd Edition. Volume 2, Sections 11 & 15. Oxford University Press, Oxford, 1996.

2 Dunnington PN, Sniederman A. *Hyperlipidaemias* (Fast Facts). Health Press, Albuquerque, USA, 2000.

References (grade I evidence and grade A recommendations in bold)

1 McDermott MM, Mehta S, Ahn H, Greenland P. Atherosclerotic risk factors are less intensively treated in patients with peripheral arterial disease than in patients with coronary artery disease. *J Gen Intern Med* 1997; 12: 209-215.

2 Anand SS, Kundi A, Eikelboom J, Yusuf S. Low rates of preventative practices in patients with peripheral vascular disease. *Can J Cardiol* 1999; 15(11): 1259-1263.

3 West JA. Cost-effective strategies for the management of vascular disease. *Vasc Med* 1997; 2(1): 25-29.

4 Sites CK. Hormone replacement therapy: Cardiovascular benefits for ageing women. *Coronary Artery Disease* 1998; 9(12): 789-793.

5 Connelly PW, Stachenko S, Maclean DR, Petrasovits A, Little JA. The prevalence of hyperlipidaemia in women and its association with use of oral contraceptives, sex hormone replacement therapy and non-lipid coronary artery disease risk factors. Canadian Heart Health Surveys Research Group. *Can J Cardiol* 1999; 15(4): 419-427.

6 **Hulley S, Grady D, Bush T, Furberg, Herrington D, Riggs B, Vittinghoff E. Randomised trial of estrogen plus progestin for secondary prevention of coronary heart disease in postmenopausal women. *JAMA* 1998; 280(7).**

7 **Hsia J, Simon JA, Lin F, Applegate WB, Vogt MT, Hunninghake D, Carr M. Peripheral arterial disease in randomized trial of estrogen with progestin in women with coronary heart disease: the Heart and Estrogen/Progestin Replacement Study. *Circulation* 2000; 102(18): 2228-2232.**

8 **Westendorp IC, in't Veld BA, Grobbee DE, Pols HA, Meijer WT, Hofman A, Witteman JC. Hormone replacement therapy and peripheral arterial disease: the Rotterdam study. *Arch Intern Med* 2000; 160(16): 2498-2502.**

9 Lassila R, Le Pantalo M, Lindfors O. The effect of ASA on the outcome after lower limb arterial surgery with special reference to smoking. *World J Surg* 1991; 15(3): 378-382.

10 Reilly M, Delanty N, Lawson JA, Fitzgerald GA. Modulation of oxidant stress in vivo in chronic cigarette smokers. *Circulation* 1996; 94(1): 19-25.

11 Klipstein-Grobusch K, den Breeijen JH, Grobbee DE, Boeing H, Hofman A, Witteman JC. Dietary antioxidants and peripheral arterial disease: the Rotterdam study. *Am J Epidemiology* 2001; 154(2): 145-149.

Chapter 2

12 Rapola JM, Virtamo J, Ripatti S, Huttunen JK, Albanes D, Taylor PR, Heinonen OP. Randomised trial of alpha-tocopherol and beta-carotene supplements on incidence of major coronary events in men with previous myocardial infarction. *Lancet* 1997; 349(9067): 1715-1720.

13 **West R, McNeill A, Raw M. Smoking cessation guidelines for health professionals: an update.** *Thorax* **2000; 55: 987-999.**

14 Wallis EJ, Ramsay LE, Ul Haq I, Ghahramani P, Jackson PR, Rowland-Yeo K, Yeo WW. Coronary and cardiovascular risk estimation for primary prevention: validation of a new Sheffield table in the 1995 Scottish health survey population. *BMJ* 2000; 320: 671-676.

15 **Leng GC, Price JF, Jepson RG. Lipid lowering for lower limb atherosclerosis (Cochrane review). In: The Cochrane Library, Update Software, Oxford, 2001.**

16 Crisby M, Nordin-Fredrikson G, Shah PK, Yano J, Zhu J, Nilsson J. Pravastatin treatment increases collagen content and decreases lipid content, inflammation, metalloproteinases, and cell death in human carotid plaques: implications for plaque stabilization. *Circulation* 2001; 103(7): 926-933.

17 **Mowat BF, Skinner ER, Wilson HM, Leng GC, Fowkes FG, Horrobin D. Alterations in plasma lipids, lipoproteins and high-density lipoprotein subfractions in peripheral arterial disease.** *Atherosclerosis* **1997; 131(2): 161-166.**

18 Khan F, Litchfield SJ, Belch JJ. Cutaneous microvascular responses are improved after cholesterol lowering in patients with peripheral arterial disease and hypercholesterolaemia. *Adv Exp Med Biol* 1997; 428: 49-54.

19 Kirk G, McLaren M, Muir AH, Stonebridge PA, Belch JJ. Decrease in P-selectin levels in patients with hypercholesterolaemia and peripheral arterial occlusive disease after lipid lowering treatment. *Vasc Med* 1999; 4:23-26.

20 **Pederson TR, Olsson AG, Faergeman O,** *et al.* **Lipoprotein changes and reduction in the incidence of major coronary heart disease events in the Scandinavian Simvastatin Survival Study.** *Circulation* **1998; 97: 1453-1460.**

21 **Elam MB, Hunninghake DB, Davis KB,** *et al.* **Effect of Niacin on lipid and lipoprotein levels and glycaemic control in patients with diabetes and peripheral arterial disease; the ADMIT Study: a randomised trial.** *JAMA* **2000; 284: 1263-1270.**

22 Heart Protection Study - http://www.hpsinfo.org.

23 Massaro M, Carluccio MA, De Caterina R. Direct vascular antiatherogenic effects of oleic acid: a clue to the cardioprotective effects of the mediterranean diet. *Cardiologia* 1999; 44(6): 507-513.

24 Woodcock BE, Smith E, Lambert WH, Jones WM, Galloway JH, Greaves M, Preston FE. Beneficial effects of fish oil on blood viscosity in peripheral vascular disease. *BMJ Clin Research Ed* 11984; 288(6417): 592-594.

25 **Effect of intensive diabetes management on macrovascular events and risk factors in the Diabetes Control and Complication Trial.** *Am J Cardiol* **1995; 75: 894-903.**

26 **UK Prospective Diabetes Study (UKPDS) Group. Intensive blood-glucose control with sulphonylureas or insulin compared with conventional treatment and risk of complication in patients with type 2 diabetes (UKPDS 33).** *Lancet* **1998; 352: 837-853.**

27 Kannel WB, Dawber TR, McGee DL. Perspectives on systolic hypertension. The Framingham Study. *Circulation* 1980; 61: 1179-1182.

28 Stamler J, Stamler R, Neaton JD. Blood pressure, systolic and diastolic, and cardiovascular risks. US population data. *Arch Intern Med* 1993; 153: 598-615.

29 Olin JW. Antihypertensive treatment in patients with peripheral vascular disease. *Cleveland Clinic J Med* 1994; 61(5): 337-344.

30 Radack K, Deck C. Beta-adrenergic blocker therapy does not worsen intermittent claudication in subjects with peripheral arterial disease: a meta-analysis of RCT's. *Arch Intern Med* 1991; 151: 1769-1776.

31 Heintzen MP, Straver BE. Peripheral vascular effects of beta-blockers. *Eur Heart Journal* 1994; 15: suppl C: 2-7.

32 **The Heart Outcomes Prevention Evaluation Study Investigators. Effects of ACE-Inhibitor, Ramipril on cardiovascular events in high-risk patients.** *N Eng J Med* **2000; 342: 145-153.**

33 Clarke R, Daly L, Robinson K *et al.* Hyperhomocysteinaemia. *N Eng J Med* 1991; 324: 1149-1155.

34 Saw SM. Homocysteine and atherosclerotic disease: the epidemiological evidence. *Ann Acad Med*, Singapore 1999; 28(4): 565-568.

35 **Collaborative overview of randomised trials of antiplatelet therapy. I. Prevention of death, MI, and CVA by prolonged antiplatelet therapy in various categories of patients.** *BMJ* **1994; 308: 81-106.**

36 Goldhaber SZ, Manson JE, Stampfer MJ, *et al.* Low dose aspirin and subsequent peripheral arterial surgery in the Physicians' Health Study. *Lancet* 1992; 340: 143-145.

37 **Yusuf S, Zhao F, Mehta SR, Chrolavicius S, Tognoni G, Fox KK. The clopidogrel in unstable angina to prevent recurrent events trial investigators. Effects of clopidogrel in addition to aspirin in patients with acute coronary syndromes without ST-segment elevation.** *N Engl J Med* **2001, 345: 494-502.**

38 **Shah, H, Gondek K. Aspirin plus extended-release dipyridamole or clopidogrel compared with aspirin monotherapy for the prevention of ischaemic stroke: a cost-effectiveness analysis.** *Clin Therap* **2000; 22(3): 362-370.**

39 CAPRIE Steering Committee. A randomised, blinded, trial of clopidogrel versus aspirin in patients at risk of ischaemic events. *Lancet* 1996; 348 (9038): 1329-1339.

Chapter 3

Exercise programmes for claudicants

Phyllida Morris-Vincent Nurse Specialist

Tina Theophilus Specialist in Therapeutic Exercise

THE ROYAL FREE HOSPITAL, LONDON, UK

Introduction

"Let us eat and drink; for tomorrow we shall die"[1] may be an apposite description of society's hedonistic inclination to "discount" particularly if smoking is added to the equation. Unfortunately, this tendency to pay tomorrow for what we have today, will result in at least half of all premature deaths in the 21st century being related to the individual's unhealthy behaviour and life-style [2].

As patients with peripheral arterial occlusive disease (PAOD) will undoubtedly play a part in realising these statistics, it is increasingly important to establish practical strategies that will enable patients and health professionals to challenge the disease process. Maximising the health potential of patients through exercise and life-style modifications that target predominate risk factors, may improve quality of life and patient outcomes by stabilising the progression of the disease. However, the difficulties lie in convincing the patient to change a lifetime of deleterious habits. The factors that affect compliance to risk modification regimes and how patients may be encouraged to co-operate with health and life-style advice form the subject of this chapter.

The health of the nation

There are strong social and economic arguments to support a pro-active stance on health education programmes particularly as heart disease, stroke and related illness are preventable and cost the National Health Service £3.8 billion every year [3]. Government initiatives are targeting four priority areas that include heart disease and stroke. The aim is to reduce the mortality from these and related illness by 40% in people under the age of 75 years by the year 2010 [4,5].

Intermittent claudication, an early manifestation of PAOD, affects 5% of the population aged between 55 to 74 years. Although this may adversely affect quality of life, there is also compelling evidence that claudicants have a 2-3 fold higher mortality than non-claudicants from cardiac and cerebrovascular disease [6,7]. Furthermore, claudicants are more likely to suffer non-fatal cardiac or cerebrovascular events. This places an enormous financial burden on the Health Service for rehabilitation and long-term care.

With the same underlying pathology as coronary heart disease the adverse effects of smoking,

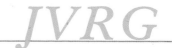

hypercholesterolaemia, stress, hypertension and diabetes mellitus are well known. Obesity and lack of exercise are also risk factors and therefore it would seem logical to accept that exercise, risk factor modification, and life-style changes should be central to the management of patients with PAOD.

Claudication and exercise

There is a wealth of evidence to suggest that exercise regimes for claudicants are beneficial, cost effective and safe [8,9,10,11]. The Cochrane review [12] **(I)** recommends that exercise should be a key constituent of claudicant management as there is evidence that it may be more effective than angioplasty after 6 months [13] **(A)**, without the attendant risks of intervention. The review concludes that an exercise programme could enable a patient to achieve a 150% improvement in walking ability. In 1995, a meta-analysis of 21 exercise training programmes demonstrated that training for at least 6 months by walking to near maximum pain tolerance produced a significant improvement in pain free and maximum walking distances [14] **(I)**. However, although exercise appears highly effective these studies were small and provided little evidence of a sustained, long-term, improvement. Thus, further studies are required to establish the optimum treatment plan for improving symptoms, quality of life and long-term outcome [15,16].

Although the ideal exercise programme has not been established it is clear that maximum benefit is achieved from supervised, structured programmes that are maintained indefinitely [17]**(A)**, with the greatest improvement occurring in patients who undertake exercise sessions of 30 minutes, at least three times a week [14] **(I)**.

The physiological benefits of exercise appear immutable but the main considerations should be in attempting to understand some of the reasons why merely advising the patients to "stop smoking and keep walking" [18] is not enough.

The nature of compliance

By definition, lifelong habits are notoriously difficult to change and human nature is such that we often have little intention of doing what is good for us, particularly if it requires sacrifice or effort. Adopting new behaviours that promote health and finding the resolution to avoid habits that may result in ill health is problematic. At a time when patients are increasingly required to take responsibility for their own health care, the relationship between the health carer and patient is also undergoing a degree of change.

It is not always an easy relationship. Quoting from Franz Kafka's "A Country Doctor", one contributor to the BMJ points out that: "to write prescriptions is easy, but to come to an understanding with people is hard" [19]. This was in response to a fellow correspondent's original quotation that replaced the preposition "with" by "of". The point being that there is every chance, although difficult, that we come to an understanding *with* patients but it is unlikely we will ever reach an understanding *of* them.

The word "compliance" has negative connotations that allude to prescription, submission, obedience, coercion and intimates that the patient is placed in a subservient position to the professional. Recently, buzzwords such as "concordance" reflect an attempt to shift the balance and place the patient in a position of collaboration and negotiation.

Several factors may predict compliance - "characteristics of the disease, characteristics of the person and characteristics of the relationship with the health care provider" [20]. Key elements relate to verbal communication, perceived level of competence of the practitioner, the amount of time between patient referral and treatment and interestingly, the length of time the patient has to wait in the waiting room. It would appear that patients are more inclined to co-operate with practitioners who are perceived as friendly, empathetic and genuinely interested in their needs [20].

Patients need a clear understanding of the purpose of change and what benefits the change will bring before attitudes and behaviour alter. Clearly, the greater the effort required for compliance or the greater the life-style change necessitated the lower the compliance is likely to be.

There is no doubt that some patients do not know when they are ill or at risk of illness and they would often rather not know. There is also a small proportion of patients who appear to enjoy ill health. Criteria such as personal philosophy, upbringing, social norm and reward can afford rationale for some behaviours. As a consequence, barriers to certain behaviours can be recognised and as health professionals we must be aware that we are often asking patients and their families to adopt certain attitudes and beliefs that are alien and unrecognisable to them.

Theories relating to patients' beliefs on how much conviction they have to change may help to explain why individuals have such different approaches to understanding their own health or illness [21]. Those with an "internal locus of control" [22] believe that health and recovery is determined through their own actions. They tend to be pro-active in their care and may already lead a relatively "healthy" life-style.

Patients with an "external" locus of control believe that they must respond to strong role models or people in authority such as doctors. They will not take the lead but are usually happy to comply with prescriptive regimes. A sub group of these patients have what is deemed a fatalistic perspective whereby fate determines ill health and outcome. These are the patients who will tend to remain passive and may be the most difficult to re-educate.

Studies on lack of compliance are well-documented [20,23]. About 75% of patients keep scheduled appointments when they initiate them, but only about 50% keep appointments that have been scheduled by the health professional. Compliance to dietary regimes range from about 30-70%. Studies of treatments in a variety of illnesses including hypertension, glaucoma, coronary heart disease and diabetes have indicated that only 40-70% of patients comply with prescriptions or advice [23].

Compliance improves when treatment involves a cure rather than prevention and shorter regimes are tolerated better than longer ones. Rates of compliance with preventative procedures are even lower [23].

Communication and levels of understanding have always been an issue between the patient and health professional. Studies on patient compliance demonstrate that 52% of patients could not correctly report what their clinician expected of them. Similarly, out-patients could not recall approximately 40% of what their clinician had told them 10-80 minutes afterwards and that over 60% of patients interviewed immediately after a visit to their doctor had misunderstood the directions concerning prescribed medication [20,24,25].

Learners remember 20% of what they hear, 30% of what they see, 50% of what they see and hear, 70% of what they say and 90% of what they say and do [26]. It would be a natural conclusion to suggest that techniques which attempt to increase patient involvement and encourage an active on going relationship are more likely to improve compliance and bring about a higher level of therapeutic success.

Compliance and exercise therapy

The Allied Dunbar National Fitness Survey reported 70-80% of men and women in Great Britain fell below their age appropriate activity level [27]. Of those people who adopt an exercise programme 50% will drop out within 6 months. It is, therefore, important for the exercise professional to get the patient past the 6-month mark [2].

The determinants of adherence to exercise can be divided into three categories: personal characteristics (physical, physiological and social), environmental factors and programme factors. Research is not conclusive but does highlight that different groups of patients may need different emphasis on these [2].

The main factors associated with poor adherence to exercise and medical regimes such as smoking cessation are perceived inconvenience, depression, low socio-economic status, obesity, poor social support and low motivation [2]. Naturally, attitudes and beliefs play an important part in predicting compliance, and there are indications that causal belief is associated with a commitment to further behaviour change.

Enjoyment is a positive emotion and a component of intrinsic motivation, and as such is one of the most important factors affecting adherence [28]. Given the

Chapter 3

choice people will not stick to anything they do not enjoy.

Factors that affect adherence negatively may be modified by giving individual counselling and support and by providing an appropriate programme in terms of mode, intensity, choice and control. Intention to exercise, attitude to exercise, subjective norm, self-efficacy and self-motivation can all be linked to adherence. Social support from family, spouse, friends, exercise group and exercise leader tends to increase adherence and enjoyment of the exercise and its social aspect is of great importance [29,30,31,32,33].

Motivational strategies

The literature is clear that simply giving information, the educational approach, is not adequate in encouraging patients to change habits and that it requires a careful combination of educational and behavioural strategies, including health education, counselling, instructional techniques and demonstration [25,34,35]. A clear understanding of how behaviour is influenced by health beliefs is also required [36].

Motivational interviewing and intervention is one example of such strategy. The technique is based on the premise that change should be instigated from the patient enabling them to be active and willing to use the information provided to a positive end. The interview, at assessment, is a powerful tool allowing patients to identify problems and means of solution [37]. The motivational approach assumes that the patient has the skills and understanding to change but is resistant and lacking motivation. A collaborative approach ensures that patients are offered options and not just given instructions.

The likelihood that patients will adopt a valued health behaviour may depend on three sets of cognitions: "the expectancy that one is at risk, the expectancy that behavioural change will reduce the threat, and the expectancy that one is capable of adopting positive behaviour patterns and attitudes" [21]. The practitioner must understand where the patient is on the continuum of change [38] as progress is unlikely if the patient is ambivalent or resistant and their perception of risk is low.

Self-efficacy is the belief and confidence of one's ability to behave in such a way as to achieve a desirable outcome [39]. The theory is widely used in areas such as cardiac rehabilitation, smoking cessation, dietary modification and physical activity. It is the connection between knowledge and action that influences choice of behaviour, the environment in which it is performed and the amount of effort required. It is important to realise that levels of self efficacy can impede as well as motivate but it is a good predictor for short and long-term adherence. Self-regulation allows the patient to make appropriate judgements and react realistically to managing problems. High degrees of decision making may be required and it could be argued that not all patients are capable of such sophisticated techniques. It is the health professional's role to identify difficulties and work on other methods of problem solving. The confidence to carry out the appropriate behaviour comes from the concept of self-efficacy. Further, partnership, collaboration and excellent communication are the keys to success of any behavioural strategy. Adequate time and commitment are vital.

Assessment

On initial referral the patient must be fully assessed to confirm the diagnosis of intermittent claudication (muscle pain, most commonly calf, thigh or buttock) due to inadequate arterial blood flow. The symptoms are quite specific:

- The pain or cramp is brought on by walking.

- The pain starts after walking roughly the same distance on each occasion.

- The pain comes on earlier when walking uphill or quickly.

- The pain takes a few minutes to resolve after ceasing exercise (it does not disappear immediately).

Before a claudicant is referred to an exercise and life-style programme alternative diagnoses such as:

- Spinal claudication (cauda equina compression): similar symptoms, tends to radiate down both legs, made worse by walking but may be brought on by standing, not relieved rapidly by rest,

- Osteoarthritis of hips and knees,

- Sciatic pain,

- Venous claudication: "bursting" sensation in calf during walking, relieved by rest or raising leg,

- Neuropathic pain,

- Myalgic syndromes,

must be excluded. However, in elderly patients one or more of these problems may co-exist increasing the difficulty in diagnosis.

Many patients may be limited by factors such as angina, dyspnoea and severe arthritic disorders and these problems may be more disabling than their claudication. However, they should not bar the patient from exercise therapy, as a chair-based programme may provide an opportunity to exercise that may otherwise be missed.

Interview and fitness assessment

The average length of first interview, including a comprehensive assessment of the patient's medical, vascular and social history, takes approximately 90 minutes. Managing clinics such as these is one area where the specialist nurse practitioner can apply principles of holistic, therapeutic nursing care, that can enable a patient to maximise his potential [40,41]. It is important that the patient becomes an active participant in his care, feels in control and fully understands what can be achieved. The key to a successful partnership is the development of trust. Patients also benefit from constant reinforcement, goal achievement and the gradual sense of well-being.

Patients express similar views and fears. Most commonly, patients display a fundamental lack of knowledge of the disease and its contributory factors. They express fears of amputation and pain. They are embarrassed by their disability, feel vulnerable, isolated and lack confidence. They are reluctant to commit to activities and generally express great dissatisfaction with their quality of life.

Reassurance is important and it is essential to stress to patients that symptoms will improve in 50% of patients; will remain unchanged in 30% and will only deteriorate in 20% of patients. Amputation is required in approximately 5% of patients [42].

By using some of the techniques discussed earlier the practitioner can gain a clear picture of the patient's knowledge and understanding and where they see themselves in terms of commitment to change [39].

Claudication and maximal walking distances are measured pre and post programme. There are many methods of assessing this although treadmill testing is unhelpful as it does not simulate normal walking and some patients find it difficult to walk on. Beep testing [43] can be stressful and confusing to the elderly patient and thus our preferred method is a simple 6 minute walk along a corridor which allows a basic assessment of claudication distance and functional ability, including balance, posture and stance.

Smoking cessation advice is paramount and nicotine replacement therapy is offered routinely if patients are seriously prepared to plan a "quit date" with the nurse. The interview and subsequent routine follow-ups also allow the nurse to monitor compliance with drug therapies, monitor blood pressure and blood glucose as well as advise on diet, foot care and any other problems the patient may be experiencing.

Once a baseline has been established and goals have been set the patient can safely commence a supervised exercise programme or be given a regime to follow at home. Home regimes are not as effective as supervised programmes either in terms of walking improvement or quality of life endpoints. However they do have a role for patients who are still working, for those who live a long way from the hospital, and for those who do not wish to attend a supervised clinic. They also provide a mechanism by which the nurse practitioner can keep in contact with the patient [44].

The exercise programme

The suggested components of an exercise programme are outlined in Tables 1 and 2. The single most important factor for success of any exercise programme is the exercise specialist or programme leader. Physiotherapists often do not have the time or special interest to lead programmes but a professional trained in therapeutic exercise therapy provides the enthusiasm, commitment and skill necessary to provide a programme that is safe, stimulating, fun and effective.

The primary aim of any exercise programme is to increase the pain-free walking distance with secondary aims being an improvement in overall function and independence in this group of predominately elderly patients. The physiological changes that occur with training include improved cardiorespiratory status, blood rheology, muscle metabolism and improvements to biomechanical status [45] (I). The possibility of an exercise associated inflammatory response is outweighed by the overall physical and psychological benefit of the exercise training [46] (II).

The ageing process is associated with a reduction in muscle strength and flexibility, reduced bone density, reduced range of movement around joints and reduced cardiovascular and respiratory capacity. Changes to the nervous system lead to slower reaction time and loss of balance. These changes can cause pain, discomfort and a gradual decline in functional fitness and independence. By incorporating certain "functional exercises" into the exercise programme we can do much to ameliorate the effects of ageing [47]. The suggested programme follows established principles of exercising the elderly that incorporates a full warm up and pulse raising, the main exercise component, and a cool down period [48,49,50,51]. A period of relaxation is added at the end of each session followed by an educational talk that serves to keep patients within the department during the vulnerable period in those with cardiovascular disease when arrythmias may occur. The programme is complemented by a commitment to undertake 3-5 independent walking sessions/week at home. Patients are advised against exercising if they are feeling unwell or have new or unstable symptoms.

Elderly patients require careful supervision and may take many weeks of repetition before they learn even the most simple of techniques. However, once they gain confidence and feel the benefits of the training they express enormous enthusiasm and desire to try more complex routines.

The American College of Sports Medicine (ACSM) recommends interval training or stair climbing three times a week at an intensity that causes pain at 3 on a 4 point scale [52] (A). The onset of pain should be within approximately 5 minutes and full recovery should be attained between intervals. They also suggest a training time and target heart rate of 20mins at 40% of heart rate reserve initially, building up to 40 minutes at 70% of heart rate reserve over 6 months [52].

In our experience the older patient rarely raises his heart rate above the suggested levels because general discomfort and claudication interfere. Cardiac medications such as beta blockers reduce resting and training heart rates and so for many patients it is not possible or even practical to set a training heart rate.

We instruct patients to exercise at a level where they feel "comfortably challenged", warm, and perspiring with a slight increase in respiratory rate. They should be slightly breathless but be able to hold a normal conversation. This level of exertion corresponds to suggested target heart rates [53].

Obviously claudication pain is a significant de-motivator. A recent study measuring the effect of upper limb aerobic interval training on lower limb claudication may provide a solution. Patients who completed a programme of exercise using an arm cycle ergometer increased pain free and maximal walking distance. This effect may be due to changes in central cardiovascular function [54] (II).

Increasingly, we have younger, slightly fitter patients on the programme. Individual adaptations are required to allow for these patients to work harder than their elderly counterparts.

Patients are encouraged to take responsibility for documenting their walking distances and many keep diaries that reflect their successes and failures, good days and bad.

Table 1 The warm-up can be divided into pulse raising, mobility and stretching activities.

Pulse raiser	**10-15 minutes of low level, rhythmic exercise using large muscle groups of buttocks, thighs and calves.**
Aim	To gently increase respiratory rate, heart rate and blood flow to muscles.
	To warm muscles prior to main activity.
	To reduce the risk of exercise induced arrythmias and the incidence of early onset fatigue and claudication pain.
Component	Stationary bike and/or seated exercise: toe taps, heel digs, alternating leg extensions and marching on the spot.
Tips	To avoid local muscle fatigue pulse raising activities should be alternated with low intensity arm movements and mobility exercises. eg. arm swings, thigh slapping, hand clapping etc.
	Attention should be paid to posture. Patients should sit towards the front of the chair, feet flat on the floor, hip width apart, lengthening through the spine and neck whilst gently pulling in the stomach muscles.
Mobility	**2-3 minutes designed to gently move joints through their full range of movement**
Aim	To prevent injury by stimulating the production of synovial fluid which cushions, protects and nourishes the joint.
	To reduce joint stiffness, improve posture and improve walking capacity and technique.
Component	Mobilise shoulder joint; shoulder girdle; trunk; hip; knee and ankle joint.
Tips	Can be performed seated or standing. Can follow a cycle pulse raiser or interspersed with a chair pulse raiser.
Stretch	**2-3 minutes of specific stretches for muscle groups to be used during the exercise session.**
Aim	To increase range of movement around specific joints and prevent injury by gently lengthening muscles prior to use.
	To enhance posture and independence in activities of living.
Component	Suggested stretches; calf; hip flexor; inner thigh; chest; side.
Tips	Stretches should be static and held for 8 seconds.

Exercise programmes for claudicants

Table 2 The main component. The training required to improve claudication walking distance and pain can be made more varied and interesting by circuit training. This involves alternating periods of exercise designed specifically to stimulate the cardiovascular system and peripheral vasculature (PV) with periods of "active rest" which can be utilised to improve upper body muscle endurance and strength. Including a few dynamic strengthening exercises in the PV component adds variety to the exercise session and also helps improve balance, strength and joint stability. Non weight bearing exercises if performed at an intensity of 40-70% heart rate reserve (11-13 Borg scale) will help improve central cardiovascular fitness and possibly improve claudication pain.

PV stations - weight bearing	walking; treadmill; stepping; alternate knee lifts; walking on mini trampolene.
Specific leg strengthening exercises	calf raises; squats. These are worthwhile but maybe not as effective as walking in improving exercise performance.
Non weight bearing cardiovascular exercise	stationary bike; rowing machine.
Active rest stations	bicep curls; wall press ups; tennis ball squeezing; seated rowing; arm raises. These suggested exercises will help strengthen muscles, joints and bones, promote good posture and independence with daily activities.
Tips and other ideas	Brisk walking as a group to invigorating music is fun and allows the leader to stress good walking technique which can prevent accidents on stairs and uneven pavement surfaces. Simple low level country dancing and line dancing is enjoyable. Simple choreographed classic dance moves are reminiscent of dance hall steps. The moves are fun and stimulate mind, body and muscle groups which may not otherwise be used.
COOL DOWN	**can be divided into cardiovascular and stretching activities**
Aim	To gradually reduce heart rate thus reducing risk of post exercise arrythmias, pooling of blood in the legs which can lead to post exercise dizziness. To reduce the accumulation of metabolic waste in the muscles causing stiffness and soreness. The stretching exercises aim to reduce muscle stiffness by returning muscles to pre exercise length and develop functional fitness by increasing range of movement in specific joints.
Component	Cardiovascular options include: easy cycling on stationary bike and seated exercises gradually decreasing in intensity, speed and resistance. Suggested stretches include: calf, hip flexors, hamstrings, adductors, chest, shoulders, triceps and side.

Figure 1 Management pathway of patient with intermittent claudication.

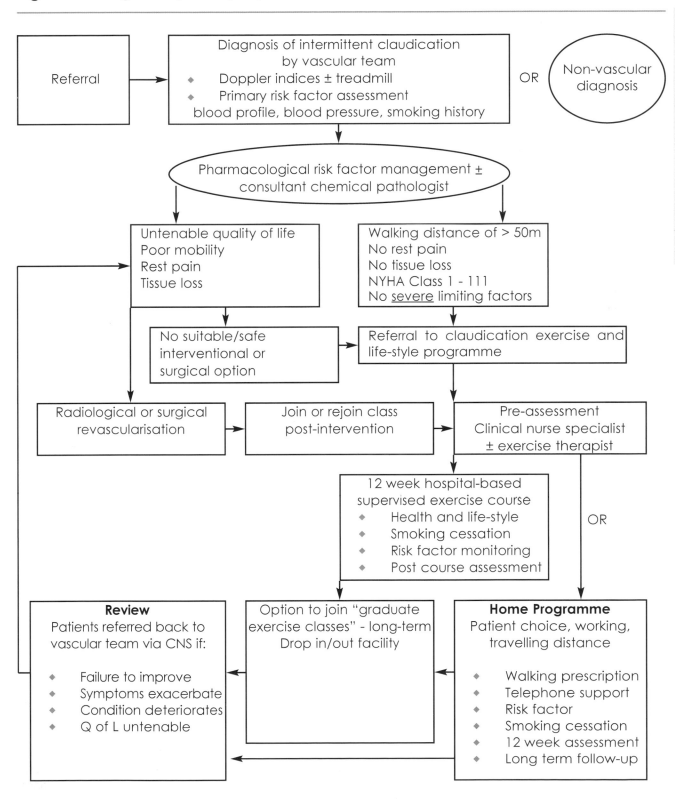

Conclusion

It is in the interests of the health service that time and effort is invested in establishing working relationships with patients to improve compliance to health regimes through improved communication, new learning and appropriately targeted educational and behavioural strategies particularly in chronic disease processes.

Exercise and life-style programmes provide the impetus and supervised environment for many patients to alter life long habits and maintain changes long-term. The psychosocial aspects of such programmes cannot be underestimated and serve both patients and their families. The message should be that exercise is therapeutic, fun and beneficial regardless of age or disability.

We must, however, be prepared to assess each patient's ability and motivation individually and be prepared to offer alternative therapies. Not all claudicants will readily accept long-term change to their life-style and these patients require the most attention. The danger is that they will fail to attend clinics and may be lost in an inflexible system that is intolerant of non-compliers. By establishing programmes, particularly in the primary care setting it is possible to involve many patients and their families in long-term life-style changes reducing the risk of interventional procedures and potentially lengthy hospitalisation.

Summary

◆ Exercise is an inexpensive, low risk treatment option for claudication **(II)**.

◆ Nurse specialists and trained exercise therapists should manage exercise and life-style programmes. They are ideally placed to establish long-term relationships and continuity of care **(B)**.

◆ By identifying the locus of control and health beliefs, patients can be encouraged to adhere to long-term life-style changes through simple motivational techniques **(A)**.

◆ Flexible, innovative and fun exercise and life-style programmes can be established with minimal resources **(B)**.

◆ Patients can be reassured and assisted in setting realistic, achievable goals to improve their health and fitness **(A)**.

◆ The optimum exercise programme is still to be established **(B)**.

Further reading

1 London Central YMCA Training and Development Department. *Exercise for the Older Person Knowledge Base.* London, 1995.

2 Dishman R, Ed. *Exercise Adherence: Its impact on public health.* Human Kinetic Books, Illinois, 1988.

3 Kenney W, Humphrey R, Bryant D, Mahler V, Froehlicher V, Miller N, York T, Eds. American College of Sports Medicine. *ACSM's guidelines for exercise testing and prescription.* 5th ed. Williams & Wilkins, Baltimore, 1995.

References (grade I evidence and grade A recommendations in bold)

1 Isaiah, Chapter 22 Verse 13. King James Bible.

2 Dishman R. *Exercise Adherence: Its impact on public health.* Human Kinetic Books, Illinois, 1988.

3 Kaplan R, Sallis J, Patterson T. *Health and Human Behaviour.* McGraw-Hill, Inc. USA, 1993.

4 Department of Health. A Vision for the Future. DOH, London, 1993.

5 Department of Health. National Service Framework for Coronary Heart Disease. DOH, London, 2000.

6 Leng GC, Fowkes FGR. The epidemiology of peripheral arterial disease. *Vascular Medicine Review* 1993; 4: 5-18.

7 Fowkes FGR, Housley E, Cawood EHH, Macintyre CCA, Ruckley CV, Prescott RJ. Edinburgh Artery Study: prevalence of asymptomatic and symptomatic peripheral arterial disease in the general population. *Int J Epidemiol* 1991; 20: 384-92.

8 Regensteiner JG, Gardner A, Hiatt WR. Exercise testing and exercise rehabilitation for patients with peripheral arterial disease: status in 1997. *Vascular Medicine* 1997; 2: 238-242.

9   Ekroth R, Dahloff A, Gundevall B, Holm J, Schersten T. Physical training of patients with intermittent claudication: indications, methods and results. *Surgery* 1978; 84(5) 640-643.

10   Larsen OA, Larsen NA. Effect of daily muscular exercise in patients with intermittent. *Lancet* ii: 1966;1093-1096.

11   Skinner JS, Strandess DE. Exercise and intermittent claudication 11. Effect of physical training. *Circulation* 1967; 36: 23-29.

12   **Leng GC, Fowler B, Ernst E. Exercise for Intermittent claudication. Cochrane Review. In: The Cochrane Library 3 200. Update Software, Oxford.**

13   **Perkins JMT, Collin J, Creasy TS, Fletcher EW, Morris PJ. Exercise Training versus Angioplasty for Stable Claudication. Long and Medium Term results of a Prospective Randomised Trial. *Eur J Vasc Endovasc Surg* 1966 11: 409-413.**

14   **Gardner AW, Poehlman ET. Exercise rehabilitation programs for the treatment of claudication pain. A meta-analysis. *JAMA* 1995; 27: 975-980.**

15   Chong P, Golledge,J, Greenhalgh R, Davies A. Exercise therapy or angioplasty? A summation analysis. *Eur J Endovasc Surg* 2000; 20: 4-12.

16   Taft C, Karlsson J, Gelin J, Jivegard L, Sandstrom R, Arfvidsson B, Dahllof A, Lundholm K, Sullivan M. Treatment efficacy of intermittent claudication by invasive therapy, supervised physical exercise training compared to no treatment in unselected randomised patients II: One year results of health related quality of life. *Eur J Vasc Surg* 2001; 22:114- 123.

17   **Tisi P, Shearman C. The impact of treatment of intermittent claudication on the subjective health of the patient. *Health Trends* 1999; 30: 109-114.**

18   Housley E. Treating claudication in five words. *Br Med J* 1988; 296: 1483-1984.

19   Bamforth I. 'Compliance and concordance with treatment'. *BMJ* 197; 314: 1905.

20   Feist J, Brannon L. *Health Psychology: an introduction to behaviour and health.* Wadsworth Publishing, USA, 1988.

21   Naidoo J, Wills J. *Health Promotion: Foundations for Practice.* 3rd ed. Bailliere Tindall, London, 1993.

22   Rotter JB. Generalised expectancies for internal versus external control of reinforcement. *Psychological Monographs* 1966; 80: 609.

23   Sackett L, Snow M. *The Magnitude of compliance and non-compliance.* John Hopkins University Press, Baltimore, 1979.

24   Gatchell R, Baum A, Krantz D. *An introduction to Health Psychology.* 2nd ed. Mc Graw and Hill, Singapore, 1989.

25   Haynes R, Taylor D, Sackett D, Eds. *Compliance in healthcare.* John Hopkins Press, Baltimore, 1979.

26   Green S, Faden R. Potential effects on the patient - 3. *Drug Information J* 1977; 645-705.

27   Allied Dunbar National Fitness Survey. The Sports Council and Health Education Authority. London, 1992.

28   Anderson K, Kirk L. Methods of improving patient compliance in chronic disease states. *Archives of Internal Medicine* 1992; 142:1673-1675.

29   Haynes R. *Strategies for improving compliance: a methodologic analysis and review.* John Hopkins University Press, Baltimore, 1976.

30   Clark N, Gong M. Management of chronic disease by practitioners and patients: are we teaching the wrong things? *BMJ* 2000 320: 572-575.

31   Wilkinson J. Understanding patient's health beliefs. *Professional Nurse* 1999;14(5): 320-322.

32   Wilkinson J. Understanding motivation to enhance patient compliance. *British Journal of Nursing* 1988; 6(15): 879-884.

33   Oldridge N. Compliance with exercise in cardiac rehabilitation. In Ed Dishman R. *Exercise Adherence: Its impact on public health.* Human Kinetic Books, Illinois. 1988; 283-304.

34   Rollnick S, Heather N, Bell A. Negotiating behaviour change in medical settings: the development of brief motivational interviewing. *Journal of Mental Health* 1992; 25-37.

35   Rollnick S, Kinnersley P, Stott N. Methods of helping patients with behaviour change. *BMJ* 1993; 307: 188-190.

36   Becker M, Maiman L. Sociobehavioural determinants of compliance with medical care recommendations. *Medical care* 1975; 1:18, 10-24.

37   Botelho R, Skinner H. Motivating Behaviour Change in Health Promotion: implications for health promotion and disease. *Primary Care* 1995; 22 (4): 565-589.

38   Prochaska J, Di Clementi C. Stages and processes of self-change of smoking: towards an integrative model of change. *Journal of Consulting and Clinical Psychology* 1983;51: 390-95.

39   Bandura A. Self-efficacy: towards a unifying theory of behavioural change. *Psychological review* 84: 192-215.

40   Binnie A, Perkins J, Hands L. Exercise and nursing therapy for patients with intermittent claudication. *Journal of Clinical Nursing* 1999; 8: 90-100.

41   Ciacca J. Benefits of a structured peripheral arterial vascular rehabilitation program. *Journal of Vascular Nursing* 1993; 11: 1-4.

42   McAllister FF. The fate of patients with intermittent claudication managed non operatively. *Am J Surg* 1976; 132: 593-595.

43   Singh SJ *et al.* Development of a shuttle walking test of disability in patients with chronic airways obstruction. *Thorax* 1992; 47: 1019-24.

44   Patterson M, Pinto B, Marcus B, Colucci R, Braun T, Roberts M. Value of a supervised exercise program for the therapy of arterial claudication. *J Vasc Surg* 1997; 25:2.

45   **Tan K, de Cossart L, Edwards R. Exercise training and peripheral vascular disease. *Br J Surg* 2000; 87 (5) 553-563.**

46   Tisi PV, Shearman CP. The evidence for exercise-induced inflammation in intermittent claudication: should we encourage patients to stop walking? *Eur J Endovasc Surg* 1998; 15: 7-17.

47   Dinan S, Sharp C. *Fitness for life.* Piatkus Ltd, London, 1996.

48   Bird SR. *Exercise Physiology for Health Professionals.* Chapman & Hall, London, 1992.

49   Keighley H, Dinan S. Exercise for the older person knowledge base. London Central YMCA Training and Development Department, 1996.

50   Wilmore JH, Costill DL. *Physiology of Sport and Exercise.* Human Kinetics, 1994.

51   Coates A, Mcgee H, Stokes H, Thompson D. BACR *Guidelines for Cardiac Rehabilitation.* Blackwell Science, Oxford, 1995.

52   **American College for Sports Medicine. *Exercise management for persons with chronic disease and disabilities.* Human Kinetics, Illinois, 1995.**

53   Borg Scale. Adapted from Wilmor J, Costill D. *Physiology of Sport and Exercise.* Human Kinetics, Illinois, 1994.

54   Walker R, Nawaz S, Wilkinson C, Saxton, J, Pockley A, Wood R. Influence of upper and lower limb exercise training on cardiovascular function and walking distances in patients with intermittent claudication. *J Vasc Surg* 2000; 31; 4 662-669.

Chapter 3

Chapter 4

Smoking cessation in the 21st century

Christine Jackson Smoking Cessation Co-ordinator [1]

Diana White Executive Nurse [2]

[1] NORTH AND EAST DEVON HEALTH AUTHORITY, EXETER, UK
[2] EXETER PRIMARY CARE TRUST, EXETER, UK

"For every thousand 20 year old smokers it is estimated that one will be murdered, six will die in a road accident and 250 will die in middle age from smoking!" [1] *(I)*.

Introduction

Each year in the UK smoking causes more than 120,000 deaths in people aged > 35 years, 20% of deaths at all ages, and more than 25% of deaths between 35 - 65. Smoking is reducing the female advantage in life expectancy and widening the social class divide in mortality. It remains the largest single preventable cause of death and disability in the UK [2].

Smoking peaked in the 1950s and 1960s [3] when it was fashionable to smoke, tobacco advertising was widespread, and the harmful effects of smoking were not widely known. Smoking rates fell steadily in the 1970s and 1980s due to the overwhelming evidence that smoking was harmful [4].

Although the prevalence of smoking in the UK has declined over the last 30 years, 27% of adults still smoke [2]. Over two thirds of smokers want to stop and about one third try to stop in any year. The unaided cessation rate in middle-aged smokers is only about 2% per annum, demonstrating that nicotine is a highly addictive drug [4].

The smoke from tobacco is estimated to contain more than 4000 chemicals, around 60 of which are suspected or known carcinogens [5]. These are released into the air as particles and gases. The three main components are **nicotine**, **carbon monoxide** and **tar**. Nicotine, an alkaloid, is a powerful, fast-acting and addictive drug. Most people who smoke are addicted to the nicotine in cigarettes [6], whilst about 7% of the population will never be addicted and will only smoke on social occasions, with no withdrawal symptoms between smoking episodes.

Improving health is a dynamic process requiring action by individuals, the community and local government in addition to Health Services. Smoking remains a prevalent habit with serious consequences for public health. There are now effective treatments for nicotine addiction and, in the UK, specialist services for the management of smoking cessation are becoming available in all areas.

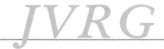

Why do people smoke?

Most smokers are nicotine addicts: they need, deserve, and increasingly expect help in stopping!

This is why many smokers need help in stopping and why treatment services have been established through the NHS, as is the case for alcohol and illicit drug dependence. It is sometimes suggested that if smokers can afford to smoke they can afford the treatment to help them stop. This misunderstands their motivation and dependence. Many cannot afford to smoke and find a way of "affording" it because they are addicted. It also discriminates against the poorer smokers, who are often the most dependent and most in need of support.

Helping people to stop smoking is fundamental to the success of the NHS plan [7], and the NHS Cancer Plan [8] provides targets for the reduction of mortality from heart disease and cancer, and for tackling inequalities. Specific milestones for smoking cessation for 2001/02 have been set in the NHS Plan Implementation Programme. Progress will be monitored under NHS performance improvement arrangements and the Local Modernisation Review is the process by which these local plans are implemented.

Since the inception of smoking cessation services in Health Action Zones in 1999/2000 there have been considerable developments in Government policy in this area. A major theme is the need to address inequalities in health, and services are increasingly focusing on disadvantaged groups. Policy changes such as the availability of nicotine replacement therapy (NRT) on NHS prescription from April 2001 have made a crucial difference to the services.

Smoking cessation services are a key part of the Government's NHS modernisation agenda and will help reduce inequalities in health.

Since 1997 The Government has been committed to the development of a comprehensive strategy to tackle smoking and has produced a number of key documents which set targets and plans to develop smoking cessation services. It sees Primary Health Care as the vehicle to delivering these services. This

is backed by a £110 million programme over 3 years. The more cynical of us, however, would point out that this equates to approximately 5 days worth of tobacco revenue received by the Government!

Key documents

- **The White Paper "Smoking Kills"** [2] sets out the Government's objectives to reduce smoking and its commitment to develop smoking cessation services.

- **The Coronary Heart Disease National Service Framework** [9] indicates that smoking causes 40,300 deaths a year in the UK from all circulatory diseases and the NSF pledged that by 2001 all health authorities would have specialist smoking cessation services.

- **The NHS Plan** [7] reinforced the Government's commitment to establish high quality smoking cessation services. It also announced that NRT would be available on NHS prescription from GP and nurse prescribers **(A)** , and that buproprion, which has been licensed for the treatment of tobacco dependence, should be available on prescription from GPs **(A)**.

- **The NHS Cancer Plan** [8] states that three out of every ten cancer deaths are caused by smoking, equivalent to 46,500 deaths/year. The cancer plan set additional targets to reduce smoking in manual workers where higher rates of smoking are matched by higher rates of cancer and heart disease.

The evidence for smoking cessation services

Smoking cessation interventions are very cost-effective compared with other medical interventions and are estimated to cost about £900 per life-year **(I)** [10]. This compares favourably with the median cost of over 310 medical interventions that were estimated at £17,000 per life-year gained [10]. Furthermore, Muir *et al* demonstrated that 80% of smokers who were prescribed statins would fall below the threshold

Chapter 4

needing statin therapy if they stopped smoking [11]. However, more is currently spent on statin therapy than smoking cessation interventions.

Thus smoking cessation interventions should result in population health gains, for relatively modest expenditure, and in the long-term they will reduce smoking related health care costs, releasing resources for other needs. The evidence base for interventions to promote smoking cessation is well established and a series of systematic reviews [12] have produced good quality evidence to support many of the approaches available to smokers (I).

Smoking cessation - practical aspects

Smoking related diseases in England cost the NHS approximately £1500 million a year [2]. Smoking fits the National Health Service Executive's (NHSE) criteria for developing clinical guidelines, and it is hoped that proposed changes will produce a climate which encourages preventive health care and more attention to evidence based medicine.

Clinical guidelines for smoking cessation published in the journal *Thorax* in December 1998 [10] and updated in December 2000 [13] reviewed the evidence base and set out recommended treatments. The guidelines were based on the evidence provided by the Cochrane Collaboration's Tobacco Addiction Review Group and other authoritative reviews. They were extensively peer reviewed, and are endorsed by a wide range of professional bodies including many Royal Colleges (I).

Traditionally smoking cessation has been viewed as a personal affair, with doctors advising patients to quit, but providing little support. However, the majority of smokers have a desire to quit, and nearly all smokers have attempted to quit at some point in their lives [14]. There does, however, appear to be a discrepancy in the success rates of quitters. 90% of those who quit do so without the help of stop smoking services or products [14] and currently some 20% of adult males are successful ex-smokers [15]. Yet it seems difficult to square this with the low rates of successful long-term abstinence reported by stop smoking clinics [16].

It would seem that smokers are not a homogenous population and that while some may find it very easy to quit the habit, others may find it nearly impossible. Clearly, identifying what categories of smokers exist, how to tell which category an individual patient will fall into, and what treatments will suit each one are vital aspects of combating smoking.

What can the health professional do to start a smoker on the road to quitting and to help them to stay tobacco free?

The first stage is to persuade smokers to start thinking about quitting. The ideal candidate for this is the patient's general practitioner (GP) who most people trust more than others on issues regarding their health. GPs also see people when they are most susceptible to health information and can personalise advice using the smoker's medical history [16]. The tone of advice is all-important. While taking opportunities to promote cessation, the GP must be careful to ensure that the locus of control remains with the patient and avoid appearing nagging and authoritative. Gentle reminders and mentions of available support will work better than scare tactics or "doctors orders" (A) [17].

Once a smoker attempts cessation regular contact with a health professional is an important determinant of success. Thus, 35% of smokers who had intensive contact with their GP were still abstinent at 12 months, compared to 8% who only received initial cessation advice [18]. However most GPs' time is limited and it is usually more practical for a nurse to undertake follow-up sessions. Advice from a nurse in addition to a GP increases the rates of cessation from 3.9% to 7.2% (I) [19]. This may be due to the fact that patients find nurses less intimidating and easier to talk to than their doctor.

Interventions to reduce cigarette smoking

Current cessation treatments fall into three broad groups:

- *Behavioural treatments* that seek to break the link between the act of smoking and the relief of craving.

◆ *Pharmaceutical agents* that aim to reduce nicotine craving after cessation.

◆ *Counselling*, where the smoker is supported by a health professional, peer group or both.

Whilst it would be ideal to offer every available treatment to every smoker, the limited nature of NHS resources means that a degree of targeting will probably be inevitable although initial cigarette smoking consumption is only one of several factors that should be taken into account.

Brief advice

Systematic reviews of randomised control trials found brief opportunistic advice results in approximately 2% of smokers quitting a year [20]. Although this may seem a very poor success rate it represents a significant public health gain when viewed incrementally. Primary health care teams should ensure that the smoking status of each patient is recorded to enable them to advise patients against smoking periodically **(A)**.

Nicotine replacement therapy (NRT)

There is a large literature demonstrating the efficacy for NRT which increases the odds of successful cessation 1.7 - 2.1 times, and reduces withdrawal discomfort **(I)** [21]. The cost effectiveness is also extremely attractive in comparison to NHS norms and other treatments. NRT became available on prescription in April 2001 and is widely used to assist cessation. It is not a "magic cure" for smokers and careful consideration needs to be made when using these products. There are cost implications to prescribing budgets (NRT costs about £18 per week, the same as the average cost of smoking) and if the patient is not committed then their quit attempt may fail.

NRT is available in six different forms: chewing gum (2 mg & 4 mg), transdermal patch (16 hour & 24 hour in varying doses), nasal spray, inhalator, sublingual tablet and lozenge. There is evidence to suggest that their efficacy is maximised when used in conjunction with behavioural support by trained health professionals and side-effects are rare **(A)** [21] (Figure 1).

There is no clear evidence that one method of nicotine delivery is more effective than another and treatment options are based on common sense and the patient's personal preference.

Buproprion

A meta analysis of two published trials confirms that quit rates are significantly increased by buproprion [22,23]. In these trials buproprion was used concurrently with behavioural support and there is no evidence that it is successful without this.

Smokers need to be carefully assessed for suitability, as there is a small risk of serious adverse effects, which is broadly similar to that of other antidepressants. It is not yet clear whether buproprion is more effective than NRT and further research is needed before any conclusions can be drawn.

Offering a prescription for NRT or buproprion increases the success rate of the quit attempt **(A)** [21,22,23] and smokers of ten or more cigarettes per day should normally be encouraged to use one of these **(A)** [21,22,23].

Smoking and pregnancy

Smoking during pregnancy harms the unborn child and leads to lower birth weight, premature birth, stillbirth, childhood asthma, cot death and the risk of miscarraige. New evidence also shows that women who smoke during pregnancy pass harmful carcinogens to their baby [24].

The White Paper "Smoking Kills" [2] targets a reduction in the percentage of women who smoke during pregnancy from 23% to 15% by 2010. The problems of smoking during pregnancy are closely related to health inequalities between those in need

Figure 1 Protocol for health professionals prescribing smoking cessation therapy with motivational support. *For North and East Devon Health Authority.*

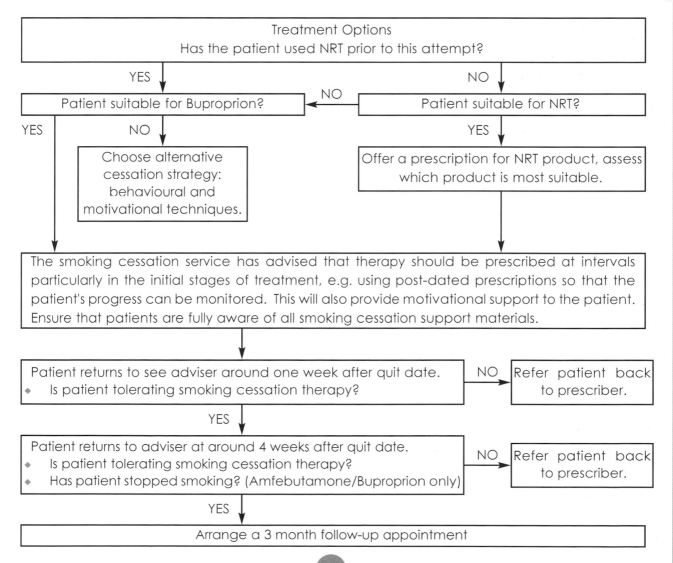

Chapter 4

Figure 2 Improvements in total cancer mortality due to specific intervention. *In persons under age 75* England by 2010.*

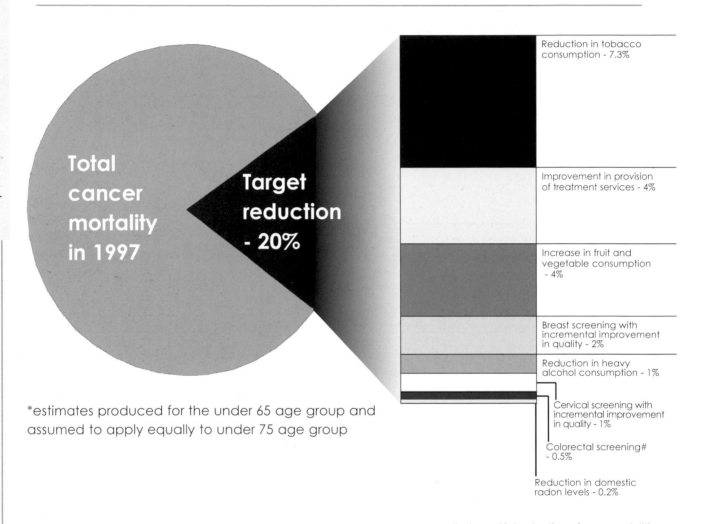

*estimates produced for the under 65 age group and assumed to apply equally to under 75 age group

Reproduced with kind permission of Professor N Day, University of Cambridge

 # phased introduction of new modalities

and the most advantaged. An additional £3m was made available in 2001 to employ local champions to co-ordinate services for pregnant women who want to give up smoking [13]. It is becoming more apparent, as the smoking cessation services develop, that women who smoke during pregnancy find it difficult to stop and often do not welcome advice from health professionals. This is confirmed by the number of monitoring forms returned to the Department of Health.

West *et al*, [13] recommended that NRT products should be available to pregnant women for whom non-pharmacological interventions have failed **(C)**. However, it is important that this is assessed during early pregnancy: the pregnant smoker should not necessarily be required to fail in an unaided quit attempt before receiving effective treatment.

Smoking and secondary care

The Government has pledged to reduce mortality from cancer by 20% by the year 2010 and a 7.3% reduction in tobacco consumption is one of the components of this target (Figure 2). The National Service Framework for Coronary Heart Disease also includes a 19% reduction in tobacco consumption. In order to maximise the benefits of available NHS resources, and for Primary Care Trusts to meet their long-term targets, smoking cessation services will need to be embedded into long-term strategic planning.

Although there is strong evidence supporting cessation help for smokers in hospital (I) [13], not all secondary care staff are aware of the resources available locally. A hospital visit should be treated as an opportunity to help smokers stop, particularly when surgery is planned since smoking may interfere with post-operative recovery. A hospital visit should establish the smoking status of all patients, and use this information to help smokers stop (A) [25].

Smoking cessation services

Initial funding was given, in the first year, to Health Action Zone areas to address inequalities in health and target the most deprived smokers in the community. This allowed GPs to do no more than give brief advice about stopping, prescribe a pharmacotherapy and/or refer to the local smoking cessation service. Training health professionals has been a major part of setting up the service [13], and in an ideal world, would be extended to enable every GP to receive smoking cessation training in order to use the five As model:

◆ **Ask** about smoking at every reasonable opportunity.

◆ **Advise** all smokers to stop.

◆ **Assess** smoker's motivation to stop.

◆ **Assist** smoker to stop.

◆ **Arrange** follow-up.

There are three broad levels of smoking cessation services, reflecting the intensity of the intervention:

◆ **Specialist intervention** smoking cessation services run by a smoking cessation specialist who has received training for this role. The clinic/service will be evidence based and offer intensive treatment in the form of group support over the course of 5 - 6 weeks, including the use of NRT. Clients may also receive one-to-one treatment if for any reason group sessions are deemed unsuitable.

◆ **Intermediate intervention** This is usually provided on a one-to-one basis by either a specialist health professional or another suitably trained individual. Professionals who have accessed the training come from a variety of different backgrounds including project workers in family centres, pharmacists, youth workers and others. These people are registered with the local smoking cessation co-ordinator, and receive regular visits, literature and resources from the service.

◆ **Brief intervention** This could be carried out by GPs, health professionals and other relevant people. This would be provided within the course of the professional's normal duties rather than comprising a "new" service, and monitoring information about clients in receipt of such interventions is not required.

The Government needs to obtain robust and reliable information about the operation of smoking cessation services in the NHS, in order to demonstrate the effectiveness of the investment it is making in these services. Each Health Authority should have individual targets for the numbers of clients setting a quit date and those successfully quitting, based on the overall national targets.

Summary

◆ Our understanding of tobacco use has increased considerably, and it is now widely recognised as a pervasive syndrome of addiction to the drug nicotine, with dependence characteristics on a par with heroin or cocaine (A).

Chapter 4

◆ It is clear that tobacco use is not a habit or a trivial indulgence that may be easily abandoned at the will of the user. Tobacco dependence should be understood as a serious medical condition, and its treatment should be seen as clearly within the remit of the NHS **(A)**.

Further reading

1   Smoking Cessation Guidelines and their Cost Effectiveness. *Thorax* 1998; (53) Supplement 5.

2   Coronary Heart Disease: Guidance for Implementing the Preventative Aspect of the National Service Framework. Health Development Agency, 2001, 2nd Edition. ISBN 1-84279-014-5.

References (grade I evidence and grade A recommendations in bold)

1   **Peto R, Lopez AD, Borham J** *et al*. **Imperial Cancer Research Fund and World Health Organisation.** *Mortality from smoking in developing countries 1950-2000*. **Oxford University Press, Oxford, 1994.**

2   DOH. Smoking Kills. A White Paper on Tobacco. The Stationery Office, London, December 1998.

3   Wald N, Nicolaides-Bouman A, Eds. *UK Smoking Statistics*. Oxford University Press, Oxford, 1988.

4   Royal College of Physicians Tobacco Advisory Group. Nicotine Addiction in Britain. Royal College of Physicians, London, 2000.

5   US Surgeon General. The Health Consequences of Smoking, Nicotine Addiction, 1988.

6   Health Education Authority. Smoking the Facts. HEA, London, 1998.

7   **DOH. The NHS Plan: A Plan for Investment. A Plan for Reform. The Stationery Office, London, July 2000.**

8   DOH. The NHS Cancer Plan. DOH, London, Sept 2000.

9   Coronary Heart Disease National Service Framework. DOH, London, March 2000.

10   **West R, McNeill A, Raw M. Smoking cessation guidelines and their cost effectiveness.** *Thorax* **Dec 1998; (53) Suppl 5.**

11   Muir J, Fuller A, Lancaster T. Applying the Sheffield tables to data from general practice. *British Journal of General Practice* 1999; 49: 218-9.

12   **Tobacco Addiction Review Group.** *The Cochrane Library*. **Update Software Ltd, Oxford, 2001; issue 2.**

13   **West R, McNeill A, Raw M. Smoking cessation guidelines for health professionals: an update.** *Thorax* **December 2000; 55: 987-999.**

14   USDHHS. Treating tobacco use and dependence. Agency for Healthcare Research Quality, Rockville MD, 2000.

15   Ogden J. *Health Psychology*. Open University Press, Buckingham, 2000.

16   Simpson D. Tobacco Control Resource Centre. *Doctors and tobacco*. BMJ Books, London, 1999.

17   **Broome A, Llewellyn S.** *Health psychology, processes and applications*. **London, 1995.**

18   Tobacco Control Resource Centre, 2000. Venables, T. 1991: NHS Centre for Reviews & Dissemination, 1998.

19   Fowler G. Smoking cessation: the role of general practitioners, nurses and pharmacists. In: *The tobacco epidemic*. Bollinger CT, Fagerstrom KO, Eds. Basel, Karger, 1997: 165-177.

20   Silagy C, Ketteridge S. The effectiveness of physician advice to aid smoking cessation. In: *Tobacco addiction module of the Cochrane database of systematic reviews*. Lancaster T, Silagy C, Eds. Updated 2 December 1996. Available in *The Cochrane Library*. Update Software, Oxford, 1996.

21   **Silagy C, Mant D, Fowler G, Lancaster T. Nicotine replacement therapy for smoking cessation. In: The** *Cochrane Library*, **Issue 1. Update Software, Oxford, 2000.**

22   **Hurt RD, Sachs DP, Glover ED,** *et al*. **A comparison of sustained release buproprion and placebo for smoking cessation.** *N Engl J Med* **1997; 337: 1195-202.**

23   **Jorenby DE, Leischow SJ, Nides MA,** *et al*. **A controlled trial of sustained-release buproprion, a nicotine patch or both for smoking cessation.** *N Engl J Med* **1999; 340: 685-91.**

24   Hecht SS, Carmella SG, Chen ML, Salzberger U, Tollner U, Lackmann GM. Metabolites of the tobacco specific lung carcinogen in the urine of newborn infants. Abstract Papers. *Am Chem Soc* 1998: 216; 32.

25   **Cromwell J, Bartosch WJ, Fiore M,** *et al*. **Cost effectiveness of the clinical practice recommendations in the AHCPR Guideline for smoking cessation.** *JAMA* **1997; 278: 1759-66.**

Chapter 5

The diabetic foot

Stephen Gough Reader in Medicine

Andrew Bradbury Professor of Vascular Surgery

UNIVERSITY OF BIRMINGHAM & BIRMINGHAM HEARTLANDS HOSPITAL, BIRMINGHAM, UK

Introduction

In the UK the prevalence of type 2 diabetes is 2-3% and this is predicted to double over the next 10 years [1]. Approximately 5% of diabetics have a foot ulcer at any point in time [2] and the "diabetic foot" leads to more amputations than any other pathology [3]. Its management is consuming a significant and increasing proportion of healthcare resources. For many years the treatment of diabetic foot disease was neglected. However, advances in management over the past 10 years, including the establishment of multidisciplinary foot clinics [4,5] and the recognition of specific diabetic foot syndromes, has made an impact on ulcer healing rates and the number of major amputations [6] **(II)**.

Diabetic foot syndromes

Although diabetics may present with "pure" ischaemia, most present with neuropathy or neuro-ischaemia [6]. The recognition of these two distinct syndromes, each with their respective management pathways, has made an important contribution to improved outcomes.

The neuropathic foot

Sensory neuropathy

There is a bilateral symmetrical sensory loss that occurs in a stocking distribution.

Motor neuropathy

Loss of the small muscles of the foot and the long extensors leads to foot deformity and abnormally situated load-bearing sites; for example, the metatarsal heads or the tips and dorsum of claw toes.

Autonomic neuropathy

The foot is warm, the skin is dry (often fissured), the pedal pulses are palpable (often bounding) and dorsal veins are distended. There may be oedema and a destructive neuro-arthropathy (Charcot's joint).

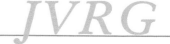

Neuropathic ulceration

Although some patients will have leg and foot pain as part of their neuropathy, the ulcer itself is usually painless and develops at a site of (abnormally) high mechanical pressure on the plantar surface of the forefoot or toes (tip or dorsum).

The neuro-ischaemic foot

The ischaemic foot is typically cold and pale with absent pedal pulses and venous "guttering". However, where there is associated neuropathy, dermal capillary vasodilatation may lead to the foot appearing deceptively "pink" and warm to the touch, with visible veins. This is especially so when the foot is dependent. Despite this, elevation is associated with pallor and venous emptying with restoration of dependency leading to a creeping rubor of the forefoot (sometimes called a "sunset" foot) due to reactive hyperaemia (Buerger's test).

Neuro-ischaemic ulceration

Ulceration typically develops on the margins of the foot and toes, heel and malleoli due to pressure necrosis. This is often related to poorly fitting shoes and, where there is neuropathy, unrecognised trauma to the insensate foot.

Prevention

The feet of all diabetics should be examined annually for the presence of pulses, testing of sensation with a 10 g monofilament or tuning fork, and inspection of foot shape and footwear (A). In March 2000 Diabetes UK (formerly the British Diabetic Association), the Royal College of General Practitioners, the Royal College of Physicians, and the Royal College of Nursing published an evidence based joint document entitled "Clinical Guidelines for Type 2 Diabetes - Prevention and management of foot problems". The review date is March 2003 and further information is available at http://www.rcgp.org.uk. The management plan was based upon the classification of patients into specific "risk" categories (A).

Low risk

Sensation is normal and pedal pulses are palpable. The patient should receive general foot care advice and be seen in a year.

At risk

There is one or more of the following present: neuropathy, absent pulses or other risk factor including old age, plantar callus, poor footwear, duration of diabetes, social deprivation, poor vision, smoking. A podiatrist should review these patients 3-6 monthly for advice on appropriate foot wear, prevention of plantar callus and nail care.

High risk

Foot as above, with the addition of a foot deformity, skin changes, or a previous ulcer. Patients in this group should receive frequent (1-3 month) specialised podiatry review, with special attention to intensified foot care education, specialised footwear and insoles, frequent nail and skin care and medical review to assess the need for a more detailed vascular assessment.

Ulcerated foot

A foot with a break in the skin or obvious infection, usually associated with the clinical features of a high risk foot. These patients require urgent (within 24 hours) referral to a hospital-based, multi-disciplinary diabetic foot clinic.

Management: the role of the multi-disciplinary foot care team

This team comprises diabetologists, specialist nurses, dieticians, orthotists, microbiologists, podiatrists, and shoe-fitters. There must be direct access to X-ray facilities, and in-patient facilities for bed rest and intravenous antibiotics. If there is a significant ischaemic component the patient should be reviewed jointly with a vascular surgeon.

The team's primary role is to provide care to the *high risk* foot that has developed an active complication such as ulceration, infection, or destructive neuro-arthropathy. Many clinics also provide a post-operative foot service with respect to wound care, specialist footwear and rehabilitation, often in conjunction with the regional limb fitting service.

According to Edmonds and Foster [6], the diabetic foot can be categorised in to one of six stages: 1 - normal, 2 - high-risk, 3 - ulcerated, 4 - cellulitic, 5 - necrotic and 6 - amputated. At each stage, six areas that require "control" should be considered: educational, metabolic, biomechanical, vascular, wound and microbiological (Figure 1). A loss of control, for example microbiological control, in the ulcerated foot will automatically move the patient from stage 3 to 4. At each stage due attention must be paid to the general medical care of the diabetic patient; this includes glycaemic control, hypertension, dyslipidaemia and advice, where necessary, on smoking. The different aspects of diabetic foot problems will now be presented with the staging of Edmonds and Foster in parenthesis.

Normal and high risk (stages 1 and 2)

These patients will be primarily managed in the community. A podiatrist should advise on footwear and deal with minor foot problems such as onychogryphosis (Ram's horn nail) onychocryptosis (ingrowing toenail), subungual haematomas, fungal infection, verrucae and corns. Biomechanical control while walking can be achieved with sensible high street shoes, ready made "off the shelf" orthopaedic shoes or customized bespoke shoes with redistributive insoles. Specific deformities in the neuropathic but not neuro-ischaemic foot, may, in certain circumstances, be managed by prophylactic surgery, particularly if it represents a site of recurrent ulceration and is difficult to accommodate in a shoe. These include clawed toes and prominent metatarsal

heads (common in the neuropathic foot) and hallux valgus. Dry skin and fissures, again common in the neuropathic foot, should be treated with a simple emollient.

Ulceration (stage 3)

It is important to differentiate between the neuropathic and neuro-ischaemic ulcer because the management of each is quite different.

Neuropathic ulcer

This usually develops at a site of high plantar pressure and is often surrounded by a "halo" of white callus. The callus may be extensive and actually hide the ulcer. The mainstay of treatment is a careful and even reduction of callus. This will facilitate the development of healthy granulation tissue and relieves the increased local pressure that leads to the build-up of callus in the first place. The ulcer must also be rendered non-weight bearing **(A)** [7]. This can be achieved with a redistributive insole although in other patients a more sophisticated orthotic advice will be required.

Neuro-ischaemic ulcer

The neuro-ischaemic ulcer usually develops on the margins of the foot, or the tips of the toes, and may be preceded by an area of redness as a result of localised pressure from the shoe. Granulation tissue is usually minimal. In contrast to the neuropathic ulcer, where the aim is to redistribute plantar pressure, the primary aim here is to protect the ulcerated area **(A)**. Furthermore, the scalpel should be used with more caution for fear of accidentally damaging neighbouring ischaemic tissue. However, limited debridement and removal of dead tissue will facilitate ulcer healing.

Dressings

There are no controlled trials to demonstrate that any particular dressing leads to more rapid healing **(I)** [8]. Generally, non-adherent, absorbent dressings are

Figure 1 The multi-disciplinary management of the diabetic foot.

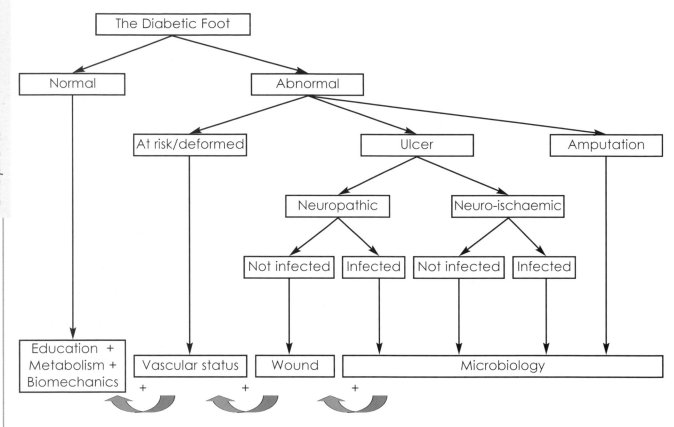

Chapter 5

preferred and these should be changed daily to permit wound inspection.

Vascular assessment and intervention

Neuropathic ulcers will usually heal without surgery. In contrast, the neuro-ischaemic ulcer may only heal once the limb has been revascularised. However, non-invasive assessment of the arterial status of the diabetic foot can be difficult. This is because arterial calcification may lead to spuriously high ankle pressures and because the segmental nature of diabetic vascular disease can lead to areas of focal ischaemia. As such, it can be difficult to determine exactly what part the ischaemia, as opposed to the neuropathy, is playing and whether the benefits of revascularisation will outweigh the risks.

Several centres, notably from the US [9], have published remarkable long-term patency and limb salvage rates for femorotibial bypass in diabetic patients. Impressive though these results are, one cannot help wondering how many of these patients would have healed their ulcers and kept their legs with best medical therapy alone. Furthermore, data collected within the more rigorous conditions of a randomised trial, national or multi-centres registries, paint a far less optimistic picture of what can be achieved by femorodistal bypass.

So, when to operate? Pragmatically, experience suggests that ulcers that show signs of healing within 4-6 weeks with good wound care, a protective orthosis and prophylactic antibiotics often go on to heal completely without revascularisation. By contrast, if the ulcer remains indolent or deteriorates despite best medical treatment, revascularisation is usually required. The threshold for surgery will depend upon many factors such as the fitness of the patient and the availability of a good quality autogenous conduit. The role of angioplasty has not been defined. However, the on-going Bypass versus Angioplasty in Severe Ischaemia of the Leg (BASIL) trial will provide randomised, controlled data on the relative merits of an angioplasty versus a bypass first strategy in patients (diabetic and non-diabetic) with severe limb ischaemia [10].

Infection (stage 4)

Infection, invariably due to a break in the skin or ulceration [11], leads to septic vasculitis and tissue necrosis. This process is, of course, exacerbated and accelerated by any co-existing ischaemia. Early, effective control of infection and necrosis is mandatory if amputation is to be prevented [12]. Unfortunately, an exaggerated fear of the complications of prolonged, combination antibiotic therapy frequently leads to the inadequate treatment of infection.

It is important to remember that symptoms (pain) and signs (rubor, color, lymphangitis, systemic upset) may be reduced, even absent, in the diabetic patient [13]. Severe pain and tenderness may indicate a collection of pus. Callus may obscure the extent of tissue infection and necrosis. Early debridement is crucial as it reveals the true extent of the infection (which is always greater than initially suspected), removes dead tissue that harbour bacteria (and can be sent for culture), and drains any collections that may be present **(A)**. Debridement of the neuropathic foot is relatively straightforward as the lack of sensation removes the need for anaesthesia, and the boundary between non-viable and healthy tissue is usually quite clear. This boundary is less obvious in the neuro-ischaemic foot and there is a natural reluctance to debride such a foot for fear of causing further damage. However, the benefits of debridement, by a suitably experienced surgeon, still outweigh the risks. In addition an assessment of tissue perfusion can be made from the extent of bleeding, and the immediate threat of rapidly spreading wet gangrene is removed. This allows time for vascular imaging and the planning of revascularisation if required. Furthermore, the presence of osteomyelitis can also be assessed at debridement **(II)** [14]. Although a foot x-ray should always be performed to look for signs of osteomyelitis, it is important to remember that the films may remain normal for 10-14 days. The x-ray should, therefore, be repeated at fortnightly intervals. Plain films may also show gas in the deep tissues and/or a foreign body (which can easily go unnoticed in the neuropathic foot).

Magnetic resonance imaging (MRI) and leucocyte labelled scans may be helpful in the detection of early change and help to show the true extent of tissue destruction. For example, an MRI that shows extensive necrosis of the posterior plantar fascia indicates a non-salvageable foot and prevents repeated well intentioned, but ultimately fruitless, surgical "nibbling". On the medical side, optimal glycaemic control is mandatory and this may require intravenous insulin.

A combination of broad spectrum antibiotics will be needed to cover what is likely to be a heavy mixture (often three to six pathogenic bacteria) of gram-positive (*Staphylococcus aureus*, *Streptococcus*, *Enterococcus*), gram-negative (*Escherichia*, *Proteus*, *Klebsiella*, *Enterobacter*, *Pseudomonas*) and anaerobic organisms (*Bacteroides*, *Clostridia*, *Peptostreptococcus*) **(II)** [10,15]. Despite the culture of both multiple swabs and surgical specimens, the precise identification of the underlying organism(s) is often difficult. This, and the lack of good trials comparing different antibiotic combinations, means that therapy is often empirical. The regimen chosen will depend upon a number of factors including the severity of the infection and, to some extent, whether there is neuropathy or neuro-ischaemia. The following are suggested as reasonable options **(C)**.

Mild cellulitis (< 2cm)

In the absence of an isolated organism the neuropathic ulcer can be treated with co-amoxyclav (625 mg t.d.s) and metronidazole (400 mg t.d.s). Trimethoprim (200 mg b.d.) can be added if gram-negative bacteria are strongly suspected. In the event of penicillin allergy, erythromycin (500 mg q.d.s.) can be used as an alternative to co-amoxyclav. If methicilin-resistant *Staphylococcus aureus* (MRSA) is isolated, and there are signs of infection, trimethoprim, rifampicin, and sodium fucidate should be considered along with topical mupirocin (2%) ointment. If the lesion is neuro-ischaemic, ciprofloxacin may be used instead of trimethoprim to provide more extensive coverage of both gram-positive and negative organisms. The patient should be reviewed daily by the district nurse and in the clinic every couple of weeks. Antibiotics should be continued until signs of infection have gone and/or the ulcer is healed.

Severe cellulitis (> 2cm)

This is a potentially limb threatening complication and requires emergency in-patient treatment with the above antibiotics administered intravenously. If deep infection is also suspected, or the cellulitis is spreading, a cephalosporin such as ceftazidime (1 g t.d.s) should be added (quadruple therapy). Patients should be reviewed on a daily basis. Failure to settle suggests underlying sepsis requiring debridement and drainage. If MRSA is isolated intravenous, vancomycin (1g b.d.) or teicoplanin (200-400 mg b.d.) should be considered. Dosing should be adjusted according to serum level.

Osteomyelitis

This does not necessarily require bone removal/amputation **(II)** [16,17]. Good tissue and bone penetration can be achieved with a combination of either ciprofloxacin (500 mg b.d.) and clindamycin (150 mg q.d.s.), or flucloxacillin (500 mg q.d.s.) and sodium fusidate (500 mg t.d.s.). Antibiotics may need to be continued for between 3 and 6 months. Surgery should be considered if, during this time, the condition deteriorates.

Necrosis and gangrene (stage 5)

Dry gangrene

This is primarily due to chronic ischaemia and is characterised by a clear line of demarcation between the dead and healthy tissues. Dry necrosis occurs in the neuro-ischaemic foot and often presents as a black toe. If there are no signs of infection and the toe is dry and mummified, the patient does not require antibiotics and the toe can be allowed to auto-amputate over a period of months. The toe should be inspected by the patient or carer every day and reviewed in the clinic every 1 to 2 weeks **(C)**. Dry gangrene does not require debridement either by surgery or the application of topical preparations by nursing staff. This may need to be stressed, particularly to community nurses. However, any signs of infection should be managed as per the infected foot to prevent cellulitis and the development of wet gangrene.

Wet gangrene

This is caused by septic vasculitis and can occur in the neuropathic and neuro-ischaemic foot. The skin or toe is bluish-purple-black with features of severe tissue infection and malodour. Intravenous antibiotics should be given as a prelude to urgent vascular referral for consideration of amputation. In this circumstance, a so-called guillotine amputation can be life-saving.

Major amputation (stage 6)

Major (transfemoral or transtibial) limb amputation may be required when there is overwhelming sepsis or non-reconstructable critical limb ischaemia that cannot be controlled medically. It is rare for patients with purely neuropathic disease to require major limb amputation although digital and partial foot amputations are not infrequent. Major limb amputation carries a high mortality and morbidity and rehabilitation can be protracted. The surviving limb is at increased risk of ulceration and amputation and appropriate care including orthotic advice and treatment should be given.

Figure 2 Rocker-bottom deformity.

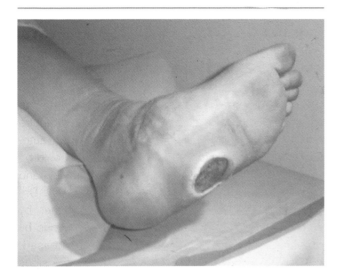

Figure 3 Aircast walker.

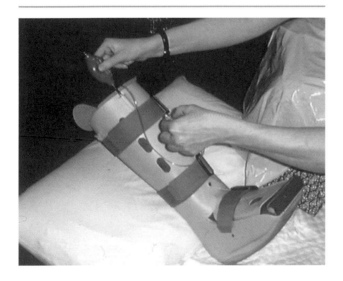

The Charcot foot: destructive neuro-arthropathy

Foot deformity due to neuro-arthropathy, is present in 10-40% of neuropathic diabetics [18]. Diagnosis of the acute, early stages of the disorder requires a high index of suspicion but can prevent subsequent deformity and ulceration. The Charcot foot usually presents with sudden onset of pain, swelling and erythema in the foot of a patient who has had diabetes

for at least 10 years. The foot may feel hot to touch and characteristically the temperature is $2^{\circ}C$ higher than that of the unaffected foot. Often there may be no, or a minimal, history of foot trauma. Without treatment, there is rapid progression to bony destruction with loss of the foot arches and the development of a "rocker-bottom" deformity (Figure 2). The patient may also notice a bony prominence developing over the medial aspect of the foot. Prior to collapse the x-ray may be normal, although a technetium methylene diphosphonate bone scan will detect early bone destruction. Once collapse has occurred the x-ray will show bone fragmentation, fracture, joint subluxation and new bone formation. The Charcot foot should be immobilised immediately, either (preferably) in a total contact cast or in an orthotic device (Aircast walker) (Figure 3), until the clinical symptoms have settled and the x-ray shows no further evidence of bone destruction **(A)**. This can take between 4 and 12 months. The use of bisphosphonates in stabilising the joint at an earlier stage is currently under investigation. Once the foot appears to have stabilised gradual rehabilitation is needed with appropriate footwear prescribed and assessed by a trained orthotist. Inadequate immobilisation or a late diagnosis will result in foot deformity that is difficult to accommodate in standard or even bespoke footwear. In the acute stage the Charcot foot may be indistinguishable from osteomyelitis. The latter, however, is unusual without a break in the skin. If there is uncertainty, the foot should be immobilised and appropriate antibiotics prescribed. A rapid improvement in symptoms with immobilisation points to the diagnosis of a Charcot's foot.

Summary

- The management of the diabetic foot requires a multi-disciplinary approach in order to reduce the morbidity and mortality associated with this condition **(II)**.

- Recognition of the different diabetic foot syndromes, in particular the neuropathic and the neuro-ischaemic foot, is important. The management of each is different and involves different care pathways within the framework of a multi-disciplinary approach **(II)**.

Chapter 5

- ◆ Infection is almost always secondary to ulceration and should be treated aggressively not just in terms of antibiotics but also pressure off-loading, surgical debridement, good wound management and where necessary revascularisation **(II)**.

- ◆ Adequate provision of these components of care may prevent tissue necrosis and amputation **(II)**.

Further reading

1 Boulton A, Connor H, Cavanagh P, Eds. *The Foot in Diabetes*. 3rd edition. John Wiley and Sons, Chichester, 2000.

References (grade I evidence and grade A recommendations in bold)

1 King H, Aubert RE, Herman WH. Global burden of diabetes, 1995-2025: prevalence, numerical estimates, and projections. *Diabetes Care* 1998; 21: 1414-1431.

2 Mason J, O'Keeffe C, McIntosh A, Hutchinson A, Booth A, Young RJ. A systematic review of foot ulcer in patients with Type 2 diabetes mellitus. I: prevention. *Diabet Med* 1999; 16: 801-812.

3 Reiber GE, Boyko EJ, Smith DG. Lower extremity foot ulcers and amputations in diabetes. In: *Diabetes in America*. Harris MI, Cowie CC, Stern MP, Boyko EJ, Bennett PH, Eds. Washington DC, U.S. Govt. Printing Office, 1995: 409-428.

4 Larsson J, Apelqvist J, Agardh CD, Stenstrom A. Decreasing incidence of major amputation in diabetic patients: a consequence of a multidisciplinary foot care team approach? *Diabet Med* 1995; 12: 770-776.

5 Holstein PE, Sorensen S. Limb salvage experience in a multidisciplinary diabetic foot unit. *Diabetes Care* 1999; 22 Suppl 2: B97-103.

6 Edmonds ME. Progress in care of the diabetic foot. *Lancet* 1999; 354: 270-272.

7 **Armstrong DG, Lavery LA. Evidence-based options for off-loading diabetic wounds. *Clin Podiatr Med Surg* 1998; 15: 95-104.**

8 **Mason J, O'Keeffe C, Hutchinson A, McIntosh A, Young R, Booth A. A systematic review of foot ulcer in patients with Type 2 diabetes mellitus. II: treatment. *Diabet Med* 1999; 16: 889-909.**

9 Pomposelli FB, Jr., Marcaccio EJ, Gibbons GW, Campbell DR, Freeman DV, Burgess AM, Miller A, LoGerfo FW. Dorsalis pedis arterial bypass: durable limb salvage for foot ischemia in patients with diabetes mellitus. *J Vasc Surg* 1995; 21: 375-384.

10 Bell JB, Papp L, Bradbury AW. Bypass or angioplasy for severe limb ischaemia of the leg: the BASIL trial. In: *Vascular and Endovascular Opportunities*. Greenhalgh RM , Powell JT, Mitchell AW, Eds. WB Saunders, London, 2000: 485-494.

11 Lipsky BA, Berendt AR. Principles and practice of antibiotic therapy of diabetic foot infections. *Diabetes Metab Res Rev* 2000; 16 Suppl 1: S42-46.

12 Reiber GE, Pecoraro RE, Koepsell TD. Risk factors for amputation in patients with diabetes mellitus. A case-control study. *Ann Intern Med* 1992; 117: 97-105.

13 Eneroth M, Apelqvist J, Stenstrom A. Clinical characteristics and outcome in 223 diabetic patients with deep foot infections. *Foot Ankle Int* 1997; 18: 716-722.

14 Grayson ML, Gibbons GW, Balogh K, Levin E, Karchmer AW. Probing to bone in infected pedal ulcers. A clinical sign of underlying osteomyelitis in diabetic patients. *JAMA* 1995; 273:721-723.

15 Lipsky BA, Pecoraro RE, Wheat LJ. The diabetic foot. Soft tissue and bone infection. *Infect Dis Clin North Am* 1990; 4: 409-432.

16 Venkatesan P, Lawn S, Macfarlane RM, Fletcher EM, Finch RG, Jeffcoate WJ. Conservative management of osteomyelitis in the feet of diabetic patients. *Diabet Med* 1997; 14: 487-490.

17 Pittet D, Wyssa B, Herter-Clavel C, Kursteiner K, Vaucher J, Lew PD. Outcome of diabetic foot infections treated conservatively: a retrospective cohort study with long-term follow-up. *Arch Intern Med* 1999; 159: 851-856.

18 Frykberg RG. Charcot foot: an update on pathogenesis and management. In: *The foot in diabetes*. Boulton AJ, Connor H, Cavanagh PR, Eds. John Wiley & Sons Ltd, Chichester, 2000: 236-260.

Chapter 6

Out-patient management of varicose veins

Daryll Baker Consultant Vascular Surgeon [1]

Janice Tsui Vascular Research Registrar [1]

Jonathan Beard Consultant Vascular Surgeon [2]

[1] DEPARTMENT OF SURGERY, THE ROYAL FREE HOSPITAL, LONDON, UK
[2] SHEFFIELD VASCULAR INSTITUTE, THE NORTHERN GENERAL HOSPITAL, SHEFFIELD, UK

Introduction

This chapter outlines the clinical decisions that need to be taken when a patient presents to the out-patient clinic (or the primary practitioner's surgery) complaining of varicose veins.

Three questions require answering:

◆ Are there varicose vein symptoms or complications?

◆ Do the varicose veins require treatment?

◆ What treatment should be undertaken?

Figure 1 outlines an algorithm for the management of such a patient. A specific varicose vein proforma recording the history, examination and results of investigations enhances the reliability and consistency of the out-patient care pathway (see website).

Are there varicose vein symptoms or complications?

Before a treatment plan can be considered it is necessary to determine the exact symptoms the patient has and exclude other causes for these symptoms. The patient needs to have leg varicose veins and appropriate varicose vein symptoms [1].

A full examination will determine the type and distribution of the superficial varicose veins as well as any signs of chronic venous insufficiency. There are three different types of superficial leg veins:

◆ True or trunk varicose veins are abnormal tortuous dilated superficial veins.

◆ Reticular veins are prominent normal superficial veins, which do not usually vary in thickness.

◆ Thread or spider veins are fine thin cutaneous veins of a millimetre or so diameter.

All types of visible superficial leg vein may be regarded as unsightly but only trunk varicose veins cause symptoms (II). The symptoms and complications of trunk varicose veins include:

◆ Aching. This is a deep, dull heaviness affecting the whole leg, but in particular that below the

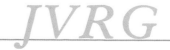

Figure 1 Algorithm for the management of varicose veins in the out-patients.

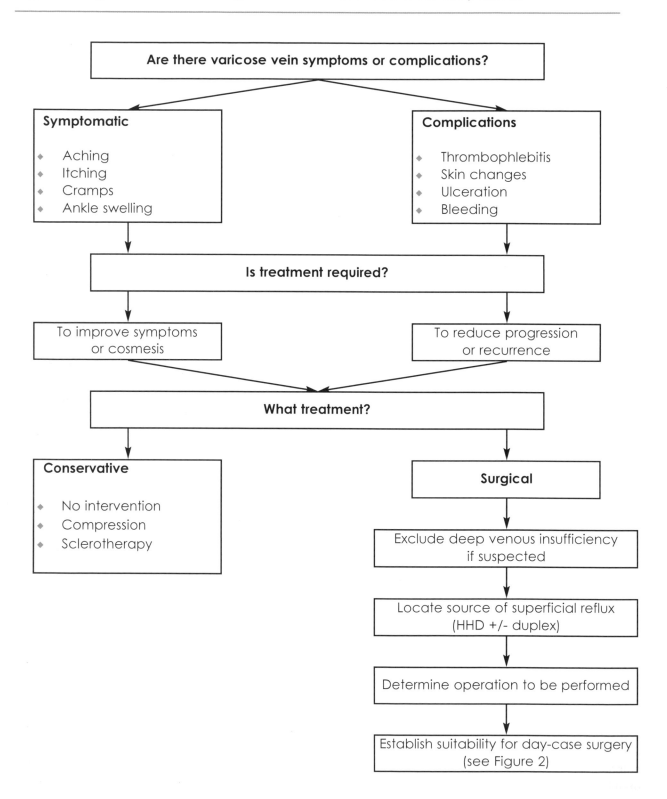

knee. It is worsened by any length of standing and eased by elevating the leg **(II)**.

- Itching. The leg may itch and feel hot, burn or occasionally throb. This is usually over the varicose veins and not a generalised sensation although occasionally it can be confined to the ankle area when skin changes are involved. It is usually worsened by standing or hot weather **(II)**.

- Ankle swelling. Mild to moderate ankle swelling is more prominent in the evenings.

- Nocturnal cramps are a common symptom but the relationship to varicose veins is unproven.

- Superficial thrombophlebitis [2]. Thrombosis of superficial varicose veins causes acute inflammation of the overlying skin. It can occur spontaneously, but is often associated with mild trauma to the vein or immobility/long-distance travel. Other causes such as occult malignancy should not be forgotten. In the acute phase the skin over the vein is erythematous, hot and exquisitely tender. After time residual haemosiderin staining is left over a hard non-tender vein. Eventually the vein recanalises and the process may then repeat itself.

- Venous ankle skin changes range from mild haemosiderin pigmentation to varicose eczema, lipodermatosclerosis and frank ulceration.

- Bleeding at the ankle following minor trauma to delicate skin when there is a high venous ankle pressure can be devastating. Likewise trauma to a prominent leg vein can result in extensive bleeding **(II)**.

If there are no leg varicose veins, superficial venous insufficiency is unlikely to be the cause of the symptoms. Many of the milder symptoms attributed to varicose veins are common in the population and can also exist in the absence of varicose veins **(II)**. Conversely, other conditions causing leg pain such as osteoarthrosis may co-exist with varicose veins. This emphasises the need for a careful history and examination.

Do the varicose veins require treatment?

Patient with uncomplicated varicose veins

Patients with asymptomatic or symptomatic, uncomplicated varicose veins are unlikely to develop significant complications of venous disease. In an 11-year observational study only 1% of patients with mild or moderate varicose veins progressed to venous ulceration [3] **(II)**.

The risk of deep vein thrombosis (DVT) or pulmonary embolism (PE) is not increased in the presence of certain other risk factors such as long-distance travel or taking the oral contraceptive pill or hormone replacement therapy [4] **(II)**. There is however some evidence that patients with varicose veins who are undergoing major surgery are at an increased risk of developing a DVT [5] **(II)**. There is no evidence that varicose vein surgery should be undertaken as a prophylaxis against DVT prior to major surgery but thromboprophylaxis with subcutaneous heparin and/or graduated compression stockings seems sensible, if only to avoid superficial thrombophlebitis **(C)**.

Treatment for varicose vein symptoms is aimed solely at improving the quality of life [6] and not to prevent the small risk of possible complications. Therefore if the symptoms are not severe interventional treatment should be withheld. If on the other hand the symptoms are severely affecting the patient's quality of life then treatment should be considered.

Treatment should only be considered after the patient has considered the potential benefits against the risks of treatment. Percentages of likelihood of each risk should be quoted e.g. 20% likelihood of some varicose veins recurring in the future [7,8] and a 10% risk of altered skin sensation post-operatively, although only 1% have a permanent dysaesthesia [9]. A wound infection rate of 3% can be expected, although many more will receive antibiotics from their general practitioner for an inflamed wound, without proven

Chapter 6

evidence of infection. All patients will have bruising but very few (< 1%) will develop a haematoma large enough to require draining. Surgery will improve most of the symptoms of varicose veins [6] (II) However, there are risks to any procedure and the patient should make an informed decision in the light of these risks especially as varicose vein surgery is the commonest cause of litigation in vascular surgery (see chapter on medico-legal issues). Most hospitals now use printed information leaflets to help inform patients and reduce the risk of litigation (see website). The notes should always record that information has been given to the patient and in what form.

Patients with complicated varicose veins

Patients who already have venous disease complications are at a higher risk of developing further complications [2] (II) and therefore treatment should be considered (Figure 2).

- **Venous skin changes at the ankle** (venous eczema, lipodermatosclerosis and venous ulceration). Colour duplex scanning will identify the sites of deep and superficial venous occlusion and incompetence. Generally if the only abnormality is superficial venous incompetence this is corrected surgically. If the deep veins are incompetent then superficial venous surgery is less likely to help and the patient should be treated with compression therapy (bandages or stockings) in the first instance [10] (A) (see chapter on leg ulcers).

- **Venous bleeding**. An acute episode can be treated with direct pressure and leg elevation. Prevention of further episodes by superficial venous surgery is advisable and if the deep veins are incompetent the patient should also wear compression hosiery [10]. In unfit patients, the bleeding point can be underun with sutures under local anaesthetic. In young active patients who are likely to be subjected to leg trauma such as sportsmen or those in the police force, prophylactic removal of varicose veins is often undertaken (III). Varicose veins are included in the exclusion criteria for entry into the British police force and recruits may request surgery for this reason.

- **Superficial thrombophlebitis.** If a duplex scan demonstrates thrombus extending up the long saphenous vein into the femoral vein, urgent saphenofemoral vein ligation should be undertaken to prevent pulmonary embolus [2] (III). Surgery, in the form of a high tie, strip and avulsions of the varicose veins during the acute phase may reduce the period of discomfort [11] (III).

Which treatment should the patient receive?

Treatment can be divided into non-operative or operative procedures.

Non-operative management of varicose veins

- **No intervention** is recommended for patients with no or minimal symptoms. These patients should be reassured that their visible leg veins are of no concern and are best left well alone.

- **Graduated compression stockings** do reduce aching, itching and ankle oedema and may be the only alternative in elderly patients who are unfit for surgery [12] (A). They are of little help with regards to cosmetic appearance. Compression reduces the symptoms of superficial thrombophlebitis (III) and is the mainstay for the conservative treatment of venous ankle skin changes (I). Most patients prefer below-knee stockings as these are self-supporting, easier to apply and more comfortable, especially in hot weather. Some patients with extensive thigh varicose veins will require full-length stockings and these are best supplied with a waistband support. Class I stockings may relieve the symptoms of mild varicose veins but most patients require the stronger class II stockings.

Figure 2 Algorithm for the selection of patients for day-case varicose vein surgery.

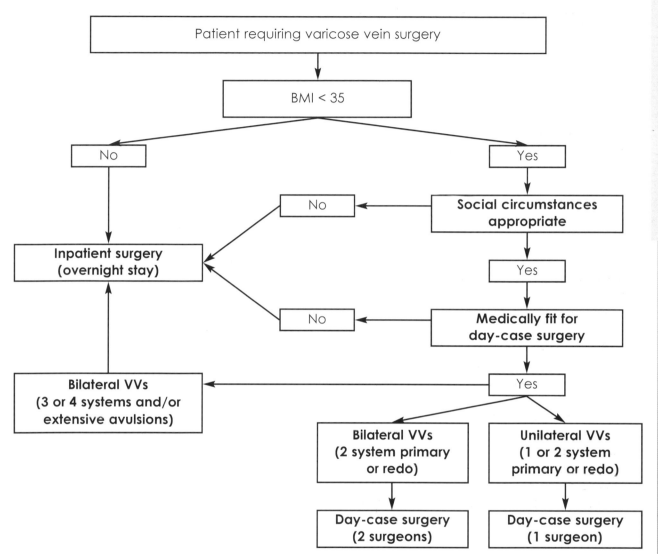

◆ **Sclerotherapy** of trunk varicose veins fails to remove the source of reflux from the deep to superficial venous systems and is thus associated with a high recurrence rate [13] **(II)**. In this country it is therefore not usually employed for varicose veins with significant long or short saphenous vein reflux [14]. Sclerotherapy for minor varicose veins, reticular veins and thread veins is performed extensively for cosmetic reasons (see chapter on sclerotherapy).

Varicose vein surgery

Once the decision to surgically treat the patient's varicose veins has been made, three further decisions are required:

◆ Are the deep veins patent and competent?

◆ What operation should be performed?

◆ Is the patient suitable for day-case surgery?

Is the deep venous system patent and competent?

Before undertaking any procedure, which involves removing superficial leg veins, it is important to confirm that the deep venous system is patent and competent. Suspicion should be raised in cases where there is a history of DVT, or fracture, clinical or venous hypertension (e.g. lipodermatosclerosis), varicose veins in atypical places (e.g. perineum) or associated congenital venous malformations (e.g. Klippel Trenaunay Syndrome). Patency of the deep venous system can be confirmed by duplex ultrasound scanning. In equivocal cases, other investigations such as contrast venography or magnetic resonance venography may be required.

Deep venous obstruction is a contra-indication to varicose vein surgery because the varicose veins may act as important collaterals. Deep venous reflux does not preclude varicose vein surgery but surgery may not be as effective in relieving symptoms or preventing recurrent complications such as ulceration. Patients should be warned of this and the likely need for long-term compression stockings

What operation should be performed?

If both trunk and thread or reticular veins are present it is usual to treat the trunk veins before managing the thread and reticular veins (see chapter on sclerotherapy).

Based on the hypothesis that trunk varicose veins develop as a result of incompetence between the deep and superficial leg venous systems, disconnecting the superficial from the deep venous systems at the site of incompetence will prevent further varicose veins from developing [7,8] (II).

Although there are several potential sites of incompetent communication between the deep and superficial venous systems, for practical purposes this is at either the groin at the saphenofemoral junction where the long saphenous vein drains into the common femoral vein or the saphenopopliteal junction where the short saphenous vein drains into the popliteal vein in the popliteal fossa. The significance of other sites of incompetence between deep and superficial venous systems is yet to be determined and the role of perforator surgery is unclear [15] (III). There are several ways to determine the site of deep to superficial leg venous system incompetence:

- **The Trendelenberg test** is often able to confirm the source of reflux at the saphenofemoral junction in the groin. A narrow tourniquet is placed tightly around the upper thigh after elevating the leg. Lack of filling of the varicose veins on standing indicates that the source of reflux is located above the level of the tourniquet. The test requires prominent varicose veins in a slim patient. A negative test has little significance.

- **The hand-held Doppler (HHD)** is a useful adjunct to determine the presence of saphenofemoral incompetence and reflux in the long saphenous vein at the level of the knee joint [16] (II). Clinicians, including trainees can quickly learn the technique which has an accuracy of > 95% [17]. However, it cannot distinguish between saphenopopliteal and deep vein reflux in the popliteal fossa (II).

- **Duplex ultrasound scanning** will accurately determine the sites of incompetence and it remains the gold standard [18]. However, it is difficult to justify the cost for all patients with varicose veins.

- **On table or pre-operative venography** now has a very limited role. It is difficult to do well, often difficult to interpret and subjects the patient to unnecessary irradiation and contrast.

Clinical examination combined with HHD will suffice for most patients with primary varicose veins in the distribution of the long saphenous vein (medial thigh and/or calf together with reflux at the saphenofemoral junction at the groin and in the LSV at the knee on hand-held Doppler examination). A duplex ultrasound scan should be performed in the following cases [19,20].

- Recurrent varicose veins (previous sapheno-femoral or saphenopopliteal ligation). The presence of persistent or recurrent junctional reflux and the presence of a refluxing long saphenous vein (even if scars suggest previous stripping) help to plan subsequent surgery.

◆ Varicose veins arising from the popliteal fossa. These may be due to saphenopopliteal reflux but some will be due to reflux down a Giacomeni vein connecting to a refluxing long saphenous vein. The site of the saphenopopliteal junction can vary considerably and requires accurate pre-operative localisation with respect to the midpoint of the skin crease.

◆ Past history of DVT or fracture to exclude deep venous occlusion/reflux.

◆ Signs of venous hypertension e.g. lipodermato-sclerosis or ulceration.

Is the patient suitable for day-case surgery?

Varicose veins are amenable to day-case surgery in over 80% of cases [21]. However, this reduces the margin for clinical error and it is important that the patient fits the criteria laid down by the particular unit. In general three things need to be considered:

◆ **The planned procedure.** Due to the duration of the procedure bilateral varicose vein operations are usually not undertaken as day-cases. Sequential unilateral procedures are usually a better option as the incidence of post-operative nausea and vomiting increases with the duration of the anaesthetic [22]. Bilateral primary procedures can be undertaken in the day unit if there are two experienced surgeons and the number of avulsions required is not excessive. Unilateral redo procedures are also suitable for day-case treatment.

◆ **Associated co-morbidity.** If the patient has significant co-morbid diseases that increase the risks of surgical (e.g. known thrombophilia) or anaesthetic (e.g. significant cardiac or respiratory disease) complications, inpatient treatment is recommended. Patients with a high body mass index (BMI > 35) are also excluded from day-case surgery because of their increased anaesthetic risk.

◆ **The patient's living/social arrangements** may be inappropriate for day-case discharge.

Figure 2 outlines an algorithm for the selection of patients for day-case surgery. This selection can be undertaken in the varicose vein clinic but is more reliably undertaken by a nurse working to protocol in a pre-assessment clinic (see relevant chapter).

Summary

◆ Thread veins are not associated with leg aching or swelling **(II)**.

◆ Only 1% of patients with mild or moderate varicose vein symptoms progress to venous ulceration **(II)**.

◆ 20% of patients with severe varicose veins develop ulcers **(II)**.

◆ The incidence of deep vein thrombosis following major surgery (abdominal or gynaecological) is higher in patients with varicose veins than in those without **(II)**.

◆ Ankle ulceration associated with superficial venous disease alone and no deep venous disease usually heals after varicose vein surgery. This is not the case if the deep venous system is diseased **(II)**.

◆ Superficial thrombophlebitis should be treated by surgical excision as this results in a significant decrease in the symptomatic period and prevents further attacks **(C)**.

◆ Hand-held Doppler evaluation is reliable for detecting saphenofemoral junction and long saphenous vein reflux **(II)**.

◆ A duplex scan is indicated for patients with suspected saphenopopliteal reflux **(B)**.

◆ Graduated compression stockings reduce the symptoms and complications of varicose veins and are recommended for those with minor varicose veins and those who are unfit for surgery **(I)**.

Chapter 6

Chapter 6

◆ Sclerotherapy of large trunk varicose veins is associated with a high incidence of recurrence **(I)**.

◆ Varicose vein surgery improves symptoms and quality of life **(II)**.

◆ Most varicose vein surgery can be performed as a day-case procedure **(B)**.

◆ All patients undergoing varicose vein surgery should be given written information that explains the procedure and the risk of complications **(A)**.

Further reading

1   Tibbs DJ, Sabiston DC, Davies MG, Mortimer PS, Scurr JH. *Varicose veins, venous disorders and lymphatic problems in the lower extremity.* Oxford University Press, Oxford, 1997.

References (grade I evidence and grade A recommendations in bold)

1   Bradbury A, Evans C, Allan P, Lee A, Ruckley CV, Fowles FGR. What are the symptoms of varicose veins? Edinburgh vein study cross sectional population survey. *BMJ* 1999; 318: 353-356.

2   Husni EA, Williams WA. Superficial thrombophlebitis of lower limbs. *Surgery* 1982; 91: 70-74.

3   Widmer LK, Holz D, Morselli B *et al.* Progression of varicose veins in 11 years. Observations on 1441 working persons in the Basle study 1992 (unpublished) Referenced in Varicose veins. Smith JJ, Davies AH. In: *Vascular Surgery Highlights.* Davies AH, Ed. Health Press, Oxford, 2000-01.

4   Campbell WB. Are patients with varicose veins at special risk of thromboembolism? In: *Inflammatory and thrombotic problems in vascular surgery.* Greenhalgh and Powell, Eds. WB Saunders Company, London, 1997; 289.

5   Sue-Ling HM, Johnston D, McMahon MJ. Pre-operative identification of patients at high risk of deep venous thrombosis after elective major abdominal surgery. *Lancet* I, 1986: 1173-1176.

6   Baker DM, Turnbull NB, Pearson JC, Makin GS. How successful is varicose vein surgery? A patient outcome study following varicose vein surgery using the SF-36 Health Assessment Questionnaire. *Eur J Vasc Endovasc Surg* 1995; 9: 229-304

7   Rutgers PH, Kitslar PJEHM. Randomised trial of stripping versus high ligation combined with sclerotherapy in the treatment of the incompetent greater saphenous vein. *Am J Surg* 1994; 168: 311-315.

8   Dwerryhouse S, Davies B, Harradine K, Earnshaw JJ. Stripping the long saphenous vein reduces the rate of reoperation for recurrent varicose veins: five-year results. *J Vasc Surg* 1999; 29: 589-592.

9   Docherty JG, Morrice JJ, Ben G. Saphenous neuritis following varicose vein surgery. *Br J Surg* 1994; 81: 695.

10   **MacKenzie RK, Bradbury AW. The management of venous ulceration. In: *The Evidence for Vascular Surgery*. Earnshaw JJ, Murie JA, Eds. Tfm Publishing UK, Shropshire, 1999; 151- 158.**

11   Lofgren EP, Lofgren KA. The surgical management of superficial thrombophlebitis. *Surgery* 1981; 90: 49-54.

12   **Travers JP, Makin GS. Reduction of varicose vein recurrence by use of post-operative compression stockings. *Phlebology* 1994; 9: 104-107.**

13   Hamilton Jacobsen B. The value of different forms of treatment for varicose veins. *Br J Surg* 1979; 66: 182-184.

14   Galland RB, Magee TR, Lewis MH. A survey of current attitudes to British and Irish vascular surgeons to venous sclerotherapy. *Eur J Vasc Endovasc Surg* 1998; 16: 43-46.

15   Stansby G, Delis K. The case for endoscopic perforator surgery. In: *The Evidence for Vascular Surgery.* Earnshaw JJ, Murie JA, Eds. Tfm publishing, Shropshire, 1999; 145-149.

16   Campbell WB, Niblett PG, Ridlow BMF, Peters AS, Thompson JF. Hand-held Doppler as a screening test in primary varicose veins. *Br J Surg* 1997; 84: 1541-1543.

17   Dawke SG, Vetrivel S, Foy DMA, Smith S, Baker S. A comparison of duplex scanning and continuous wave Doppler in the assessment of primary and uncomplicated varicose veins. *Eur J Vasc Endovasc Surg* 1997; 14: 457-461.

18   Mercer KG, Scott DJA, Berridge DC. Preoperative duplex imaging is required before all operations for primary varicose veins. *Br J Surg* 1998; 85: 1495-1497.

19   Kent PJ, Weston MJ. Duplex scanning may be used selectively in patients with primary varicose veins. *Ann R Coll Surg Engl* 1993; 80: 388-389.

20   Lees TA, Beard JD, Ridler BMF, Szymanska T. A survey of the current management of varicose veins by the members of the Vascular Surgical Society. *Ann R Coll Surg Engl* 1999; 81: 407-417.

21   Ramesh S, Umeh HN, Galland RB. Day case varicose vein operations: patient suitability and satisfaction. *Phlebology* 1995; 10: 103-105.

22   Onuma OC, Beam PE, Khan U, Malluci P, Adiseshiah M. The influence of effective analgesia and general anaesthesia on patients' acceptance of day case varicose vein surgery. *Phlebology* 1993; 8: 29-31.

Chapter 7

Sclerotherapy

Claire Judge Vascular Research Sister

DEPARTMENT OF SURGERY, THE ROYAL FREE HOSPITAL, LONDON, UK

Introduction

This chapter discusses sclerotherapy and provides a basic care pathway for patients undergoing this treatment (Figure 1). It should serve as a tool for identifying, evaluating and then modifying processes of care delivery.

Sclerotherapy aims to ablate superficial veins in the legs by the introduction of a sclerosing agent into the vein. Although primarily devised as a treatment for varicose veins, being inexpensive, safe and greatly appreciated by those treated, it is now used less frequently for this because of the high recurrence rate in patients with sapheno-femoral or sapheno-popliteal incompetence. Thus the majority of vascular surgeons reserve sclerotherapy for patients without proximal incompetence and for residual varicose veins following surgery [1]. However, it is increasingly used for ablation of veins < 1mm in diameter in order to improve cosmesis. Visible leg veins can be classified according to their size into thread veins, reticular veins, and varicose veins (see Table 1 and Chapter 6).

"Thread veins" is the lay term for telangiectasia, which are small, unsightly, superficial veins usually seen in clusters on the face and legs. They are a common cosmetic problem occurring in 50% of the population [2].

Genetic predisposition, hyperoestrogenic states, standing vocations and obesity are thought to be the major predisposing factors [3].

Sclerotherapy for thread veins is regarded as a cosmetic treatment and as such is not covered by the majority of private health insurance companies, nor is it widely available within the NHS.

Approximately 100,000 operations for varicose veins are performed in the UK each year [4]. Whilst the number of treatment episodes for injection of minor veins can only be guessed because of lack of data, it is likely to be a similarly large figure.

There is very little established evidence as regards the techniques employed for sclerotherapy and there are no professionally accredited training courses for practitioners [5]. The most appropriate technique will depend on the expertise and the preference of the operator.

In the current era of litigation, it is important that the techniques and sclerotherapy agents used are researched fully to enable evidence-based practice. Thus, there is a need for randomised controlled trials comparing these aspects of treatment for both efficacy and cost effectiveness.

JVRG

Figure 1 Sclerotherapy flow chart.

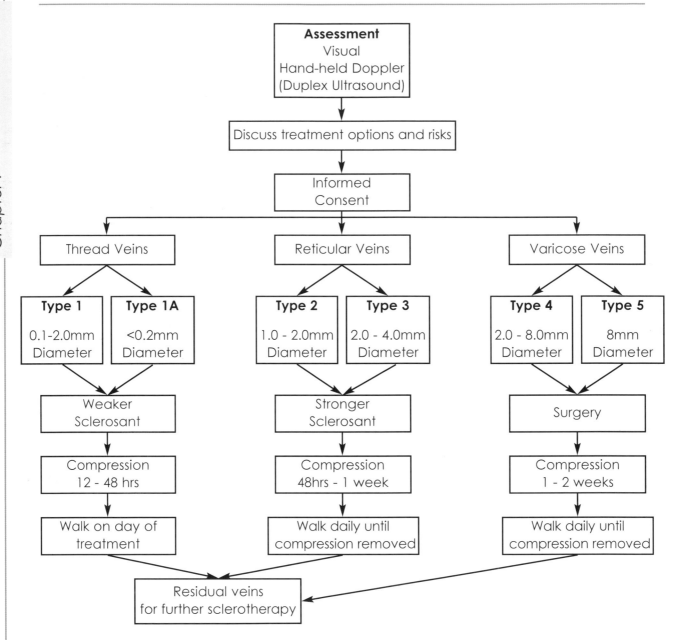

Evidence for pathways of care

Clinical assessment

Sclerotherapy may be ineffective in the presence of superficial or deep venous reflux and this should be excluded prior to treatment.

In a nurse-led clinic the majority of patients will have been referred by a vascular consultant having already had full assessment of their venous and arterial circulation. If this is not the case then the Nurse Practitioner should be trained to assess the patient's suitability and must rule out any signs of chronic venous or arterial insufficiency [2] **(A)**.

Chapter 7

The patient should be assessed whilst standing to inspect and palpate the paths of the long and short saphenous veins and their major tributaries. At this time the sites of common perforators, as well as all areas in which the spider veins are present are assessed to rule out the presence of bulging varices.

The majority of patients presenting with thread veins have no clinical evidence of either varicose veins or deep venous insufficiency, and apart from the cosmetic impact of their veins will be asymptomatic.

Investigations

Venous reflux is most commonly assessed using a hand-held Doppler, although some vascular surgeons prefer patients to undergo duplex scanning to assess the superficial and deep veins.

In a nurse-led clinic if the patient appears to have superficial or deep venous insufficiency further non-invasive investigation should be considered. This may require referral back to the family doctor or, with their permission, an appointment with a vascular surgeon for full assessment.

Consultation

This is the most important factor in the preparation of the patient. Information is often given prior to their appointment explaining the procedure and its potential side-effects.

At assessment there is ample opportunity for the patient to exhibit the areas causing concern and to discuss the procedure. The therapist should be honest about the results that might be achieved, quoting their own percentage risk of side-effects, the probable number of treatment sessions required, the potential recovery period, and post-procedural restrictions (patient information sheet on www.jvrg.org.uk). False optimism will heighten patients' expectations and affect their perception of the eventual result [6] (I). Pre-treatment photographs may provide a useful comparison with the appearance after therapy. A typical patient consent form is available at www.jvrg.org.uk.

Patients should be made aware that thread veins recur over an unspecified period of time and that they are likely to require further treatment.

History

A full medical history (specimen history sheet available on www.jvrg.org.uk) is required to exclude conditions that could precipitate a serious adverse event or which might jeopardise treatment success. Possible exclusion criteria include:

Absolute contraindications

◆ Pregnancy or breast feeding: risk of foetal damage, drug transfer in breast milk.

◆ Immobility: increased risk of deep vein thrombosis.

◆ Ischaemia and diabetic neuropathy: risk of non-healing of "injection site" ulcers.

◆ Known allergy to sclerosing agents.

◆ Asthma: some sclerosants may increase risk of allergic asthma.

Relative contraindication

◆ History of thrombophlebitis: increased risk of underlying venous insufficiency.

◆ History of deep vein thrombosis: risk of recurrence unknown.

◆ Type 4 and Type 5 veins (Table 1): require surgical intervention.

◆ Acute or severe heart disease: some sclerosants alter cardiac perfusion.

◆ Hypercoagulability (eg. Protein C and S deficiency, lupus anticoagulant): risk of DVT.

◆ Local or general infection: exacerbation of sepsis.

◆ Diabetes Mellitus: need to exclude neuro-vascular complications.

Chapter 7

Table 1 Classification of varicose veins.

TYPE	TYPE 1	TYPE 1A	TYPE 2	TYPE 3	TYPE 4	TYPE 5
Size	0.1- 2.0mm in diameter	< 0.2mm diameter	1.0-2.0mm diameter	2.0-4.0 diameter	2.0-8.0mm diameter	>8mm diameter
Colour	Usually red, May rarely be cyanotic.	Network bright red	Violaceous, cyanotic	Cyanotic to blue	Blue to blue/green	Blue to blue/green
Description	Telangiectasia 'spider veins'	Telangiectatic matting	Venulectasis (usually protrudes)	Reticular veins (minor or feeder varicose)	Varicose veins usually related to an incompetent perforator	Varicose veins due to groin reflux

Drugs

Currently available sclerosing agents have both advantages and disadvantages. In addition there is no comprehensive evidence base comparing these drugs and practitioner's preference usually dictates the sclerosing agent used.

All sclerosing agents, classified according to their mode of action as detergent, osmotic or irritant, cause inflammation of the intimal lining of the veins, and a local, adhesive, thrombosis in the area of the damaged endothelium. The thrombus becomes organised so that conversion to a fibrous scar takes place [7].

The drugs listed below are those most commonly used in the UK (see Table 2 for dose).

Polidocanol (Sclerovein)

A detergent-based urethane anaesthetic agent that alters surface tension around endothelial cells causing vascular injury.

Advantages

♦   Available in various strengths: 0.5 - 3%.

♦   Reduced pain on injection: it is a local anaesthetic.

♦   Intradermal injection does not cause necrosis [8].

♦   A very low incidence of allergic reactions [9].

♦   Extensively studied and shown to have a high therapeutic index

Disadvantages

♦   Not licensed in the UK; not approved by FDA as a sclerosing agent.

♦   Occasional anaphylaxis.

♦   Some risk of hyperpigmentation, although less than with many other agents.

♦   Risk of post-sclerotherapy telangiectasia (matting) similar to other agents.

Table 2 Dose of sclerosants.

GENERIC NAME	COMMON TRADE NAME	VEIN TYPE 1 & 1A	VEIN TYPE 2	VEIN TYPE 3	MAXIMUM DOSE PER SESSION
Polidocanol	Sclerovein	0.5%	0.5 & 1%	1%	2mg/kg
Sodium tetradecyl sulphate	Fibrovein	0.2%	0.5 & 1%	3%	10ml of 1% or 3%
Chromated glycerine	Scleremo	Dilute with 1% lignocaine/ saline 4:1 or 1:1	undiluted	Too mild to be effective	5ml
Hypertonic saline	Hypertonic saline	11.7% diluted with 0.4% lignocaine/ saline or heparin	18.7% diluted with 0.4% lignocaine/ saline or heparin	23.4% diluted with 0.4% lignocaine/ saline or heparin	6-10ml

Sodium tetradecyl sulphate (Fibrovein)

A long chain fatty acid with detergent properties.

Advantages

◆ Available in different strengths (0.2 - 3%).

◆ A safe, effective, agent holding a UK drug license and approved by FDA.

Disadvantages

◆ Hyperpigmentation in up to 30% of patients.

◆ Occasional anaphylaxis.

◆ Significant risk of epidermal necrosis following extravasation.

◆ Risk of allergic reaction after repeated treatment; may require intervals of several years between courses of injections [10].

Chromated glycerin (Scleremo)

A chemical irritant causing cell surface protein denaturation.

Advantages

◆ Rarely causes hyperpigmentation or matting.

◆ Rarely causes extravasation necrosis [8].

Disadvantages

◆ Not licensed as a sclerosing agent in UK nor FDA approved.

◆ A weak sclerosant (approximately 25% the "strength" of polidocanol at same concentration and volume) [7].

◆ Only effective in small vessels.

◆ Extremely viscous and thus hard to use.

◆ May be painful on injection.

◆ Chromate moiety highly allergenic.

◆ Occasionally causes ureteric colic and haematuria.

Hypertonic Saline

An osmotic agent (10% - 30% concentration), causing damage by a gradient dehydration effect. Desired concentrations achieved by diluting with local anaesthetic or bacteriostatic water.

Advantages

◆ Used for years.

◆ Non-allergenic.

Disadvantages

◆ Not approved for sclerotherapy by FDA.

◆ Dilution makes it difficult to achieve sclerosis of large vessels without exceeding an excessive salt load.

◆ May cause significant pain on injection, and cramping after treatment.

◆ Extravasation invariably causes necrosis [8].

◆ Poor cosmesis due to marked haemosiderin staining.

◆ Patient satisfaction lower than with some other available agents.

Techniques for sclerotherapy

No specific evidence-based technique has been described and practice depends on practitioner preference. Needles vary in size from 30-33G and may be part of a specific microsclerotherapy set or used with a syringe with the needle bent at an angle of 10°-30°.

◆ Performed with the patient lying supine, both for comfort and to reduce the risk of syncopal attacks.

◆ Larger veins: section of vein isolated using the ring and index finger, skin stretched, slow injection 0.25-0.5ml into isolated segment.

◆ Treat feeding reticular veins prior to thread veins [11] **(A)**.

◆ Smaller veins: skin stretched, slow injection 0.2ml (maximum) of sclerosant and observing blanching [8] **(A)**.

◆ Immediate compression with cotton wool ball/ dental roll.

◆ Compression applied with stocking, bandaging or tubigrip.

The role of compression

There are theoretical as well as clinical reasons for applying post-treatment compression. It allows direct contact of the drug with the inner walls of the veins, causing more effective occlusion, and should lead to diminished retrograde blood flow, which could damage the deep venous system. It also improves calf muscle pump function, preventing stasis of sclerosant in the deep venous system [9]. These effects reduce the risk of deep vein thrombosis. Further, thrombus formation is minimised in both reticular and thread veins, resulting in a smaller area of inflammation (phlebitis), and a lower risk of recanalisation. This diminishes the risk of pigmentation.

These beneficial effects are dependent upon the duration of compression, with 3 weeks compression appearing to produce the best results. However, even a 3-day period of compression is better than none at all [12] **(I)**.

Side-effects

Pigmentation

Although the reported frequency varies widely it is likely that 10-30% of patients will develop post-sclerotherapy staining as a result of thrombus formation [8]. Fortunately, haemosiderin stains invariably fade over 6-24 months, this being enhanced by avoiding exposure to sunlight.

As discussed earlier, hyperpigmentation is reduced by the use of compression stockings although there is no consensus regarding the strength of stocking applied, this varying from low-compression TED stockings to 30-40mmHg graduated compression stockings **(III)**.

The type and concentration of sclerosing agent may also affect the severity of pigmentation. Thus, when using 0.5% polidocanol instead of the 1% solution, the incidence of staining is more than halved [8].

Blistering

Cutaneous necrosis is uncommon after sclerotherapy of spider veins. It can occur following inadvertent perivascular infiltration of the sclerosant or after injection of an arteriovenous anastomosis. Reactive vasospasm of small vessels or excessive compression are other mechanisms that might precipitate blistering.

The risks are also higher when treating veins over bony prominences, particularly in the distal areas of the leg. This may be due to a more precarious blood supply to skin around the ankle.

Although some sclerosants carry a greater risk of blistering than others, most provide adequate sclerosing power, with a low risk of necrosis if the dose is kept sufficiently low.

Patients should be made aware that their cosmetic treatment might leave a permanent scar if ulceration occurs. In the event that secondary infection occurs antibiotic treatment and dressings may be required. The ulcer should heal over a period of about 6 weeks.

Telangiectasia (matting)

Telangiectatic vessels (< 0.2mm diam) causing a red blush may appear after sclerotherapy. The mechanisms responsible for this remain unknown although it has been suggested that angiogenic and inflammatory processes may cause dilation of existing sub-clinical blood vessels by promoting collateral flow through arteriovenous anastomoses [8].

It has been suggested that minimal sclerosant concentrations and limiting the area of blanching on injection to 1-2 cm reduce the risk of matting. Areas at higher risk, particularly the inner thighs, should have low-pressure injections. Patients who are obese or using contraceptive therapy are also considered at higher risk and should be warned accordingly [11] **(II)**. Matting can be treated by laser therapy.

Bruising and tenderness

Tender or nodular thrombi are more likely to develop, particularly in the popliteal fossa, after treatment of larger reticular veins. The incidence is reported as being approximately 5% [2]. This tenderness may last for several days or, possibly weeks. However, if clots are evacuated by piercing the overlying skin with a needle and applying pressure, the tenderness settles and the risk of haemosiderin staining is reduced.

Superficial thrombophebitis may also occur after sclerotherapy and ambulation, aspirin, warm compresses and compression hosiery provide symptomatic relief.

Allergy

Allergic reactions are very rare and are classified as mild (rash, hives, itching), moderate (stridor, wheezing, facial/tongue swelling) or severe (anaphylactic shock). Occasional deaths have occurred with the latter. Rapid access to the necessary drugs required for treatment is therefore vital. Thus the clinic equipment should include:

- Adrenaline, hydrocortisone and antihistamine injections.

- Oxygen, endotracheal tube.

- Intravenous lines and fluids.

Post-procedural care

Patients should be given written advice covering their post-procedural care. As discussed earlier, most patients will be wearing some form of compression and the length of time that this should remain in place should be stated. The advice should also include a description of the symptoms (swelling, paraesthesia, dusky toes) that may occur if the compression bandaging is too tight and instructions as to what to do should this happen. Patients should also be advised that:

♦ Walking, prior to driving, is vital post sclerotherapy. This reduces the risk of deep vein thrombosis by exercising the calf muscle pump and promotes venous drainage or flushing away of sclerosant. There is no fixed time limit although a minimum of 15 minutes is suggested.

♦ They should refrain from vigorous pounding activities for 24 - 72 hours post-treatment.

♦ That prolonged standing or sitting will increase the venous pressure in the legs.

On removal of the compression, patients should be made fully aware that their veins will look unsightly and bruised and this could last for up to 2 weeks. They should not expect to see the final result of their sclerotherapy for at least 2 to 3 months although further fading of their veins and any haemosiderin staining may continue over a longer period.

Patients may be seen on a weekly basis whilst undergoing treatment for extensive thread veins although follow-up visits should occur less often so that bruising settles and the success of previous sclerotherapy is evident.

Summary

♦ Sclerotherapy has been practiced for many years with great success **(A)**.

♦ There is no evidence with regard to most of the practices in current use **(A)**.

♦ Patients need to be fully aware of the potential risks of this cosmetic procedure **(II)**.

Further reading

1 Vitale-Lewis V. *Sclerotherapy of Spider Veins*. Butterworth-Heinemann, Oxford, 1995.

2 Sadick NS. *Manual of sclerotherapy*. Lippincott Williams & Wilkins, Philadelphia, 2000.

References (grade I evidence and grade A recommendations in bold)

1 Galland RB, Magee TR, Lewis MH. A survey of current attitudes of British and Irish vascular surgeons to venous sclerotherapy. *Eur J Vasc Endovasc Surg* 1998; 16: 43-46.

2 Vitale-Lewis V. *Sclerotherapy of spider veins*. Butterworth-Heinemann, Oxford, 1995.

3 Sadick NS. Predisposing factors of varicose and telangiectatic leg veins. *J Derm Surg Oncology* 1992; 18: 883-6.

4 Goodwin H. General and Vascular surgery review. *Journal of the Medical Defence Union* 1999; 15(1): 15.

5 Baccaglini U, Spreafico G, Castoro C, Sorentino P. Sclerotherapy of varicose veins of the lower limbs - consensus paper. *Dermatol Surg* 1996; 22: 883-9.

6 Tennant WG, Vaughn Ruckley C. Causes of legal action following treatment for varicose veins. *Clinical Risk* 1997; 3: 52-54.

7 Drug insert - Sclerovein®. Resinag AG, 6430 Schwyz/Switzerland, 1996.

8 Conrad P, Malauf GM, Stacey MC. The Australian Polidocanol Study. Results at 2 years. *Dermatol Surgery* 1995; 21: 334-336.

9 Sadick NS. *Manual of sclerotherapy*. Lippincott Williams & Wilkins, Philadelphia, 2000.

10 Feied CF. Sclerosing Solutions. In: *The Basic Phlebology Primer*. The American College of Phlebology. http://www.phlebology.org.

11 Weiss RA, Sadick NS, Goldman MP, Weiss MA. Post-sclerotherapy compression: controlled comparative study of duration of compression and its effects on clinical outcome. *Dematol Surg* 1999; 25: 105-8.

12 Goldman MP, Sadick NS, Weiss RA. Cutaneous necrosis, telangiectatic matting, and hyperpigmentation following sclerotherapy. *Dermatol Surgery* 1995; 21:19-29.

Chapter 8

Leg ulcer clinics

Timothy Beresford Research Fellow in Vascular Surgery

Angela Williams Vascular Nurse Specialist

Alun H Davies Reader in Surgery & Consultant Surgeon

DEPARTMENT OF VASCULAR SURGERY, CHARING CROSS HOSPITAL, LONDON, UK

Introduction

The overall prevalence of leg ulceration is approximately 1.5 per 1000 of the population. This increases with age such that in octogenarians it is estimated that around 20 per 1000 will suffer this problem [1-4]. In the UK about 25% of these ulcers (approximately 100,000) require treatment at any point in time. Thus leg ulceration presents a major financial burden and in 1997 it was estimated that venous ulceration alone consumed some 2% of the NHS budget [5]. This cost includes materials, personnel, and medications. With an increasingly large elderly population this burden will continue to grow.

The impact of leg ulceration is not purely financial. Recently, methods that identify the physical and psychosocial effects on patients demonstrate considerable morbidity that is directly attributable to this pathology [6-8].

Development of leg ulcer clinics

The development and use of compression by three and four-layer bandaging, Unna's boot, short stretch bandaging and compression hosiery for the treatment of venous ulceration has resulted in improved healing rates compared to non-compressive treatments. Prior to the development of these techniques, as now, the majority of leg ulcers were treated by overworked district nurses in the community using bandaging incapable of sustaining pressure for a sufficient length of time. Frequent visits to change dressings were required and it was estimated that 25 - 65% of district nurses' time was involved in either travelling to or treating leg ulcers [9].

Despite the good intentions of community nurses, treatment is often ineffective. Often there are inadequate facilities to treat ulcers appropriately and some ulcers, particularly those due to arterial insufficiency, are misdiagnosed, and compression bandaging applied to the detriment of the patient.

Community leg ulcer clinics were first introduced in the late 80s [10] following the pioneering study into their role within the Riverside Health Authority. These clinics aimed to provide optimum care for every leg ulcer patient, to improve healing rates, to rationalise available facilities and to reduce the costs to the Health Service. They were linked to the Vascular

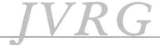

Surgical Unit at Charing Cross Hospital, establishing strong lines of communication, support and co-operation between district staff and specialists within the hospital. Inherent in this development was the education of community nursing staff in the diagnosis and treatment of leg ulcers. Central to this was the use of Doppler for assessment of arterial perfusion and training in the application of four-layer bandaging. Rapid access to expert opinion was available for complex ulcers and those of non-venous origin whilst patients with intractable venous ulceration were sometimes admitted to hospital to induce healing through bed rest, compression, and occasionally skin grafting.

Advantages of a leg ulcer clinic

Leg ulcer treatment requires significant resources and these can be provided more easily, and used more efficiently, in a centralised unit. Although this results in less movement of staff and equipment it may increase the demand on patient transport services. However, transport costs to community clinics may be offset by a reduction in similar costs for hospital visits.

Specialised clinics also provide a controlled environment, freed from the general household detritus, where effective treatment can be undertaken with a uniform standard of cleanliness. Equally clinics, compared to the independent district nurse, are more likely to have the appropriate facilities for patient evaluation (Doppler probes and pressure cuffs for ABPI measurement, access to duplex ultrasound for venous assessment) and ulcer treatment. Furthermore, protocols will normally exist for rapid referral to an appropriate consultant for non-healing ulcers or atypical presentations (Figure1).

Simon et al [11] assessed ulcer-healing rates (at 3 months) in two adjacent health authorities (similar population and socio-economic profile) before and after one of them introduced community leg ulcer clinics. In the district that developed community clinics healing rates improved from 26% to 42% whilst remaining static (23% and 20%) in the district where ulcer management continued along standard lines. This difference was highly significant. Furthermore the community clinics resulted in a 9% reduction in the number of ulcers requiring treatment.

Most of the studies assessing the benefit of community ulcer clinics have compared their results to those achieved by domicillary care. This comparison may be unfair because, until recently, the use of four-layer bandaging by district nurses was restricted. Now that the components for four layer bandaging are available on prescription, it is conceivable that the remarkable advantage of ulcer clinic treatment may be less, and merely reflects more appropriate investigation and treatment facilities.

Costs

Several studies have assessed the cost effectiveness of community ulcer clinics compared to the traditional domicillary approach [11-18].

Many of these suggest that although the costs of setting-up and running a dedicated ulcer clinic are high, perhaps higher than that of domicillary care, the costs are recouped by improved ulcer healing rates. Thus, in the long-term, it is suggested that considerable savings can be made.

Simon's study [11] also assessed the costs of ulcer care in community clinics demonstrating that the total annual cost of leg ulcer care fell by 38.2% one year after their introduction, compared to an increase of 21.1% in the neighbouring district during the same period. This reflected a highly significant reduction in dressing costs, staff costs and inpatient care despite an increase in patient transport cost. This was largely achieved by a reduction in the frequency of dressings from 2.55 per week to 1.01 per week.

In contrast, Morrell et al published the results of a randomised-controlled trial that also examined the cost effectiveness of community ulcer clinics compared to care from a district nurse [16]. The mean cost per visit was calculated as £29.90 for community clinics and £10.60 for home treatment. However, after taking into account additional NHS expenditure (general practitioner and hospital visits) and ulcer duration the annual cost for treatment by community clinics was only £14.51 more per annum per patient.

In neither of these studies were 4-layer bandages used as frequently during domicillary care and since

Figure 1 Protocol for referral of leg ulcer patients to a vascular surgical service.

All Ulcers
◆ Ankle-brachial pressure index < 0.5. Patients seen within one week No compression applied
◆ Ankle-brachial pressure index 0.5-0.8 ABPI 0.6-0.7: can use reduced compression
◆ Ulcers failing to improve Referred for arterial/venous assessment
◆ All non-venous ulcers Referred for full investigation

Venous Ulcers
◆ Recurrent ulcers Referral for full venous assessment Considered for possible surgery
◆ Young, mobile patients Referred for full venous assessment Corrective venous surgery if appropriate

the most effective way of cutting costs is to improve ulcer healing rates both may be biased in favour of the community clinics.

Patients

For patients attending a dedicated leg ulcer clinic there may be hidden benefits. Many of those suffering leg ulceration are elderly and have significant co-morbidities. They are often lonely and isolated and anecdotal evidence suggests that a regular activity and social interaction has a life-enhancing effect. The interaction with others suffering from the same condition reduces the feeling of isolation and allows patients to rationalise and compare their condition in terms of severity, treatment and progress with their peers. Frequently, an element of peer support and even competitiveness develops.

Conversely domicillary care may also have some benefits. The district nurse can make an assessment of home circumstances, instigate appropriate social service packages and attend to other concurrent conditions from which the patient may be suffering. Regular home visits from a health professional provide

reassurance and a confidence that there is a continuous interest in the patient's welfare.

Ulcer clinics have the added benefit of structured treatment within a clinical environment at predictable times. There is no requirement to act as a host and no perception of invasion of privacy, which is often a cause for non-compliance in patients treated at home.

For some, however, attendance at a community clinic is either not possible (through immobility or infirmity) or not desirable, often because there is an unpleasant odour from the ulcer. Such patients may prefer to have their wounds dressed at home where this, and other stigmata of chronic ulcerative disease, can be addressed in privacy. For district nurse treatment to be successful the appropriate diagnostic tools and dressings must be made available.

Staff

Treatment at a dedicated leg ulcer clinic eliminates nurse travelling time and avoids the practical difficulties of ulcer debridement, wound cleansing, and applying bandages within a domestic environment, thus reducing treatment times by up to two-thirds. Staff also benefit from initial education and in-service training in the assessment and treatment of leg ulcers. Opportunities for research and treatment evaluation are also presented when the majority of leg ulcers are treated and followed-up at a clinic.

Finally, staff work within an environment where there is a high level of clinical support from co-workers and, with adequate lines of communication, good access to additional backup from hospital specialists.

Standardised care

In 1998, the Royal College of Nursing published "Clinical Practice Guidelines: The Management of Patients with Venous Leg Ulceration" [19]. This was based on a literature review and an earlier publication on the use of compression therapy for venous ulcers (Effective Healthcare Bulletin, 1997). The guidelines presented a comprehensive review of ideal modern management of leg/venous ulcers although they did not specifically recommend the establishment of either community or hospital-based ulcer clinics.

The assessment and treatment of leg ulceration should be standardised to give the highest possible quality of care. The establishment of care plans and leg ulcer protocols greatly facilitates the management of these patients. A suggested pathway, based on perceived best practice is shown in Figure 2.

Practical aspects of management

History and examination

Initial assessment should be undertaken by a health care professional with specialist training in the diagnosis and treatment of leg ulceration [20,21] (III). The history and examination should identify whether the patient has had a previous ulcer or varicose veins, deep vein thrombosis, phlebitis, pulmonary embolus, lower limb fractures, diabetes, peripheral vascular disease, heart disease, hypertension, or a hyperlipidaemia. A history of tobacco use may also be relevant [1,20,21] (III).

A written or photographic record, of the ulcer, its size and characteristics, together with those of any associated skin changes should be made at the first visit (III).

Clinical investigation

Doppler assessment of the lower limbs should be made by trained staff at the first visit [10,22,23] (I) and should be repeated if the ulcer has not healed within 12 weeks or if there is any deterioration in its appearance [22-25] (II). Patients with a reduced ankle-brachial pressure index should be referred to a vascular clinic (Figure 1).

Baseline measurements of pulse, blood pressure, blood glucose and BMI are also made (III). Routine microbiological swabs are not required unless there is surrounding soft tissue infection [26,27] (I).

Ulcer management

Specialist medical opinion should be sought if there is evidence of peripheral vascular disease, if the ulcer has an atypical appearance, or if it increases in size, suggesting the possibility of malignancy. Referral should also be made if the ulcer fails to heal after 3 months adequate treatment or if there is evidence of significant infection (C). Similarly newly diagnosed diabetics, patients with rheumatoid disease, skin sensitivity to dressings, excessive pain or a requirement for orthotic equipment, require hospital referral (C).

High compression dressing systems capable of sustaining compression for at least 1 week should be the first line of treatment for ulcers considered to be venous in origin [28-34] (A). Four layer bandaging provides improved healing compared to non-compression or short stretch bandaging [30,32,35] (II). These should be applied by trained staff who also have knowledge of, and are able to monitor patients for, the potential adverse consequences of high compression bandaging [36,37] (B).

After healing of a venous ulcer has been achieved the use of compression stockings should be

Figure 2 A flow diagram summarising community clinic ulcer management and referral recommendations.

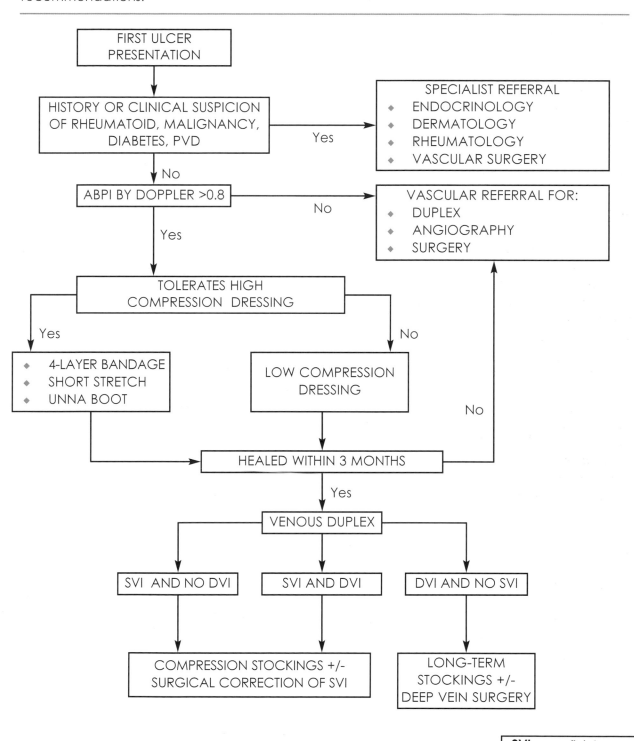

Table 1 Leg ulcer dressing.

		Venous	Arterial	Mixed	Other
Compression	ABPI measured prior to application	ABPI >0.9 4 layer bandaging or Class III stocking	ABPI <0.5 No Compression	Level of compression dependent on ABPI and clinical tolerance	Some compression (as tolerated) for reactive oedema
Granulation	Heavy Exudate	Low adherent contact layer + polyurethane foam	Alginate dressing +/- polyurethane foam	Alginate dressing +/- polyurethane foam	Low adherent contact layer + polyurethane foam
		Hydrocolloid sheet	Hydrocolloid sheet	Hydrocolloid sheet	Hydrocolloid sheet
	Light Exudate or Epithelialising	Low adherent contact layer (especially silicone based)	Low adherent contact layer +/- PFAD	Low adherent contact layer +/- PFAD	Low adherent contact layer (especially silicone based)
		PFAD	Hydrocolloid sheet	Hydrocolloid sheet	PFAD
		Semipermeable adhesive film			Semipermeable adhesive film
Slough (Heavy slough or necrotic tissue may require mechanical debridment)	Dry / Necrotic	Hydrogel + hydrocolloid sheet	Hydrogel + hydrocolloid sheet	Hydrogel + hydrocolloid sheet	Hydrogel + hydrocolloid sheet
		Hydrogel + PFAD	Hydrocolloid sheet	Hydrocolloid sheet	Hydrogel + PFAD
	Moist	Hydrocolloid sheet	Hydrogel + semipermeable adhesive film dressing	Hydrocolloid sheet	Hydrocolloid sheet
		Hydrogel + PFAD	Hydrocolloid sheet	Hydrogel + PFAD	Hydrogel + PFAD
Infected	Culture swabs	Iodinated low adherance contact layer + PFAD	Iodinated low adherance contact layer + PFAD	Iodinated low adherance contact layer + PFAD	Iodinated low adherance contact layer + PFAD
	Hypersensitivity can occur with antiseptic dressings	Flamazine cream + PFAD	Activated charcoal dressings for odour control +/- fluid absorption	Activated charcoal dressings for odour control +/- fluid absorption	Flamazine cream + PFAD
	Systemic antibiotics should be considered	Activated charcoal dressings for odour control +/- fluid absorption			Activated charcoal dressings for odour control +/- fluid absorption

PFAD - perforated film adherent dressing

encouraged to reduce the risk of recurrence [38,39] **(C)**. Following appropriate investigation patients with a healed venous ulcer may be considered for varicose vein surgery if they have superficial venous incompetence. If this is not the case, or if the patient is not suitable for surgery then lifetime use of compression stockings should be advised [40-44] **(B)**.

Dressings and ulcer care

Cleansing of the ulcer should be performed using simple tap water or saline irrigation and a clean technique employed for dressing changes to minimise cross infection [45] **(C)**. Dressings should be simple, have low adherence, and be well tolerated by the patient [45] **(A)**. In addition, the topical application of lanolin or antibiotics should be avoided [45] **(C)**. A suggested protocol for ulcer dressings is shown in Table 1.

Summary

◆ Treatment of leg ulcers consumes 2% of the NHS budget.

◆ Community ulcer clinics with appropriate facilities, resources and expertise improve ulcer healing rates and cost effectiveness when compared to domicillary care provided by district nurses when compression bandaging is not used **(II)**.

◆ Clinic staff require specific training in patient and ulcer assessment and should use these skills to define the cause of the ulcer **(A)**.

◆ Specific training is also required in the choice and application of dressings and bandages according to pre-defined protocols **(B)**.

◆ Protocols should be defined to reduce the risk of recurrence following ulcer healing and to identify patients who should be referred for a specialist medical opinion **(C)**.

References (grade I evidence and grade A recommendations in bold)

1   Cornwall JV, Dore CJ, Lewis JD. Leg ulcers: epidemiology and aetiology. *Br J Surg* 1986; 73: 693-6.

2   Nelzen O, Bergqvist D, Lindhagen A, Hallbook T. Chronic leg ulcers: an underestimated problem in primary health care among elderly patients. *J Epidemiol Community Health* 1991; 45: 184-7.

3   Lees TA, Lambert D. Prevalence of lower limb ulceration in an urban health district. *Br J Surg* 1992; 79: 1032-4.

4   Marklund B, Sulau T, Lindholm C. Prevalence of non-healed and healed chronic leg ulcers in an elderly rural population. *Scand J Prim Health Care* 2000; 18: 58-60.

5   Ruckley CV. Socioeconomic impact of chronic venous insufficiency and leg ulcers. *Angiology* 1997; 48: 67-9.

6   Walters SJ, Morrell CJ, Dixon S. Measuring health-related quality of life in patients with venous leg ulcers. *Qual Life Res* 1999; 8: 327-36.

7   Mathias SD, Prebil LA, Boyko WL, Fastenau J. Health-related quality of life in venous leg ulcer patients successfully treated with Apligraf: a pilot study. *Adv Skin Wound Care* 2000; 13: 76-8.

8   Smith JJ, Guest MG, Greenhalgh RM, Davies AH. Measuring the quality of life in patients with venous ulcers. *J Vasc Surg* 2000; 31: 642-9.

9   Peters J. A review of the factors influencing nonrecurrence of venous leg ulcers. (Review) (21 refs). *J Clin Nurs* 1998; 7: 3-9.

10   **Moffatt CJ, Oldroyd MI. A pioneering service to the community. The Riverside Community Leg Ulcer Project. *Prof Nurs* 488; 9: 486.**

11   Simon DA *et al*. Community leg ulcer clinics: a comparative study in two health authorities. *BMJ* 1996; 312: 1648-51.

12   Bosanquet N *et al*. Community leg ulcer clinics: cost-effectiveness. *Health Trends* 1993; 25: 146-8.

13   Ohlsson P, Larsson K, Lindholm C, Moller M. A cost-effectiveness study of leg ulcer treatment in primary care. Comparison of saline-gauze and hydrocolloid treatment in a prospective, randomized study. *Scand J Prim Health Care* 1994; 12: 295-9.

14   Freak L *et al*. Leg ulcer care: an audit of cost-effectiveness. *Health Trends* 1995; 27: 133-6.

15   Morrell CJ, King B, Brereton L. Community-based leg ulcer clinics: organisation and cost-effectiveness. *Nurs Times* 1998; 94: 51-4.

16   Morrell CJ *et al*. Cost effectiveness of community leg ulcer clinics: randomised controlled trial. (see comments). *BMJ* 1998; 316: 1487-91.

17   Carr L, Philips Z, Posnett J. Comparative cost-effectiveness of four-layer bandaging in the treatment of venous leg ulceration. *J Wound Care* 1999; 8: 243-8.

Chapter 8

18   Marston WA, Carlin RE, Passman MA, Farber MA, Keagy BA. Healing rates and cost efficacy of outpatient compression treatment for leg ulcers associated with venous insufficiency. *J Vasc Surg* 1999; 30: 491-8.

19   McInnes E, Cullum N, Nelson A, Duff L. RCN guideline on the management of leg ulcers. *Nurs Standard* 1998; 13: 61-3.

20   Elliot E, Russell B, Jaffrey G. Setting a standard for leg ulcer assessment. *J Wound Care* 1996; 5: 173-5.

21   Stevens J, Franks PJ, Harrington M. A community/hospital leg ulcer service. *J Wound Care* 1997; 6: 62-8.

22   **Simon DA, McCollum CN. Approaches to venous leg ulcer care within the community: compression, pinch skin grafts and simple venous surgery.** *Ostomy Wound Management* **1940; 42: 34-8.**

23   **Scriven JM, Hartshorne T, Bell PR, Naylor AR, London NJ. Single-visit venous ulcer assessment clinic: the first year. (see comments).** *Br J Surg* **1997; 84: 334-6.**

24   Feuerstein W. Importance and indications for Doppler ultrasonic diagnosis in chronic venous insufficiency. *Hautarzt* 1981; 32: 1-7.

25   Fisher CM *et al*. Variation in measurement of ankle-brachial pressure index in routine clinical practice. *J Vasc Surg* 1996; 24: 871-5.

26   **Trengove NJ, Stacey MC, McGechie DF, Mata S. Qualitative bacteriology and leg ulcer healing.** *J Wound Care* **1996; 5: 277-80.**

27   **Hansson C, Hoborn J, Moller A, Swanbeck G. The microbial flora in venous leg ulcers without clinical signs of infection. Repeated culture using a validated standardised microbiological technique.** *Acta Dermato-Venereologica* **1995; 75: 24-30.**

28   **Nelson EA. Compression bandaging for venous leg ulcers. (Review) (22 refs).** *Prof Nurs* **1997; 12: S7-S9.**

29   Palfreyman SJ, Lochiel R, Michaels JA. A systematic review of compression therapy for venous leg ulcers. *Vasc Med* 1998; 3: 301-13.

30   **Scriven JM *et al*. A prospective randomised trial of four-layer versus short stretch compression bandages for the treatment of venous leg ulcers.** *Ann R Coll Surg Eng* **1998; 80: 215-20.**

31   **Reichardt LE. Venous ulceration: compression as the mainstay of therapy. (Review) (30 refs).** *J Wocn* **1999; 26: 39-47.**

32   **Cullum N, Nelson EA, Fletcher AW, Sheldon TA. Compression bandages and stockings for venous leg ulcers. (Review) (30 refs).** *Cochrane Database of Systematic Reviews* **(computer file) 2000; CD000265.**

33   **Bergan JJ, Sparks SR. Non-elastic compression: an alternative in management of chronic venous insufficiency. (Review) (28 refs).** *J Wocn* **2000; 27: 83-9.**

34   **Kramer SA. Compression wraps for venous ulcer healing: a review. (Review) (29 refs).** *J Vasc Nurs* **1999; 17: 89-97.**

35   Danielsen L, Madsen SM, Henriksen L. Healing of venous leg ulcers. A randomized prospective study of a long-stretch versus short-stretch compression bandage. (Danish). *Ugeskrift for Laeger* 1999; 161: 6042-5.

36   Nelson EA, Ruckley CV, Barbenel JC. Improvements in bandaging technique following training. *J Wound Care* 1995; 4: 181-4.

37   Stockport JC, Groarke L, Ellison DA, McCollum C. Single-layer and multilayer bandaging in the treatment of venous leg ulcers. *J Wound Care* 1997; 6: 485-8.

38   Nelson EA, Bell-Syer SE, Cullum NA. Compression for preventing recurrence of venous ulcers. (Review) (24 refs). *Cochrane Database of Systematic Reviews* (computer file) 2000; CD002303.

39   O'Hare L. Scholl compression hosiery in the management of venous disorders. (Review) (15 refs). *Br J Nurs* 1997; 6: 391-4.

40   Taylor P. Assisting patients to comply with leg ulcer treatments. (Review) (22 refs). *Br J Nurs* 1360; 5: 1355-8.

41   Chen CJ, Guo SG, Luo D, Huang YQ. Full-valve annuloplasty in treatment of primary deep venous valvular incompetence of the lower extremities. *Chin Med J (Engl)* 1992; 105: 256-9.

42   Pierik EG, Wittens CH, van Urk H. Subfascial endoscopic ligation in the treatment of incompetent perforating veins. *Eur J Vasc Endovasc Surg* 1995; 9: 38-41.

43   Puonti H, Asko-Seljavaara S. Excision and skin grafting of leg ulcers. *Ann Chir Gynaecol* 1998; 87: 219-23.

44   Barwell JR *et al*. Surgical correction of isolated superficial venous reflux reduces long-term recurrence rate in chronic venous leg ulcers. *Eur J Vasc Endovasc Surg* 2000; 20: 363-8.

45   **Bradley M, Cullum N, Sheldon T. The debridement of chronic wounds: a systematic review. (Review) (62 refs).** *Health Tech Assess* **(Rockville, Md) 2001; 3: iii-iiv.**

46   Lambourne LA, Moffatt CJ, Jones AC, Dorman MC, Franks PJ. Clinical audit and effective change in leg ulcer services. *J Wound Care* 1996; 5: 348-51.

47   Chaloner D, Noirit J. Treatments and healing rates in a community leg ulcer clinic. *Br J Nurs* 1997; 6: 246-2.

48   Vowden KR, Barker A, Vowden P. Leg ulcer management in a nurse-led, hospital-based clinic. *J Wound Care* 1997; 6: 233-6.

49   Thorne E. Community leg ulcer clinics and the effectiveness of care. (Review) (51 refs). *J Wound Care* 1998; 7: 94-9.

50   Liew I, Sinha S. A leg ulcer clinic: audit of the first three years. *J Wound Care* 1998; 7: 405-7.

51   Carrington C. A nurse-led clinic for managing venous leg ulcers. *Nurs Standard* 1999; 13: 42-6.

Chapter 8

Chapter 9

Management of lower limb lymphoedema

Alok Tiwari Clinical Research Fellow
George Hamilton Consultant Vascular Surgeon
Fiona Myint Consultant Vascular Surgeon

UNIVERSITY DEPARTMENT OF SURGERY, THE ROYAL FREE HOSPITAL &
UNIVERSITY COLLEGE MEDICAL SCHOOL, LONDON, UK

Introduction

Lymphoedema refers to swelling of the limbs due to the accumulation of protein rich interstitial fluid within the skin and subcutaneous tissue, secondary to an abnormality of lymphatic structure or impaired lymphatic function. Thus, this term should only be used if all the other causes of limb swelling can be excluded. The incidence is not known but is much more common in females.

Lymphoedema is classified on the basis of age at which symptoms start and on the aetiology. It may be either primary (a developmental abnormality of the lymphatics) or secondary to a known and confirmed cause. Primary lymphoedema is further divided into congenital, praecox and tarda, depending on whether the initial presentation is in the first year of life, between the ages of 1-35 years, or after 35 years respectively.

The commonest site for lymphoedema is the lower limb, accounting for 80% of cases of which 2/3 are unilateral [1]. Other sites include the arms, face, trunk and external genitalia. Upper limb lymphoedema is often a sequela of breast cancer or its treatment, and is usually managed by the breast care team. In this chapter we discuss the differential diagnosis, investigation and current management of lower limb lymphoedema in the Western population.

Diagnosis of lymphoedema

The diagnosis of lymphoedema is based on the history, clinical examination, and the results of appropriate investigations. The latter serve to both confirm the diagnosis and to exclude other causes of limb swelling.

Differential diagnosis

Before considering the history and clinical examination, it is important to know the common differential diagnoses for these patients. The causes of lower limb swelling include lymphoedema, medical causes, venous disease, abnormal fat distribution and idiopathic [1,2]. Common medical causes of lower limb swelling are cardiac failure, hypoalbuminaemia, protein losing nephropathy and renal failure. Deep vein thrombosis and other venous disease, including varicose veins, are also common.

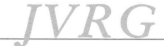

Management of lower limb lymphoedema

Lipoedema is an abnormal, symmetrical distribution of fat found exclusively in females. Here, the fat is distributed around the thighs and legs but with sparing of the feet. This condition persists following weight loss [3,4]. Figures 1 (bilateral lymphoedema) and 2 (bilateral lipoedema) demonstrate the typical appearances of these two conditions.

Other causes of lower limb swelling include post-operative oedema following major limb surgery (including vascular reconstruction), arterio-venous malformation, cellulitis, ruptured Baker's cyst, ruptured tendo-Achilles, pregnancy and cyclical oedema related to the menstrual cycle [1,2,5].

Secondary lymphoedema is usually the result of limb trauma, recurrent infection, primary malignancy (usually pelvic) or metastatic disease. Malignancy may also be responsible for phlegmasia caerulea dolens, which is a venous cause of leg swelling. World-wide, the most common cause of secondary lymphoedema is infection from filariasis but this is rarely seen in the UK.

History and clinical examination

In the history, it is important to enquire about the age at onset and any previous medical history including malignancy, pelvic surgery, groin dissection, deep vein thrombosis, varicose vein surgery or trauma to the limbs.

The general examination should exclude congestive cardiac failure, and possible venous disease. In patients with lymphoedema, there is a gradual swelling of the limb which starts from the feet and progresses proximally. It is usually asymmetrical thus differentiating it from lipoedema [6]. There may however be signs of concurrent venous disease in patients with lymphoedema. The oedema is initially pitting but becomes harder as the disease progresses. The typical skin changes seen with late cases of lymphoedema are increased skin turgor, hyperkeratosis and papillomatosis. Stemmers's sign (the inability to pinch the skin of the second toe with the fingers) is positive in lymphoedema but absent in lipoedema.

Figure 1 Bilateral lymphoedema.

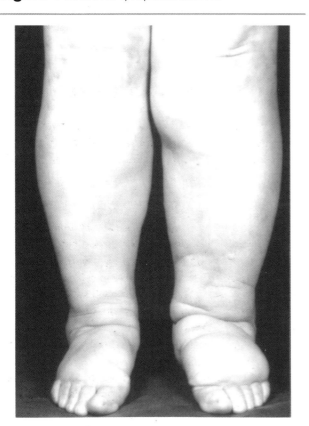

Figure 2 Bilateral lipoedema.

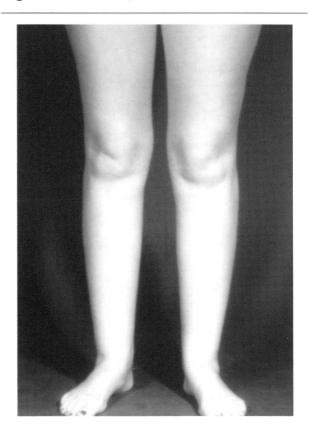

The severity of lymphoedema, when unilateral, can be assessed with a tape measure, comparing the circumference of the affected leg with that of the contralateral leg. However, this is not a reliable technique because there is normally a difference in the leg volume in normal individuals [2,7] and the condition may be bilateral. It may, however, be used to monitor progress once treatment has been commenced. Other non-invasive assessments include water displacement volumetry and tissue tonometry, though these are not used routinely [7].

Investigations

The gold standard for the confirmation of lymphoedema is a lymphoscintigram. This not only confirms the diagnosis but should also exclude venous disease and lipoedema as causes of limb swelling [1,6] (A). However, Bilancini and co-workers have suggested that the lymphoscintigraphic abnormality in lipoedema may be similar to lymphoedema [3]. It is important to realise that in patients with venous disease, there may be lymphatic insufficiency secondary to the venous disease and that patients with lymphatic disease can have impaired venous return caused by the lymphoedema [8,9].

The diagnosis of lymphoedema may be missed if the lymphoscintigraphic films are not taken early enough following injection or, in some cases, if delayed films are not taken up to 2-24 hours after the injection of contrast [10,11] (B). The sensitivity may be increased by using a two-compartment lymphoscintigram [12] (B). A lymphoscintigram is particularly important if any surgical options are being considered though in these patients a combination of both contrast lymphography and isotope lymphoscintigram may be necessary to achieve an accurate diagnosis and formulate a treatment plan [13].

Other investigations available to confirm the diagnosis of lymphoedema include ultrasound, magnetic resonance imaging (MRI) and computed tomography (CT) scanning. Ultrasound may visualise the soft tissue changes that are typical of the diagnosis although it does not give any information on the anatomical abnormality. CT can differentiate between lymphoedema, lipoedema and DVT [14]. DVT is, however, only excluded by CT if there is significant limb swelling [2]. The CT findings in patients with lymphoedema are an increase in the thickness of the skin and subcutaneous tissue the latter having a "honeycomb" appearance [14].

MRI may similarly confirm the diagnosis of lymphoedema, again showing the characteristic "honeycomb" appearance in the majority of the patients thus allowing differentiation from lipoedema and lymphoedema [5,15-17]. None of these investigations visualise the lymphatics however.

Duplex ultrasound is used to exclude DVT and superficial venous disease. In patients where no clinical cause of the limb swelling is evident, a combination of lymphoscintigram and duplex may be enough to diagnose the cause in 82% of patients [18] (II). Thus, in a series of 32 patients, 50% had an abnormal lymphoscintigram, 53% had an abnormal duplex scan whilst in 15% both investigations were abnormal.

All the above investigations can be used either to exclude potentially fatal or treatable disorders such as deep vein thrombosis or to confirm the diagnosis of lymphoedema and plan any surgical intervention.

Treatment of lymphoedema

The treatment of lymphoedema can be divided into conservative, medical and surgical. Treatment is undertaken to reduce swelling or prevent its worsening, to prevent recurrent infection, and rarely to treat lymphangiosarcoma.

Conservative management

This is the mainstay of treatment in lymphoedema and involves a combined approach between doctors, district nurses and most importantly a dedicated lymphoedema physiotherapist.

The treatment centres on combined physical therapy, also known as complex physical therapy (CPT) over a period of 4-6 weeks. CPT is a combination of skin care, manual lymphatic drainage, active exercise and compression by bandages and subsequently stockings [19,20] (A). The skin care involves treatment of any infection and educating the patient about hygiene to prevent further sepsis. Manual lymphatic drainage involves massage that starts from the normal areas and moves on to the swollen areas. This takes about 1 hour per day per patient and encourages drainage by the superficial skin lymphatics. Compression stockings should usually give compression in the region of 40-

Figure 3 Assessment and management of lower limb swelling.

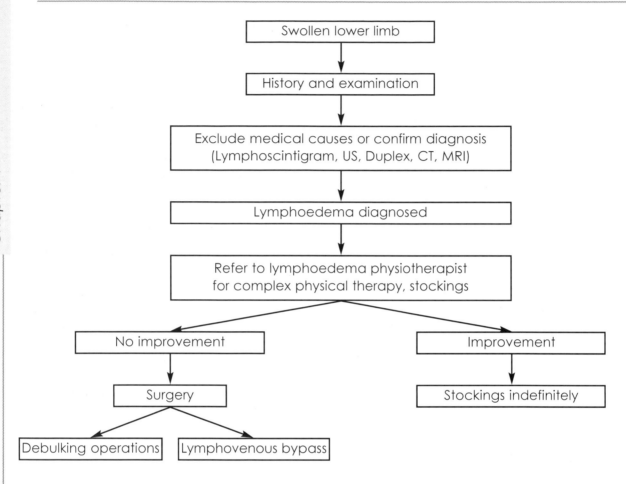

60mmHg. CPT should result in a 57-81% reduction in lower limb oedema [19] and is associated with a reduction in mean lymph capillary pressure [20].

Badger and co-workers compared the use of multilayered bandaging and subsequent hosiery with hosiery alone in the treatment of lymphoedema [21]. The group who used multilayered bandaging first achieved a significant reduction in limb volume (twice as much) **(A)**. Even in patients who have previously used stockings, multilayered bandaging will still improve lymphoedema [22] **(A)**.

There has been some interest in the use of intermittent pneumatic compression (Flowtron®) for the conservative management of lymphoedema although the majority of reports have focused upon its use in the upper limb in patients with breast cancer.

There is no evidence to indicate whether it is more or less effective than CPT.

Weight loss will also effect a reduction in lymphoedema though as mentioned earlier, this is not the case for lipoedema [6].

Medical management

The benzopyrones comprise a large group of drugs including the coumarins and flavonoids. These drugs provide a path separate from the lymphatics for the removal of proteins from the tissues by increasing macrophage-induced proteolysis [23]. The drug reduces leg volume, circumference and skin temperature, and increases tonometry [23-25] **(I)**. There are reports of transient liver dysfunction from the oral preparation of the coumarin form and the drug is unlicensed in the UK. The benzopyrones are slower to act than CPT and they are best used as an adjunct to this. In a randomised trial, the use of benzopyrones and microwave heat treatment was significantly better than placebo and microwave therapy [24] **(II)**.

Surgical management

Possible surgical management comprises either bypass surgery or debulking procedures.

Surgery is only undertaken as a last resort after all conservative measures have failed and swelling cannot be controlled **(A)**.

Debulking operations

In debulking therapy the subcutaneous tissue is excised along with a portion of the skin [26,27] **(B)**. It is done in stages, excising the medial tissue first followed by the lateral excision 3 months later. Such surgery is not universally successful and in a series of 38 patients, 30 patients experienced improvement, two were unchanged and six were worsened. However, in some patients surgery can lead to the development of new lymphatic channels. Complications of this type of surgery include impaired skin sensation and skin flap necrosis, though these are uncommon. Liposuction techniques have also been explored as a less invasive method of debulking lymphoedematous tissue. The authors' experience however is that it is associated with a relatively high incidence of bleeding and infection.

Lymphovenous shunts

Before this type of surgery is undertaken, lymphoscintigraphy, lymphography, and Doppler venous and arterial flowmetry are essential. The end-to-side lymphatic venous anastomosis is the preferred technique [28] **(B)**. The vein used for the anastomosis is that found nearest to the lymphatic collectors. In a series of 664 patients undergoing surgery for lymphoedema, 488 were treated with end-to-side lymphovenous anastomosis. Of these 200 (41%) had marked improvement, 202 (41.4%) had moderate improvement, 75 (15.4%) had mild improvement. The remainder (11, 2.2%) did not improve. If there is co-existing venous disease, autologous vein lymphatic-venous lymphatic interpositional shunting may be undertaken [29]. This can lead to a moderate to marked improvement in 90% of selected patients.

Other procedures

Two others types of surgery have been advocated for lymphoedema: enteromesenteric bridge bypass and omental bypass. The results of these are variable and are only suitable in a small number of patients and have the added complications associated with a laparotomy [30].

In patients with both varicose veins and lymphoedema, surgical removal of the varicose veins has been shown to worsen the swelling in 70.6% patients with only 1.5% patients improving [31]. In patients with lipoedema and varicose veins, venous surgery also leads to a worsening of symptoms in 58.2% with only 9.9% experiencing an improvement. It should be emphasised that this study was retrospective and the changes in swelling were based on the patient's perception **(III)**.

Figure 3 summarises the suggested pathway of care in patients presenting with lower limb oedema.

Summary

- Complex physical therapy and long-term stockings can effectively improve lymphoedema. **(A)**.

- Benzopyrones may have a role in the medical management of lymphoedema. Their efficacy requires evaluation in a large randomised trial **(II)**.

- Surgery is only indicated for failed complex physical therapy if normal activity is impaired. In these patients an end-to-side lymphovenous bypass shows promising results **(A)**.

- The role of early surgery compared to complex physical therapy has not been evaluated **(A)**.

- Surgery for varicose veins in patients with lymphoedema increases lower limb swelling in the majority of patients **(III)**.

Chapter 9

Further reading

1   Twycross R, Jenns K, Todd J, Eds. *Lymphoedema*. Radcliffe Medical Press Ltd, Oxford, 2000.

2   Consensus Document: www.lymphovenous-canada.ca/consenupdate.

References (grade I evidence and grade A recommendations in bold)

1   **Cambria RA, Gloviczki P, Naessens JM, Wahner HW. Noninvasive evaluation of the lymphatic system with lymphoscintigraphy: a prospective, semiquantitative analysis in 386 extremities. *J Vasc Surg* 1993; 18: 773-82.**

2   Vaughan BF. CT of swollen legs. *Clin Radiol* 1990; 41: 24-30.

3   Bilancini S, Lucchi M, Tucci S, Eleuteri P. Functional lymphatic alterations in patients suffering from lipedema. *Angiology* 1995; 46: 333-9.

4   Rudkin GH, Miller TA. Lipedema: a clinical entity distinct from lymphedema. *Plast Reconstr Surg* 1994; 94: 841-7.

5   Haaverstad R, Nilsen G, Myhre HO, Saether OD, Rinck PA. The use of MRI in the investigation of leg oedema. *Eur J Vasc Surg* 1992; 6: 124-9.

6   **Harwood CA, Bull RH, Evans J, Mortimer PS. Lymphatic and venous function in lipoedema. *Br J Dermatol* 1996; 134: 1-6.**

7   Stanton AW, Badger C, Sitzia J. Non-invasive assessment of the lymphedematous limb. *Lymphology* 2000; 33: 122-35.

8   Kim DI, Huh S, Hwang JH, Kim YI, Lee BB. Venous dynamics in leg lymphedema. *Lymphology* 1999; 32: 11-4.

9   Mortimer PS. Evaluation of lymphatic function: abnormal lymph drainage in venous disease. *Int Angiol* 1995; 14: 32-5.

10   Larcos G, Foster DR. Interpretation of lymphoscintigrams in suspected lymphoedema: contribution of delayed images. *Nucl Med Commun* 1995; 16: 683-6.

11   Ter SE, Alavi A, Kim CK, Merli G. Lymphoscintigraphy. A reliable test for the diagnosis of lymphedema. *Clin Nucl Med* 1993; 18: 646-54.

12   Brautigam P *et al.* Analysis of lymphatic drainage in various forms of leg edema using two compartment lymphoscintigraphy. *Lymphology* 1998; 31: 43-55.

13   Burnand KG *et al.* Value of isotope lymphography in the diagnosis of lymphoedema of the leg. *Br J Surg* 2002; 89: 74-8.

14   Hadjis NS, Carr DH, Banks L, Pflug JJ. The role of CT in the diagnosis of primary lymphedema of the lower limb. *AJR Am J Roentgenol* 1985; 144: 361-4.

15   Astrom KG, Abdsaleh S, Brenning GC, Ahlstrom KH. MR imaging of primary, secondary, and mixed forms of lymphedema. *Acta Radiol* 2001; 42: 409-16.

16   Werner GT, Kaiserling E, Scheck R. MR imaging of edematous limbs. *Acta Radiol* 1996; 37: 972-3.

17   Haaverstad R, Nilsen G, Rinck PA, Myhre HO. The use of MRI in the diagnosis of chronic lymphedema of the lower extremity. *Int Angiol* 1994; 13: 115-8.

18   Wheatley DC, Wastie ML, Whitaker SC, Perkins AC, Hopkinson BR. Lymphoscintigraphy and colour Doppler sonography in the assessment of leg oedema of unknown cause. *Br J Radiol* 1996; 69: 1117-24.

19   **Casley-Smith JR, Casley-Smith JR. Treatment of lymphedema by complex physical therapy, with and without oral and topical benzopyrones: what should therapists and patients expect. *Lymphology* 1996; 29: 76-82.**

20   **Franzeck UK *et al.* Combined physical therapy for lymphedema evaluated by fluorescence microlymphography and lymph capillary pressure measurements. *J Vasc Res* 1997; 34: 306-11.**

21   **Badger CM, Peacock JL, Mortimer PS. A randomized, controlled, parallel-group clinical trial comparing multilayer bandaging followed by hosiery versus hosiery alone in the treatment of patients with lymphedema of the limb. *Cancer* 2000; 88: 2832-7.**

22   **Yasuhara H, Shigematsu H, Muto T. A study of the advantages of elastic stockings for leg lymphedema. *Int Angiol* 1996; 15: 272-7.**

23   **Casley-Smith JR, Morgan RG, Piller NB. Treatment of lymphedema of the arms and legs with 5,6-benzo-[alpha]-pyrone. *N Engl J Med* 1993; 329: 1158-63.**

24   **Chang TS, Gan JL, Fu KD, Huang WY. The use of 5,6 benzo-[alpha]-pyrone (coumarin) and heating by microwaves in the treatment of chronic lymphedema of the legs. *Lymphology* 1996; 29: 106-11.**

25   **Casley-Smith JR, Casley-Smith JR. Modern treatment of lymphoedema. II. The benzopyrones. *Australas J Dermatol* 1992; 33: 69-74.**

26   Miller TA, Wyatt LE, Rudkin GH. Staged skin and subcutaneous excision for lymphedema: a favorable report of long-term results. *Plast Reconstr Surg* 1998; 102: 1486-98.

27   Kim DI *et al.* Excision of subcutaneous tissue and deep muscle fascia for advanced lymphedema. *Lymphology* 1998; 31: 190-4.

28   Campisi C, Boccardo F, Alitta P, Tacchella M. Derivative lymphatic microsurgery: indications, techniques, and results. *Microsurgery* 1995; 16: 463-8.

29   Campisi C, Boccardo F, Tacchella M. Reconstructive microsurgery of lymph vessels: the personal method of lymphatic-venous-lymphatic (LVL) interpositioned grafted shunt. *Microsurgery* 1995; 16: 161-6.

30   Carrell T, Burnand KG. In: *Lymphoedema*. Twycross R, Jenns K, Todd J, Eds. Radcliffe Medical Press Ltd, Oxford, 2000.

31   Foldi M, Idiazabal G. The role of operative management of varicose veins in patients with lymphedema and/or lipedema of the legs. *Lymphology* 2000; 33: 167-71.

Chapter 10

Day case angiography and intervention

Trevor Cleveland Consultant Vascular Radiologist [1]
Sumaira Macdonald Endovascular Fellow [1]
Robert Morgan Consultant Vascular Radiologist [2]
Peter Gaines Consultant Vascular Radiologist [1]

[1] SHEFFIELD VASCULAR INSTITUTE, THE NORTHERN GENERAL HOSPITAL, SHEFFIELD, UK
[2] DEPARTMENT OF RADIOLOGY, ST GEORGE'S HOSPITAL, LONDON, UK

Introduction

For a variety of reasons there has been a general shift towards the provision of healthcare procedures on a day case basis. This particularly applies to procedures and operations, which have traditionally been regarded as minor. However with advances in techniques and technology available, there has been a further move towards more invasive operations being safely performed and the patient allowed home the same day. Also the development of endovascular techniques has made minimally invasive treatments a viable option for conditions which previously required substantial open operations. This chapter considers why day case angiography and intervention may be desirable, the technologies which are making the procedures less invasive, the facilities which are needed to perform the procedures and the data to support the practice. Care pathways for diagnosis and intervention will be identified as well as issues which these raise and the relationship to alternative imaging modalities.

Why consider day case procedures?

The concept of a visit to the hospital for a procedure with discharge the same day has attractions for the patient, the radiologist and the hospital.

Patients prefer this option because:

◆ There is less disruption to their daily activities.

◆ Hotel comfort is generally more suited to an individual at home rather than in hospital.

◆ Ambulatory care is perceived as advantageous for both surgical and radiological procedures.

Radiologists and radiology nurses may find day case angiography and intervention advantageous because:

◆ The radiology department can take ownership of these episodes of the patients' management increasing responsibilities and satisfaction of performing that defined episode. Similarly if an

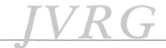

individual has a diagnostic angiogram and subsequently returns for intervention, the same personnel will probably be caring for that patient, with the familiarity and confidence which this engenders.

◆ Preassessment for suitability for day case procedures may be performed in the day case unit, allowing the patient and staff to become familiar prior to any procedure.

◆ Preassessment arrangements may be streamlined with nurse-led clinics, which generally improves the quality of assessment as suitably experienced nursing staff may improve the continuity of assessment, as the turnover of medical staff may be high.

The hospital sees benefit from day case procedures resulting from:

◆ More rapid turnover of Finished Consultant Episodes (FCEs), which generate revenue from purchasers and allows for negotiated contracts to be fulfilled.

◆ There is huge pressure on inpatient beds in most institutions, particularly during the winter months. However day case facilities are not suitable for use as inpatient back-up, therefore, even at times of bed shortage, the day unit beds are still available for treatment. This results in less problems with having to cancel routine and urgent procedures because of emergency admissions. This feeds back positively for patients who have much more confidence that their day case procedure is less likely to be cancelled.

◆ The transfer of procedures to day case from inpatient results in a general reduction of Reference Costs, improving the hospital's position in published league tables.

There are concerns with day case procedures from the above groups:

◆ Patients may be concerned about analgesia after discharge and advice in the immediate post

procedure period. Both of these can readily be addressed by appropriate discussion, and by the provision of information sheets.

◆ In a recent BSIR (British Society of Interventional Radiologists) survey [1], the main objection to day case activity was the paucity of data in support of this activity. This will be discussed later. In addition it is not the usual practice for radiologists to take direct responsibility for patient care outside the radiology department. This is an issue of culture change for both radiologists and other clinicians, which can be partly overcome by the development of a dedicated vascular (or vascular radiology) day case unit, which may be located close to the interventional suite.

◆ Efficient day case facilities are available in many hospitals, but not all. However in many these are already fully utilised by other surgical specialities and are therefore not available for vascular and endovascular procedures. If the facilities are available, then the addition of radiology patients will enable fuller utilisation of the facility, which is advantageous. Alternatively a smaller unit can be fashioned from much smaller amounts of space, either adjacent to or within the radiology department. This will require some development of the existing facilities and a business justification will be necessary.

Technological advances

Diagnostic angiography has developed over the years with improvements in convenience, safety and applicability. Translumbar aortography required large catheter systems to be introduced, under general anaesthesia, blindly into the abdominal aorta from the back. Modern angiography is performed mainly from the transfemoral route, with access to the femoral artery aided by ultrasound control in difficult circumstances. This is a much safer and more controllable access point and, with the advent of smaller catheter systems (usually 4F or 3F), day case diagnostic angiography can be performed in many patients, even if they are anticoagulated (provided that their anticoagulation is within the therapeutic range).

Contrast media advances have reduced the toxicity of these substances with reduction in both dose related and idiosyncratic contrast reactions. In addition a variety of imaging advances, including such techniques as subtracted bolus chase, have reduced both the volume and concentration of contrast media needed to produce images of diagnostic quality.

The above advances have made day case diagnostic angiograms possible, and indeed have been routine in many centres for some years. However there have been a number of advances made which now make many endovascular interventions possible on a day case basis:

♦ It has become clear that the widespread use of effective antiplatelet agents, such as aspirin and clopidogrel, reduces the need for post procedure anticoagulation. In combination with modern techniques for angioplasty and stenting, this has resulted in a low thrombosis rate immediately after the procedure, obviating the need for many patients to remain under close medical supervision in the first day or two following their angioplasty.

♦ Low profile angioplasty and stent combinations (e.g. balloon catheters requiring 4F and 5F sheaths for iliac and femoral PTA, and 6F stent systems) has made the need for large access arterial holes to be obsolete.

♦ Arterial closure devices. A number of these devices are available allowing almost instant haemostasis with sheaths up to 8F and larger, which potentially allows day case access for most endovascular devices (with the exception of some stent grafts). Closure devices are discussed in more detail in the chapter on the investigation and management of false femoral aneurysms.

Facilities

As noted above, the facilities for day case surgery are available in most hospital environments. However these may already be fully committed, without spare capacity for vascular radiology patients. In addition,

historically, radiologists have not taken primary responsibility of care for such patients and it is likely that such an addition will have low priority within the existing facility. Should such a situation exist then consideration should be paid to setting up a dedicated vascular radiology facility (this could be in combination with other interventional radiology procedures such as biopsy, drainage and endoscopic procedures). If such an arrangement is considered, then the following issues need to be taken into account:

Space

This is at a premium in most centres. However, there are continuous service developments and alterations in need for equipment. As a result, as some x-ray equipment is decommissioned, the room where it has been housed may be suitable for the development of a day case facility.

Cost

There is no doubt that the cost of interventional procedures is increased if closure devices are used. However, if their use allows for a patient to be discharged home the same day, then the cost of overnight stay is saved. In addition the inpatient bed which would otherwise have been occupied by the endovascular patient can be used for another surgical procedure, which in turn generates revenue from purchasers, and helps achieve contractual obligations.

Size

A dedicated day unit need not be large, as it will be expected to deal with a relatively small number of cases. For example, if the unit is supporting a single angiography room, which is being used for a full day, approximately 40% of the diagnostic and interventional cases will be suitable as day case [2]. On average it would be expected that 6-7 cases would be performed in a single day, approximately three of which would be day case. If one or two diagnostic angiograms were performed first on the list, followed by one or two interventional cases (with closure devices applied, allowing ambulation in 3 hours), then a maximum of three beds would be needed, with comfortable chairs for patients when ambulant, but awaiting transport home. Such an arrangement, along with a nursing station and toilet facilities, would comfortably fit into many existing rooms.

Equipment

As with all hospital facilities, a day unit needs:

◆ A nursing station.

◆ Access to kitchen facilities.

◆ Connection to the hospital information system.

◆ Resuscitation equipment, including piped oxygen and suction.

◆ Portering facilities.

◆ Toilets/sluice.

Assessment

In common with all medical procedures, patient selection is vital to ensure that only appropriate patients have their procedures performed on a day case basis. The assessment for suitability is best performed using protocols, and this can be most efficiently carried out by a specialist group of nurses, preferably those who care for the patients when they are having their day case procedure. In this way nurses and patients become familiar with each other, engendering a confidence which might otherwise not be built up. In addition the nursing staff who accompany and care for these patients are the best qualified to ensure that cases are selected appropriately. The criteria detailed in Figure 1 are assessed at the Sheffield Vascular Institute by the nurse specialists and a decision made by them as to the suitability, or otherwise, for a day case procedure. These criteria are the same irrespective of whether the patient is to have a diagnostic angiogram or an interventional procedure (but not all procedures are considered suitable for day case). Patients are issued

with written and verbal instructions and given contact telephone numbers should there be any delayed complications following discharge. Subjective nurse review remains an important aspect of assessment for suitability.

All patients are instructed to eat and drink normally prior to their angiogram or interventional procedure.

Safety data

As stated previously, one of the major objections to the adoption of day case endovascular procedures, was the perceived lack of data to support its use. Despite these reservations data do exist which justifies day case intervention. These are summarised in Table 1.

The patient's ability to recognise complications and obtain appropriate emergency care is vital. Most complications occur during or immediately after the procedure, including embolus, dissection and thrombosis at the angioplasty or puncture site [3] (II). Haematoma and bleeding are the most frequent problems and are likely to arise shortly after the procedure. A recent prospective analysis of 266 angioplasties and 51 stent placements in 240 consecutive patients demonstrated that 12 of 14 (86%) of complications were evident before the patient left the angiography suite. The additional two complications were evident within 4.5 hours of the procedure [4] (II). One study reported that all complications were noted at the time of angioplasty [5] (II) and one further study reported 21 major complications of which only one was diagnosed after discharge [6] (II). A recent assessment of 144 puncture site complications following early mobilisation after PTA has demonstrated that all major complications were detected within the first 4 hours but that 10% may require more prolonged bed rest [7] (II). Complications occurring following discharge are relatively rare and it has been stated that overnight hospitalisation does not influence outcome, including complications [6,8] (II). Late rebleeding from the groin (for example longer than 24 hours post procedure) would not be avoided with conventional inpatient care as the majority of vascular interventions are discharged after an overnight stay. Of the delayed

Figure 1 Day case nursing pre-assessment.

Patient Sticker	Creatinine.............................. (refer to protocol)	Date...................
	INR.. (refer to protocol)	Date....................
	LMP... (if appropriate)	Date...................

Information sheet given? ☐ Yes ☐ No

Answers 1-5 must be YES to be suitable for Day Case	**Yes**	**No**
1 Responsible, fit adult at home for 24 hours after procedure. OR	☐	☐
Responsible, fit friend / relation can stay with patient 24 hours after procedure.	☐	☐
OR		
Patient can stay with responsible, fit friend / relation for 24 hours after procedure.	☐	☐
2 Access to telephone at discharge address	☐	☐
3 Usual systolic BP <200	☐	☐
4 Usual diastolic BP <110	☐	☐
5 BMI <40	☐	☐

Answers 6-7 must be no to be suitable for Day Case

		Yes	No
6	Had previous contrast reaction	☐	☐
7	MRSA positive	☐	☐
8	Taking metformin	☐	☐
9	Taking anticoagulant therapy	☐	☐

10 Patient can be at hospital by: ☐ 8am ☐ 9am ☐ 10am ☐ 11am ☐ 12 noon

11 Transport requirements : ☐ Own ☐ Medicar ☐ Ambulance

Other medical history to contra-indicate Day Case. Describe. ☐ ☐

DAY CASE ☐ Yes ☐ No Assessor:.....................................

Table 1 Literature Review: results of contemporary day case vascular interventional practice.

Author (reference)	Year	No. of patients (procedures)	Clinical spectrum	Intervention	Sheath size	Heparin	Closure	Major complications	Minor complications	Delayed complications
Manashil (8)	1983	75 (81)	Iliofemoral, renal, subclavian	PTA	unknown	5000 u	20 min pressure	3/81 procedures (3.7%) (2 acute occlusions, 1 contrast reaction) requiring intervention	None	None
Lemarbre (13)	1986	64 (79)	Aortoiliac, fempop, bypass graft	PTA	5-9 F external balloon diameter	5000 u reversal at completion	20 min pressure	None	1.5%	1/64 (0.2%); 1 admission to exclude femoral PA (?time interval)
Rogers (14)	1990	106 (149)	Aortoiliac, renal, fempop, crural, celiac, SMA	PTA	Up to 9 F external balloon diameter	5-7000 u reversal at completion in some	10-15 min pressure	1/149 (0.7%) (femoral PA requiring surgery)	9/149 (6%) (hematoma)	1/149 (0.7%) femoral PA at 3 days requiring surgery
Struk (6)	1993	141 (141)	Aortoiliac, fempop, tibioperoneal	PTA	5-8F dilatation catheters	3000 u	10-15 min pressure	5% overall complication rate 7/141 hematomas, 1/141 dissection		None
Payne (5)	1997	168 (139)	Iliofemoral, vein graft	PTA	5 F balloon catheter	5000 u	Manual pressure then pressure dressing	4/168 (2.4%) four puncture-site bleeds, three vein patch, one transfusion		None
Craido (11)	1998	134 (151)	Iliofemoral, subclavian	PTA/stents	7 F sheaths	2-3000 u in 69% iliacs all fempop intervention	Femstop device	1/151 procedures (0.6%) one acute stent thrombosis	4/151 (2.6%). 1 hematoma-observed, and 3 delayed complications	3/151 (1.9%) 2 hematomas, 1 femoral PA (within 30 days-conservatively managed)
Mathie (10)	1999	28 (29)	Iliac	Stents	6-8 F sheaths	3000 u in some	AngioSeal in 21%	None	2/29 (7%) hematomas admitted for observation	None
Kruse (15)	2000	203 (239)	Iliofemoral	PTA, stents, lysis, stent-graft, atherectomy	6-7 F sheaths	48% heparinised	Manual pressure	1/239 procedures (0.4%), one ▲BP (post SFA angioplasty) requiring medical treatment	37/239 (15%)-hematomas	None
Peterson (16)	2000	53 (62)	Renal	PTA	6 F sheaths	3000 u	Manual pressure	1/162 (1.6%)-femoral PA requiring surgical repair	2/62 (3.2%) one hematoma conservatively treated and one contrast reaction (observed)	2/62 (3.2%): 1 RA rupture (6 hours), 1 peripheral thromboembolism (20 days)

Key: Fempop: femoropopliteal segment; SMA: superior mesenteric artery; RA: renal artery, SFA: superficial femoral artery, PA: pseudoaneurysm
Note: "Reversal at completion" indicates that an appropriate dose of protamine sulfate was administered at the end of the procedure. Classification of complications in this table is based on the SCVIR guidelines. Modified from MacDonald et al [2] with permission.

complications, only bleeding from a puncture site or the rare delayed contrast reaction would be immediately life threatening. The potential risk of the latter also present following out-patient intravenous urography or contrast-enhanced computed tomography (CT). Contrast-induced renal failure, arteriovenous fistula and pseudoaneurysm take time to develop, are unlikely to be recognised even during a period of overnight observation and are unlikely to be immediately life-threatening.

Complication rates of conventional inpatient peripheral angioplasty as high as 33% have been reported [9] (II). However, in a meta-analysis of 4662 non-coronary angioplasties, the overall complication rate was 10.5%, with a 5% puncture site haematoma rate as the most common isolated complication [3] (II). Again, comparison of complication rates between inpatients and out-patients may be invalid because these groups comprise different patient populations. For out-patient vascular intervention, literature review indicates a major complication rate ranging between 0-3.7%, a minor complication rate between 0-15% and a delayed complication rate of 0-3.2%. It may still be difficult to compare the complication rates of published out-patient series because of disparate definition of major complication, differences in case selection and wide variation in sample size. For example, two minor haematomas in Mathie's series of 29 [10] (II) iliac stents (28 patients) gives a minor complication rate of 7%, whereas three delayed complications in Craido's series of 151 angioplasties/stents (134 patients) gives a delayed complication rate of 1.9% [11].

Data therefore exists to support the safety of day case angiography and intervention, the majority of complications would appear to occur within the first 4 hours following the procedure which would be fully assessable on the day care unit. The number of problems which occur outside this period but within a 24-hour period would appear to be very small and those which occur in general are non-life threatening.

Post procedure care

Following all diagnostic and interventional procedures, careful and regular observations of the pulse rate, blood pressure, limb vascularity and groin puncture site should be performed. This is no different for day case and non-day care patients.

The period of bed rest required depends upon the size of the access puncture site and the presence or otherwise of a haematoma following the procedure. Again the practice in the authors' hospital is that for procedures utilising 4F and 5F sheaths, the patient is kept on flat bed rest for 2 hours and then is allowed to sit for an hour prior to mobilisation. Patients who have had a 6F sheath and no closure device has been used are kept on flat bed rest for an hour longer before being allowed to sit up. For all procedures where a closure device has been used, the mobilisation depends on the type of device used. At the Sheffield Vascular Institute, Angioseal (St Jude Medical) or Closer (Perclose) devices are used. Patients are allowed to sit up in bed after 20 minutes with both devices. With the Angioseal the patient stays in bed for 3 hours before mobilisation; this is reduced to 1 hour for the Perclose. In reality, whilst patients may be mobilised earlier with the Perclose, most patients would prefer a period of rest after their procedure.

All patients are allowed, and encouraged, to eat and drink normally after their angiogram or interventional procedure.

Provided that patients have a normal renal function Metformin therapy is not altered. If their creatinine is raised, then this is a contra-indication to Metformin and alternative therapy or imaging is investigated as described by Nawaz [12] (I).

Care pathways

Patients who are considered for day case angiography and intervention raise a number of issues, which should be addressed during their assessment for suitability. Figures 2, 3 and 4 illustrate pathways developed at the Sheffield Vascular Institute, to facilitate this assessment.

Anticoagulation

If the patient is taking warfarin the pathways illustrated in Figures 3 and 4 are applicable.

Chapter 10

Figure 2 One stop clinic.

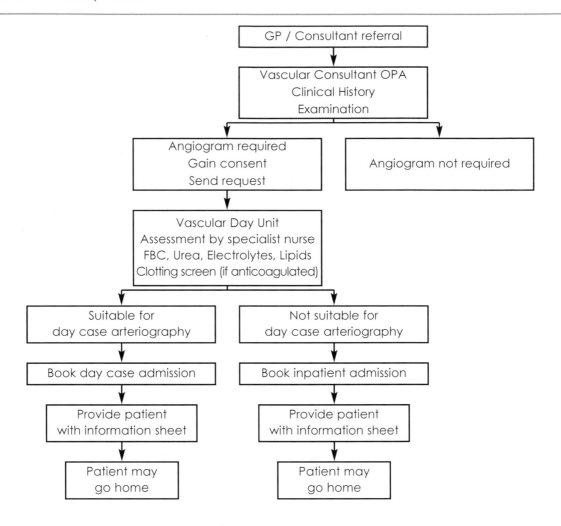

Figure 3 Anticoagulation with *investigative* procedure only.

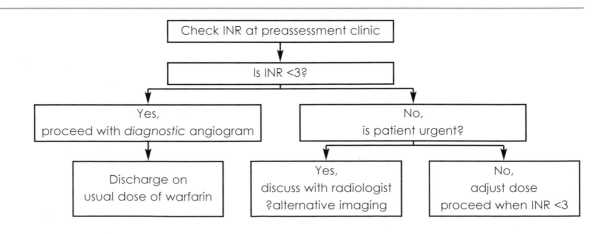

Figure 4 Anticoagulation with *interventional* procedure.

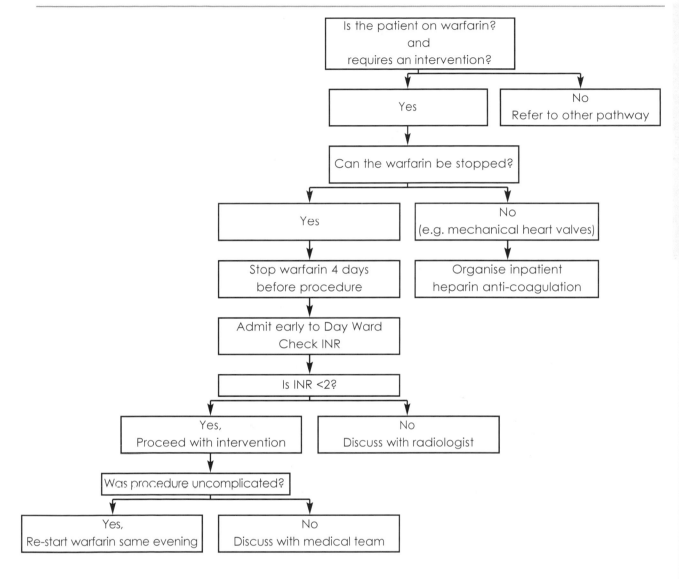

Patient with abnormal renal function

Iodinated contrast media is potentially nephrotoxic, the level of risk being directly related to the degree of renal impairment present prior to angiography. Whilst measurement of serum creatinine is a crude measure of renal function, it is a practical measurement which can be made in all patients prior to angiography. If renal function is abnormal consider again if alternative imaging not using iodinated contrast may achieve the clinical need. If not, then the maximum manifestation of contrast nephrotoxicity is likely to be seen at 48-72 hours after injection. Depending on the patients' creatinine level measured prior to angiography the following guidelines **(B)** can be used:

◆ **Creatinine 120-150 µmol/L.** These patients require no specific prophylaxis but their renal function should be checked 72 hours after the procedure. If their creatinine has changed little (e.g. less than 20µmol/L) no action is needed. If there is a moderate rise in creatinine (e.g. 20-50 μmol/L) then their creatinine should be rechecked at day seven to check that there is not a continued rise. If the creatinine rises significantly then nephrological advice should be sought.

♦ **Creatinine greater than 150 μmol/L.** These patients should probably have their angiography performed as an inpatient, with appropriate fluids, fluid balance control and alteration in medication.

Summary

♦ Day case angiography and intervention has been shown to be safe for appropriately selected patients **(II)**.

♦ Patients' quality of care may be improved in the day care environment **(III)**.

♦ Preassessment is essential and probably best performed by Nurse Specialists working to agreed protocols **(B)**.

♦ Interventional radiologists should play a primary role in day care **(A)**.

♦ Trusts benefit from out-patient intervention by the reduction of costs and reduced inpatient bed pressures **(B)**.

♦ A dedicated day unit, close to the angiography suite is ideal.

References (grade I evidence and grade A recommendations in bold)

1   Paul HJ, Moss JG. Day case lower limb angioplasty: A postal survey amongst members of the British Society of Interventional Radiologists and review of the literature. *J Interv Radiol* 1997; 12: 103-105.

2   Macdonald S, Thomas SM, Cleveland TJ, Gaines PA. Day-case Interventional Practice. *Intervention* 2000; 4(3): 72-77.

3   Becker GJ, Katzen BT, Dake MD. Noncoronary angioplasty. *Radiology* 1989; 170: 921-40.

4   Burns BJ, Phillips AJ, Fox A, Boardman P, Phillips-Hughes J. The Timing and Frequency of Complications After Peripheral Percutaneous Transluminal Angioplasty and Iliac Stenting: Is a Change from Inpatient to Out-patient Therapy Feasible? *Cardiovasc Intervent Radiol* 2000; 6: 452-456.

5   Payne SPK, Stanton A, Travers P. Out-patient angioplasty: 4-year experience in one practice. *Ann R Coll Surg Engl* 1997; 79: 331-334.

6   Struk DW, Rankin RN, Eliasziw M, Vellet AD. Safety of out-patient peripheral angioplasty. *Radiology* 1993; 189:193-196.

7   Butterfield JS, Fitzgerald JB, Razzaq R, Willard CJ, Ashleigh RJ, England RE, Chalmers N, Andrew HM. Early Mobilisation Following Angioplasty. *Clin Radiol* 2000; 55: 874-877.

8   Manashil GB, Thunstrom BS, Thorpe CD, Lipson SR. Out-patient transluminal angioplasty. *Radiology* 1983; 147: 7-8.

9   Hasson JE, Acher CW, Wojtowycz M, McDermott J, Crummy A, Turnipseed WD. Lower extremity percutaneous transluminal angioplasty: multifactorial analysis of morbidity and mortality. *Surgery* 1990; 108: 748-754.

10   Mathie AG, Bell SD, Saibil EA, Magissano R, Kucey DS. Safety of out-patient arterial stenting. *Can Assoc Radiolol J* 1999; 50(4): 268-271.

11   Craido FJ, Abdul-Khoudoud O, Twena M, Clark NS, Patten RN. Out-patient endovascular intervention: is it safe? *J Endovasc Surg* 1998; 5: 236-239.

12   **Nawaz S, Cleveland T, Gaines PA, Chan P. Clinical risk associated with contrast angiography in metformin treated patients: a clinical review. *Clinical Radiology* 1998; 53 (5): 342-324.**

13   Lemarbre L, Hudon G, Coche G, Bourassa MG. Oupatient peripheral angioplasty: survey of complications and patients' perceptions. *AJR* 1987; 148: 1239-1240.

14   Rogers WF, Kraft MA. Out-patient Angioplasty. *Radiology* 1990; 174: 753-755.

15   Kruse JR, Cragg AH. Safety of short stay observation after peripheral vascular intervention. *J Vasc Intervent Radiol* 2000; 11: 45-49.

16   Peterson RA, Baldauf CG, Millward SF *et al*. Out-patient percutaneous transluminal renal artery angioplasty: a Canadian experience. *JVIR* 2000;11: 327-32.

Chapter 11

False femoral aneurysms

Frank CT Smith Consultant Senior Lecturer in Vascular Surgery
Vikram Vijayan Vascular Research Fellow
Peter M Lamont Consultant Vascular Surgeon

VASCULAR SURGERY UNIT, BRISTOL ROYAL INFIRMARY, BRISTOL, UK

Introduction

A false aneurysm occurs when discontinuity of an arterial wall or vascular anastomosis permits extravasation of blood into surrounding tissues, with persisting flow within the contained space. An enveloping fibrous capsule of inflammatory tissue forms around the affected region in response. This capsule lacks inherent strength, predisposing to the common clinical manifestations of enlargement with pain, inflammation with threat to the overlying skin, local pressure effects on surrounding structures, including veins and nerves, and potential for rupture.

Aetiological factors implicated in false aneurysm formation have changed over the last three or four decades. Trauma, formerly the most common causative factor gave way to a period between the 1960s and 1980s when anastomotic false aneurysms became prevalent, often as a consequence of aorto-bifemoral bypass for occlusive arterial disease. As vascular sutures and prosthetic materials have improved, numbers of extra-anatomic bypasses carried out for occlusive disease have diminished. At the same time the volume of diagnostic and interventional cardiac and peripheral endovascular procedures performed has significantly increased. Iatrogenic false aneurysms arising as a consequence of femoral artery catheterisation are now the group most commonly encountered by vascular teams.

Socio-economic factors have also played their part in terms of the aetiology of infected false aneurysms. False aneurysms in drug abusers now dominate this latter group. Vasculitides including lupus erythematosus, giant cell arteritis, polyarteritis nodosa, Behcet's, Marfans and Kawasaki Syndrome are more commonly associated with true aneurysms, but all have also been implicated as rare causes of false aneurysms.

This chapter summarises the aetiology, investigation and current methods of treatment of false aneurysms. Since the majority of false aneurysms involve the femoral artery, emphasis is placed on management of false aneurysms in this anatomical region. A pathway of care for management of false aneurysms is provided at the end of the chapter (Figure 4).

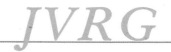

Diagnosis

False femoral aneurysms usually present as an expansile mass in the groin. Examination may reveal a palpable thrill and a bruit may be present on auscultation. A recent history of endovascular catheterisation, previous surgery or intravenous drug abuse should be sought. The aneurysm may be asymptomatic or may cause symptoms of femoral nerve or vein compression. Other potential sequelae include distal embolisation or thrombotic occlusion of the femoral artery resulting in acute limb ischaemia. Rupture with haematoma tracking into the retroperitoneal space or into the thigh occurs infrequently.

Diagnostic investigations include duplex Doppler ultrasound, contrast-enhanced computed tomography (CT) scanning, magnetic resonance angiography (MRA) and conventional angiography. Ankle Doppler pressures are helpful in establishing the severity of limb ischaemia when this is a cause for concern.

Figure 1 Duplex Doppler image of an anastomotic false femoral aneurysm.

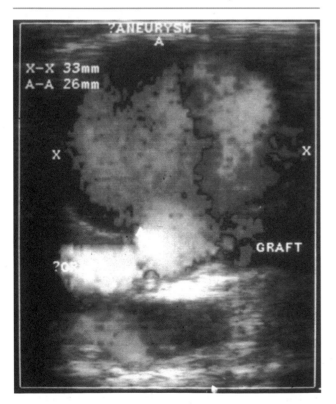

Colour flow duplex ultrasound is the most useful non-invasive modality for identifying the presence, size and extent of a false femoral aneurysm **(A)**. This technique is also helpful in distinguishing an aneurysm from a haematoma, and for locating the jet of blood filling the sac (Figure 1). Diagnosis may be combined with ultrasound-guided compression treatment or thrombin injection. Contrast CT scanning is valuable in determining the extent of haematoma particularly if this tracks into the retroperitoneal space and may detect aneurysms at other sites **(A)**. MRA is also useful in this role, avoiding the need for contrast. Digital subtraction angiography is often only necessary when there is concern about the inflow tract or the extent of peripheral embolisation, suspicion of infection, or to clarify the nature of previous surgery **(B)**.

When infection is suspected, non-specific haematological findings including leucocytosis, elevated ESR, and CRP increase the index of suspicion [1]. Positive blood cultures in a patient with a false aneurysm should be regarded as diagnostic of an infected aneurysm until proven otherwise **(A)**. Conversely, negative blood cultures do not rule out the possibility of infection. In rare cases a radio-labelled white cell scan may help detection of sub-clinical infection in an anastomotic false aneurysm [2] **(II)**.

Anastomotic false aneurysms

The incidence of anastomotic false aneurysms is between 1 and 5 % and these occur most commonly at the femoral anastomotic site of aorto-bifemoral bypass grafts [3,4] (Figure 2). Both late degenerative changes and technical problems contribute to false aneurysm formation. Progression of atherosclerotic disease may weaken the host arterial wall leading to gradual anastomotic dehiscence. False aneurysms may also result from excessive tension on the graft, suture fracture or laxity, inappropriate suture spacing and weakness of the arterial wall following endarterectomy [5] **(II)**. The presence of a false femoral anastomotic aneurysm is a potential marker of other graft problems. Shellack *et al* report a high incidence of synchronous contralateral femoral and proximal aortic anastomotic aneurysms [6].

Figure 2 Bilateral false femoral anastomotic aneurysms in a patient who had undergone aorto-bifemoral bypass 9 years previously.

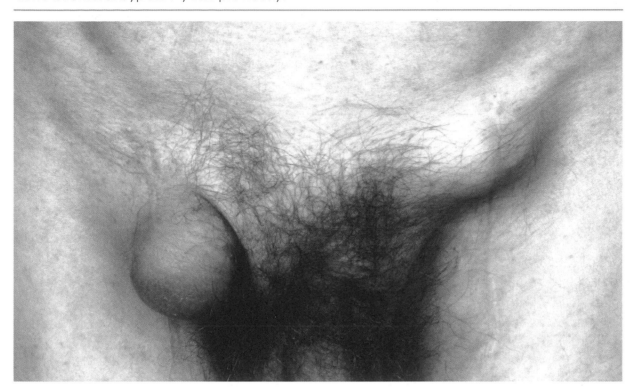

Surgical repair forms the mainstay of treatment for anastomotic false femoral aneurysms because of the associated risk of thrombosis or embolus [4] **(II)**. It is generally accepted that these sequelae are less likely to occur if the false aneurysm is less than 2 cm in diameter and is otherwise asymptomatic [7]. Proximal and distal arterial control is essential. Surgical dissection may be difficult and tedious because of fibrosis and the condition of the arterial wall is often poor. Simple resuturing of a graft anastomosis is associated with high risk of aneurysm recurrence [4,8,9] **(II)**. Definitive treatment usually involves resection of the affected portion of graft, debridement of the native arterial wall back to healthy tissue and replacement of the excised segment with an appropriate interposition graft [4,7,8,9] **(II)**. In some cases, when less extensive repair is indicated, it may be appropriate to use a patch of either prosthetic material or autogenous vein to fix a defect. This technique is often employed when the anastomotic aneurysm occurs at the proximal anastomosis of a femoro-distal graft (Figure 3).

Occult infection should always be suspected, particularly when an anastomotic false aneurysm

occurs soon after arterial reconstruction [10] **(A)**. When graft infection is encountered basic surgical principles are employed. Remote proximal and distal arterial control is obtained and the infected graft excised. The graft and aneurysm thrombus should be sent for microscopy and gram-staining, (although these are often not diagnostic at the time of surgery), and for subsequent cultures and sensitivities **(A)**. The most common infecting organisms are *Staphylococcus aureus*, *Staphylococcus epidermidis* and *Escherichia coli* [11] but in recent years the impact of methicillin-resistant *Staphylococcus aureus* (MRSA) has also become a cause for concern [12] **(I)**.

Localised wound debridement and drainage of the groin should be undertaken as necessary. Restoration of distal limb blood flow is limited only by the ingenuity of the surgeon and availability of inflow and run-off tracts. Obturator, lateral femoral and axillo-popliteal extra-anatomic bypasses have all been employed to revascularise an ischaemic leg, avoiding the infected groin region **(II)**. Although evidence from prospective randomised control trials is scanty due to difficulty in recruiting homogenous populations of graft infections,

Figure 3 Suture line dehiscence at the proximal anastomosis of a femoro-distal graft resulting in a false aneurysm (a). In the absence of infection, the defect was repaired with a Dacron® patch (b).

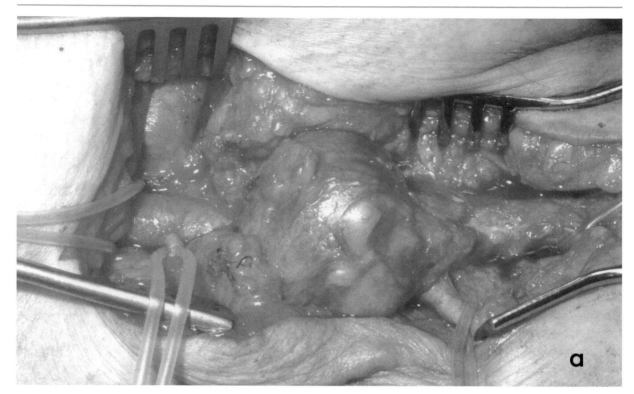

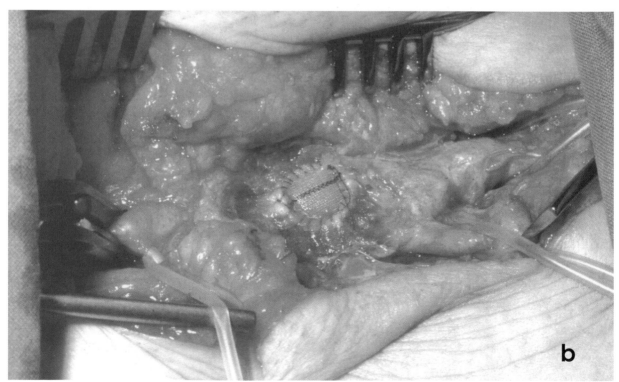

use of Rifampicin-soaked [13] or silver-impregnated grafts for secondary reconstruction, and employment of gentamycin-impregnated beads may be helpful in reducing risk of recurrent graft infection [14,15] **(C)**.

Infected false femoral aneurysms

The term "mycotic" false aneurysm is a misnomer since false aneurysms are rarely associated with fungal infection. Factors predisposing to secondary infection of an existing false aneurysm include diabetes, immuno-suppression and treatment with steroids.

The prevalence of infected false femoral aneurysms is now highest among intra-vascular drug abusers [16,17]. Although the femoral vein is usually the target for vascular access sought by these patients, the femoral pulse offers a more reliable indicator of vessel position and is often inadvertently injured. Patients present with a variety of vascular injuries including infected false aneurysms, arterio-venous fistulae, venous and arterial thrombosis, femoral abscesses and septic embolisation. Local suppuration, induration and a "herald bleed" are commonly encountered [18]. Suspicion should always be entertained that a lesion initially diagnosed as a "femoral abscess" in these patients is in fact a false aneurysm **(B)**. This has particular implications for planning surgical intervention. Because of the potentially litigious nature of the situation patients should be warned at an early opportunity of the high risk of limb loss **(B)**.

In emergency situations proximal vascular control can be achieved by a retroperitoneal approach through an oblique supra-inguinal incision. After vascular isolation, test clamping of the distal iliac artery can be undertaken and the pedal pulses examined with continuous wave Doppler. If a signal persists after distal external iliac artery or common femoral artery occlusion then ligation of the common femoral artery and drainage/debridement of the false aneurysm is undertaken.

Reddy *et al* described surgical treatment of 54 false femoral aneurysms in drug addicts with an overall amputation rate of 11% and no mortality [18]. However

the data was also analysed by subset according to involvement of various components of the femoral arterial complex. Twenty-six of 54 aneurysms involved an isolated segment of the femoral artery, which was excised without limb loss. Twenty-eight aneurysms involved the femoral bifurcation. When triple vessel ligation was undertaken in 18/28 patients, 6 (33%) subsequently required amputation. Six out of 28 patients underwent arterial reconstruction with autogenous saphenous vein, and three with prosthetic grafts. All the prosthetic grafts became re-infected and required excision. On this basis Reddy *et al* argued for a policy of selective revascularisation **(II)**.

Similar results were obtained by Padberg *et al* [19]. These authors followed up a group of 24 drug abusers with false aneurysms for up to 66 months following surgical treatment. In 12/18 patients who underwent revascularisation, significant complications necessitated three amputations and 13 secondary arterial operations in addition to skin grafts and debridement. No amputations were necessary in six patients in whom primary femoral artery ligation and debridement was undertaken.

Debate over whether to treat these patients conservatively or whether to carry out arterial reconstruction using autogenous tissue continues [18,19,20]. Despite IV drug abuse, most patients have mid-thigh saphenous vein suitable for bypass, and if reconstruction is contemplated, this remains the conduit of choice **(B)**. Some authors recommend comprehensive debridement of infected tissue, treatment with intravenous antibiotics, and reconstitution of the arterial circulation using autogenous vein, achieving graft cover with a sartorius muscle flap if necessary. However, even after aggressive post-operative drug rehabilitation there is a high incidence of persistent narcotics abuse. The authors of this chapter are reluctant to revascularise the limb where there is high likelihood that a vascular graft will provide a convenient conduit through which a patient continues to "mainline". Most patients will not require reconstruction to avoid amputation, and the collateral circulation is usually sufficient to maintain limb viability **(II)**.

Penetrating trauma

False aneurysms from non-iatrogenic penetrating trauma should be repaired surgically because the extent of the vessel wall disruption is often extensive and blood loss may be significant **(II)**. Evacuation of a large haematoma promotes soft tissue healing. Autogenous vein is preferred for repair because of the potential of contamination from the injury **(A)**.

Iatrogenic post-catheterisation false aneurysms

Angiography and cardiac catheterisation are now the predominant causes of false femoral aneurysms [21, 22]. Dorfman reviewed complications following 10,589 invasive diagnostic and therapeutic radiological procedures and found a puncture site complication in 0.44% of cases [23]. Complication rates were significantly higher in patients undergoing cardiac catheterisation (0.55%) than in those undergoing peripheral angiography (0.17%). Similar findings have been reported by Messina et al, who noted a 3.4% incidence of complications in patients undergoing therapeutic angiographic procedures [24], of which 16% were false aneurysms. Diagnostic studies were associated with a lower rate of complications (0.7%), of which 32% comprised false aneurysms. Over a 13-year period during which 24,033 radiological procedures were undertaken in our department, 63 (0.25%) patients required surgical or minimally invasive intervention for vascular complications [25]. False aneurysms accounted for 28 (0.11%) of these cases. In other studies using duplex surveillance, the incidence of false femoral aneurysms after femoral catheterisation has been reported to be as high as 14% [22].

Low entry of the catheter into the superficial rather than the common femoral artery is probably the most common cause of catheter-induced false aneurysms [26]. Other factors include "through and through" punctures of both anterior and posterior arterial walls and damage to the profunda vessels which cannot always be adequately compressed. Calcification of the vessel wall and anticoagulation are further contributory factors. Risk of aneurysm formation also relates to catheter size. Femoral artery injury has been described in up to 15% of patients requiring insertion of intravascular devices such as intra-aortic balloon pumps and endovascular stents because of the large calibre of these devices [27,28] **(I)**. False aneurysms account for approximately 44% of these injuries [27].

Non-operative treatment

Although many catheter-induced false aneurysms will require treatment this is not so in all cases. Spontaneous thrombosis has been described in some patients, particularly when the aneurysm is small. In a prospective series Kresowic et al followed up seven patients with post-catheterisation false aneurysms (1.3-3.5cm) by serial duplex Doppler ultrasound scans [29]. All seven aneurysms occluded spontaneously within 4 weeks. In another non-randomised prospective observational study, 5 iatrogenic false aneurysms showed resolution of flow after a mean of 18 (range 7-42) days [30]. Toursarkissian et al reported on approximately 300 femoral false aneurysms [31]. Fifty percent of these required immediate surgical intervention on the basis of size, symptoms or previous surgery at the same site. Fifty percent were observed. In the latter group 86% of these lesions closed spontaneously within 23 days.

Duplex follow-up may provide a viable alternative to intervention and small or asymptomatic false aneurysms can often be followed up in this way for several weeks without adverse sequelae **(B)**. This approach may be particularly valuable in early management of the increasing number of post-cardiac catheterisation aneurysms in infants.

Compression ultrasonography

Compression ultrasonography was first employed as a technique to treat false aneurysms by Fellmeth et al [32]. Duplex ultrasonography is used to accurately localise the arterial defect and "jet" of blood perfusing the extra-luminal aneurysmal sac. Visualisation of this jet allows accurate compression by the duplex probe at the neck of the false aneurysm, occluding blood flow and promoting sac thrombosis (Figure 1). Colour flow duplex further facilitates localisation of the jet of blood. Compression ultrasonography is a useful and effective non-invasive modality for dealing with patients with relatively small aneurysms with small necks (I). However the procedure is uncomfortable for the patient often necessitating sedation and parenteral analgesia. The technique usually involves repeated periodic applications of pressure to the neck of the aneurysm sac employing a 5 MHz or 7.5 MHz probe until thrombosis is complete. Sometimes more than one session of compression is required to achieve occlusion.

Cox *et al* employed the technique in 100 consecutive patients with catheter-induced false femoral aneurysms [33]. Compression was immediately successful, inducing thrombosis in 94 patients, with effective obliteration of the aneurysm sac in 30 out of 35 (86%) of anti-coagulated patients and 64 out of 65 (98%) of non-anti-coagulated patients. Recurrent false aneurysms occurred in 20% of patients who continued to receive anti-coagulation but in only 6% of those who did not (P=0.074). False aneurysm size, size of arterial sheath and duration of the primary radiological procedure did not influence success. In a recent retrospective study, Lange *et al* noted that 0.5% of patients undergoing cardiac catheterisation developed false femoral aneurysms [34]. The incidence was significantly higher after therapeutic (1.5%) compared to diagnostic procedures (0.3%). Forty-eight patients were treated by ultrasound-guided compression with an 88% success rate and successful compression was unrelated to aneurysm diameter.

Anticoagulation as a cause of failed ultrasound-guided compression has been noted in various studies [35,36,37]. Other factors implicated in failed compression include a long time interval between the original catheter injury and compression, a wide aneurysm neck or jet, and obesity preventing adequate compression. Where false aneurysms recur following compression this tends to be an early phenomenon, the majority representing within 24 hours after apparently successful primary compression [33]. For this reason follow-up duplex scanning is advocated at 24 hours (B).

Ultrasound-guided thrombin injection

When duplex-guided ultrasound compression of an iatrogenic false femoral aneurysm fails, percutaneous ultrasound-guided thrombin injection is now accepted as a useful alternative treatment [38-45] (I). Some authors recommend thrombin injection as first-line therapy. The technique involves using real time B-mode duplex ultrasound to position a 20-22G needle accurately into the aneurysm sac. A dilute solution of bovine thrombin (1000u/ml) is injected slowly into the sac under aseptic conditions with the tip of the needle angled away from the neck of the aneurysm if possible. Injection is titrated against cessation of blood flow and thrombus formation within the sac, which is evaluated by continuous Doppler monitoring.

Success rates for aneurysm thrombosis of 90-100%, employing doses of thrombin ranging from 50-2500u have been reported [38-46]. In a refinement to the procedure the neck of the aneurysm can be occluded with a balloon catheter to promote stagnation of blood flow within the sac and to prevent thrombin escape with attendant risk of systemic arterial thrombosis. Use of low dose thrombin (50-450u) has been described as effective in conjunction with balloon occlusion [46]. Fibrin tissue adhesive injection has also been employed successfully as an alternative to thrombin [47].

Failure of thrombin injection to obliterate an aneurysm appears to be independent of false aneurysm duration and size and the technique has been described as achieving success in anti-coagulated patients and in those taking aspirin and clopidogrel. In a non-randomised prospective study, Ouriel *et al* described successful treatment of 66/70 (94%) false aneurysms [42]. Failure of thrombin injections in two patients was attributed to short wide false aneurysm necks following aortic stent grafting and these aneurysms required surgical intervention. Repeated thrombin injections may also be necessary in patients who have complex or multi-lobed false aneurysms.

In rare reports where clot embolisation or distal thrombosis has occurred as a complication of thrombin injection, thrombolysis has proved a useful and effective adjuvant salvage treatment [48]. The possibility of anaphylaxis must be considered however, in patients with previous exposure to thrombin [49].

Percutaneous arterial closure devices

Despite advances in other aspects of cardiac catheterisation and peripheral interventional radiology, manual or mechanical compression followed by 4-8 hours of bed rest remains the mainstay of management for the post catheterisation femoral puncture site (II). Inadequate compression or technical problems with continued bleeding may result in haematoma or false aneurysm formation. The advent of percutaneous endovascular aortic aneurysm stent grafting using relatively large bore devices has also resulted in increased numbers of complications. These problems and a trend towards day-case angiography have spawned development of a variety of commercially available devices designed to seal the femoral artery puncture site, allowing early mobilisation. Broadly speaking these work by three separate methods.

- Percutaneous suture closure (e.g. Perclose®).

- Deployment of a biodegradable anchor and collagen plug (e.g Angio-seal®).

- Occluding balloon catheter and coagulant (e.g Duett® closure device).

Almost all trials evaluating these devices have concentrated on early ambulation and discharge as primary endpoints. The majority of such trials have been non-randomised or retrospective and the extent and quality of follow-up varies considerably (III).

Dangas et al followed a group of 5093 patients after percutaneous coronary intervention (PCI) using univariate and multivariate analysis to identify predictors of vascular complications associated with

use of arteriotomy closure devices (ACD) or manual compression [50] (I). Use of ACDs was associated with a significantly higher occurrence of haematoma compared to manual compression (9.3% vs 5.1%, P<0.001). The rate of significant haematocrit drop (>15%) was also greater in the ACD group, and vascular surgical intervention was required more frequently (2.5% vs 1.5%, P=0.03). However similar rates of false aneurysm and arteriovenous fistula formation were noted with both techniques. These results may have been skewed by the nature of patient selection for treatment with ACDs.

In contrast, Resnic et al, in a retrospective analysis of 3151 patients, (1485 of whom were treated with ACDs), reported significantly lower complication rates associated with use of closure devices (3.03% vs 5.52%, P=0.002) [51]. For a sub-group of patients treated with glycoprotein IIb-IIIa receptor antagonists, ACDs showed an even greater benefit in terms of reduced risk of vascular complications.

Specific complications encountered with percutaneous suture-mediated closure devices have included device malfunction, deployment failure, trapped closure devices, and sutures pulling through the vessel wall resulting in bleeding. False aneurysm formation, femoral artery occlusion or stenosis, intimal dissection and groin wound infections have also occurred [50-54]. Similar complications have arisen with collagen plug closure devices with the added potential risk of plug embolisation. When complications occur the need for operative intervention is frequent and the overall morbidity is significant.

Whilst there is probably a role for these devices in situations where the patient is at high risk of bleeding complications (e.g., the anti-coagulated patient), there is currently little evidence to support routine prophylactic deployment when adequate post-interventional pressure on the femoral artery is likely to be as effective at preventing complications, without the extra expense (III).

Figure 4 Care pathway for management of false femoral aneurysms.

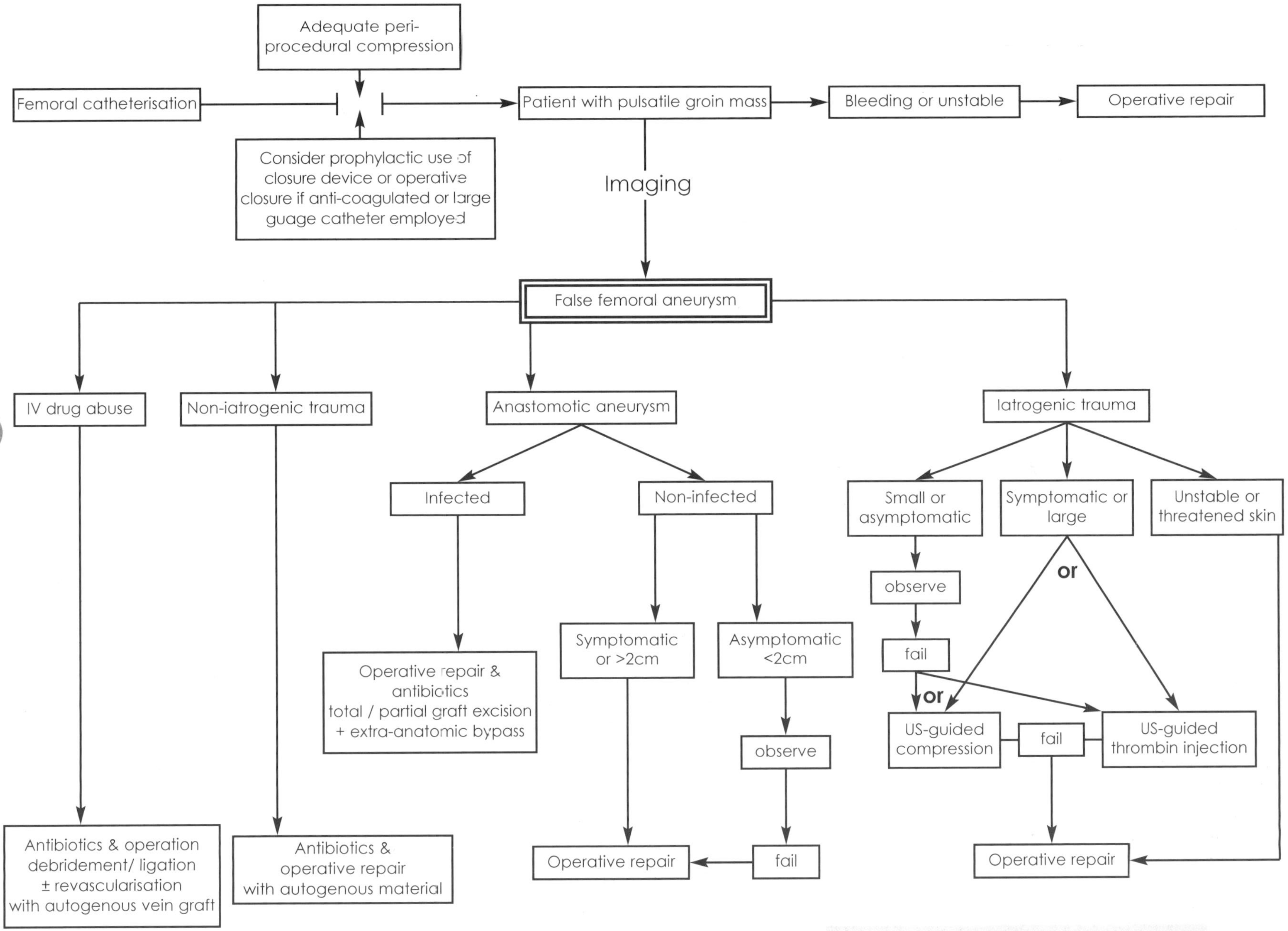

Chapter 11

Summary

♦ The management of false femoral aneurysms is dependent on aetiology and the nature of the presenting symptoms.

♦ The most frequently encountered false aneurysms are iatrogenic.

♦ Adequate compression at time of radiological intervention is probably the most important preventative manoeuvre likely to reduce the prevalence of iatrogenic false aneurysms.

♦ False aneurysms may be managed by:

  • duplex surveillance with the hope of spontaneous thrombosis;
  • intervention by ultrasound compression;
  • intervention by thrombin injection;
  • surgery should be reserved for trauma, for large or expanding false aneurysms, for those aneurysms presenting with the complications of arterial thrombosis or embolism, for anastomotic aneurysms at the site of previous vascular reconstructions and for infection.

References (grade I evidence and grade A recommendations in bold)

1 Reddy DJ, Ernst CB. Infected aneurysms. In: *Vascular Surgery.* Rutherford RB, Ed. 1995 (4th Edition) Ch 82; 1139-53.

2 Brunner MC, Mitchell RS, Baldwin JC, James DR, Olcott C 4th, Mehigan JT, McDougall IR, Miller DC. Prosthetic graft infection: limitations of indium white cell scanning. *J Vasc Surg* 1986; 3: 42-8.

3 Szilagyi DE, Elliott JP, Smith RF, Reddy DJ, McPharlin M. A thirty year survey of the reconstructive surgical treatment of aortoiliac occlusive disease. *J Vasc Surg* 1986; 3: 421-36.

4 Clarke AM, Poskitt KR, Baird RN, Horrocks M. Anastomotic aneurysms of the femoral artery: Aetiology and treatment. *Br J Surg* 1989; 76; 1014-16.

5 Ernst CB, Elliott JP Jr, Ryan CJ, Abu-Hamad G, Tilley BC, Murphy RK, Smith RF, Reddy DJ, Szilagyi DE. Recurrent femoral anastomotic aneurysms. A 30-year experience. *Ann Surg* 1988; 208: 401-9.

6 Shellack J, Salam A, Abouzeid MA, Smith RB, Stewart MT, Perdue GD. Femoral anastomotic aneurysms: a continuing challenge. *J Vasc Surg* 1987; 6: 308-17.

7 Ochsner JL. Management of femoral pseudoaneurysms. *Surg Clin North Am* 1982; 62: 43-40.

8 Millili JJ, Lanes JS, Nemir P. A study of anastomotic aneurysms following aortofemoral prosthetic bypass. *Ann Surg* 1980; 192: 69-73.

9 Sharma NK, Chin KF, Modgill VK. Pseudoaneurysms of the femoral artery: recommendation for a method of repair. *J R Coll Surg Edinb* 2001; 46: 195-7.

10 Seabrook R, Schmitt DD, Bandyk DF, Edmiston CE, Krepel CJ, Towne JB. Anastomotic femoral pseudoaneurysms: an investigation of occult infection as an etiologic factor. *J Vasc Surg* 1990; 11: 629-34.

11 Bunt TJ. Vascular graft infections: an update (Review). *Cardiovasc Surg* 2001; 9: 225-33.

12 Naylor AR, Hayes PD, Darke S. A prospective audit of complex wound and graft infections in Great Britain and Ireland: the emergence of MRSA. *Eur J Vasc Endovasc Surg* 2001 Apr; 21(4): 289-94.

13 Braithwaite BD, Davies B, Heather BP, Earnshaw JJ. Early results of a randomized trial of rifampicin-bonded Dacron grafts for extra-anatomic vascular reconstruction. *Br J Surg* 1998; 85: 1378-81.

14 Benaerts PJ, Ridler BM, Vercaeren P, Thompson JF, Campbell WB. Gentamicin beads in vascular surgery: long-term results of implantation. *Cardiovasc Surg* 1999 Jun; 7(4):447-50.

15 Nielsen OM, Noer HH, Jorgensen LG, Lorentzen JE. Gentamycin beads in the treatment of localised vascular graft infection - long term results in 17 cases. *Eur J Vasc Surg* 1991 Jun; 5(3): 283-5.

16 Blair SD. Intra-arterial drug injection. In: *Emergency Vascular Surgery.* Greenhalgh RM, Hollier LH, Eds. WB Saunders 1992; 377-85.

17 Patel KR, Semel L, Clauss RH. Routine revascularization with resection of infected femoral pseudoaneurysms from substance abuse. *J Vasc Surg* 1988; 8: 321-8.

18 Reddy DJ, Smith RF, Elliot JP Jr, Haddad GK, Wanek EA. Infected femoral artery false aneurysms in drug addicts: evolution of selective vascular reconstruction. *J Vasc Surg* 1986; 3: 718-24.

19 Padberg F, Hobson R II, Lee B, Anderson K, Manno J, Breitbart G, Swan K. Femoral pseudoaneurysm from drugs of abuse: ligation or reconstruction. *J Vasc Surg* 1992; 15: 642-8.

20 Pasic M, Segesser L, Turina M. Implantation of antibiotic-releasing carriers and in situ reconstruction for treatment of mycotic aneurysm. *Arch Surg* 1992; 127: 745-6.

21 Yao JST. Iatrogenic arterial injuries: damage to femoral artery. In: *Emergency Vascular Surgery.* Greenhalgh RM, Hollier LH, Eds. WB Saunders 1992; 365-76.

22 Katzenschlager R, Ururluoglu A, Ahmadi A, Hulsmann M, Koppensteiner R, Larch E, Maca T, Minar E, Stumpflen A, Ehringer H. Incidence of pseudoaneurysm after diagnostic and therapeutic angiography. *Radiology* 1995; 195: 463-6.

23 Dorfman GS, Cronan JJ. Postcatheterisation femoral artery injuries: is there a role for non-surgical treatment? *Radiology* 1991; 178: 629-30.

24 Messina LM, Brothers TE, Wakefield TW, Zelenock GB, Lindenauer SM, Greenfield LJ, Jacobs LA, Fellows EP, Grube SV, Stanley JC. Clinical characteristics and surgical management of vascular complications in patients undergoing cardiac catheterisation: interventional versus diagnostic procedures. *J Vasc Surg* 1991; 13: 593-600.

25 Lewis DR, Bulbulia RA, Murphy P, Jones AJ, Smith FCT, Baird RN, Lamont PM. Vascular surgical complications of cardiovascular radiology: 13 years' experience in a single centre. *Ann R Coll Surg Engl* 1999; 81: 23-26.

26 Altkin RS, Flicker S, Naidech HJ. Pseudoaneurysm and arteriovenous fistula after femoral artery catheterisation: association with low femoral punctures. *Am J Roent* 1989; 152: 629-31.

27 Skillman JJ, Kim D, Bain DS. Vascular complications of percutaneous femoral cardiac interventions. *Arch Surg* 1988; 123: 1207-12.

28 **Lumsden AB, Miller JM, Kosinski AS, Allen RC, Dodson TF, Salam AA, Smith RB 3rd. A prospective evaluation of surgically treated groin complications following percutaneous cardiac procedures. *Am Surg* 1994; 60: 132-7.**

29 Kresowik TF, Khoury MD, Miller BV, Winniford MD, Shamma AR, Blecha MB, Corson JD. A prospective study of the incidence and natural history of femoral vascular complications after percutaneous transluminal coronary angioplasty. *J Vasc Surg* 1991; 13: 328-35.

30 Johns JP, Pupa LE Jr., Bailey SR. Spontaneous thrombosis of iatrogenic femoral artery pseudoaneurysms: documentation with color Doppler two-dimensional ultrasonography. *J Vasc Surg* 1991; 14: 24-29.

31 Toursarkissian B, Allen BT, Petrinec D, Thompson RW, Rubin BG, Reilly JM, Anderson CB, Flye MW, Sicard GA. Spontaneous closure of selected iatrogenic pseudoaneurysms and arteriovenous fistulae. *J Vasc Surg* 1997; 25: 803-8.

32 Fellmeth BD, Roberts AC, Bookstein JJ, Freischlag JA, Forsythe JR, Buckner NK, Hye RJ. Postangiographic femoral artery injuries: non-surgical repair with US-guided compression. *Radiology* 1991; 178: 671-75.

33 Cox GS, Young JR, Gray BR, Grubb MW, Hertzer NR. Ultrasound-guided compression repair of postcatheterization pseudoaneurysms: results of treatment in one hundred cases. *J Vasc Surg* 1994; 19: 683-86.

34 Lange P, Houte T, Helgstrand UJ. The efficacy of ultrasound-guided compression of iatrogenic femoral pseudoaneurysms. *Eur J Vasc Endovasc Surg* 2001; 21(3): 248-50.

35 Lewis DR, Davies AH, Irvine CD, Morgan MR, Baird RN, Lamont PM, Smith FCT. Compression ultrasonography for false femoral aneurysms: hypocoagulability is a cause of failure. *Eur J Vasc Endovasc Surg* 1998;16:427-28.

36 Davies AH, Hayward JK, Irvine CD, Lamont PM, Baird RN. Treatment of iatrogenic false aneurysm by compression ultrasonography. *Br J Surg* 1995; 82:1230-31.

37 Perkins JMT, Magee TR, Gordon AC, Hands LJ. Duplex-guided compression of femoral artery false femoral aneurysms reduces the need for surgery. *Ann R Coll Surg Engl* 1996; 78: 473-75.

38 **Paulson EK, Sheafor DH, Kliewer MA, Neelson RC, Eisenberg LB, Sebastian MW, Sketch MH Jr. Treatment of iatrogenic femoral arterial pseudoaneurysms: comparison of US-guided thrombin injection with compression repair. *Radiology* 2000; 215: 403-8.**

39 **Paulson EK, Nelson RC, Mayes CE, Sheafor DH, Sketch MH, Kliewer MA. Sonographically guided thrombin injection of iatrogenic femoral pseudoaneurysms: further experience of a single institution. *Am J Roentgenol* 2001; 177(2): 309-16.**

40 **Gale SS, Scissons RP, Jones L, Salles-Cunha SX. Femoral pseudoaneurysm thrombin injection. *Am J Surg* 2001; 181(4): 379-83.**

41 **Lennox AF, Delis KT, Szendro G, Griffin MB, Nicolaides AN, Cheshire NJ. Duplex-guided thrombin injection for iatrogenic femoral artery pseudoaneurysm is effective even in anticoagulated patients. *Br J Surg* 2000; 87(6): 796-801.**

42 **La Perna L, Olin JW, Goines D, Childs MB, Ouriel K. Ultrasound-guided thrombin injection for the treatment of postcatheterization pseudoaneurysms. *Circulation* 2000; 102(19): 2391-5.**

43 **Owen RJ, Haslam PJ, Elliott ST, Rose JD, Loose HW. Percutaneous ablation of peripheral pseudoaneurysms using thrombin: a simple and effective solution. *Cardiovasc Intervent Radiol* 2000; 23(6): 441-6.**

44 **Sackett WR, Taylor SM, Coffey CB, Viers KD, Langan EM, Cull DL, Snyder BA, Sullivan TM. Ultrasound-guided thrombin injection of iatrogenic femoral pseudoaneurysms: a prospective analysis. *Am Surg* 2000; 66(10): 937-40.**

Chapter 11

45 **Sheiman RG, Brophy DP. Treatment of iatrogenic femoral pseudoaneurysms with percutaneous thrombin injection: experience in 54 patients.** *Radiology* **2001; 219(1): 123-7.**

46 Reeder SB, Widlus DM, Lazinger M. Low-dose thrombin injection to treat iatrogenic femoral artery pseudoaneurysms. *Am J Roentgenol* 2001; 177(3): 595-8.

47 Matson MB, Morgan RA, Belli AM. Percutaneous treatment of pseudoaneurysms using fibrin adhesive. *Br J Radiol* 2001; 74(884): 690-4.

48 Sadiq S, Ibrahim W. Thromboembolism complicating thrombin injection of femoral artery pseudoaneurysm: management with intraarterial thrombolysis. *J Vasc Interv Radiol* 2001; 12: 633-6.

49 Pope M, Johnston KW. Anaphylaxis after thrombin injection of a femoral pseudoaneurysm: recommendations for prevention. *J Vasc Surg* 2000; 32: 190-1.

50 Dangas G, Mehran R, Kokolis S, Feldman D, Satler LF, Pichard AD, Kent KM, Lansky AJ, Stone GW, Leon MB. Vascular complications after percutaneous coronary interventions following hemostasis with manual compression versus arteriotomy closure devices. *J Am Coll Cardiol* 2001; 38(3): 642-4.

51 Resnic FS, Blake GJ, Ohno-Machado L, Selwyn AP, Popma JJ, Rogers C. Vascular closure devices and the risk of vascular complications after percutaneous coronary intervention in patients receiving glycoprotein IIb-IIIa inhibitors. *Am J Cardiol* 2001; 88(5): 493-6.

52 Sprouse LR 2nd, Botta DM Jr., Hamilton IN Jr. The management of peripheral vascular complications associated with the use of percutaneous suture-mediated closure devices. *J Vasc Surg* 2001 33(4); 688-93.

53 Fram DB, Giri S, Jamil G, Mitchel JF, Boden WE, Din S, Kiernan FJ. Suture closure of the femoral arteriotomy following invasive cardiac procedures: a detailed analysis of efficacy, complications, and the impact of early ambulation in 1200 consecutive cases. *Catheter Cardiovasc Interv* 2001; 53(2): 163-73.

54 Nehler MR, Lawrence WA, Whitehill TA, Charette SD, Jones DN, Krupski WC. Iatrogenic vascular injuries from percutaneous vascular suturing devices. *J Vasc Surg* 2001; 33(5): 943-7.

Chapter 12

Management of acute leg ischaemia

Birgit Whitman Research Co-ordinator
Donna Parkin Consultant Nurse
Jonothan J Earnshaw Consultant Vascular Surgeon

DEPARTMENT OF VASCULAR SURGERY
GLOUCESTERSHIRE ROYAL HOSPITAL, GLOUCESTER, UK

Introduction

Acute leg ischaemia is a dangerous condition associated with significant loss of limb, and even life. In a recently published survey of 539 episodes of acute leg ischaemia produced by the Vascular Surgical Society of Great Britain and Ireland, the leg salvage rate was only 70% and 22% of the patients died during their hospital admission [1]. Accurate and speedy diagnosis is essential, but is complicated by the widely differing presentations. Assessment by a vascular specialist appears to be an advantage, as is a multi-disciplinary approach to the treatment, including input from a vascular surgeon, radiologist and nurse specialist.

There are two principal strategies for dealing with acute leg ischaemia: surgery or thrombolysis. Several randomised trials comparing these therapies exist, but in truth, they have added little to the debate. Consensus statements reviewing all the available evidence have been helpful [2] **(B)**. Acute leg ischaemia lends itself to protocol-driven care; this should be based at individual unit level and take into account the expertise and facilities available in the local hospital. A strategy must consider on-call arrangements for vascular surgery and radiology, together with the provision of critical care facilities [3].

Diagnosis

Acute native vessel arterial ischaemia is caused either by an arterial embolus from a proximal source, or *in situ* thrombosis of a native vessel. A significant workload also derives from occlusion of existing bypass grafts. It may be important to distinguish between the two principal causes of native vessel acute ischaemia as the outcome is different, and the best results are achieved if the treatment is prescribed according to aetiology. Unfortunately it is not always easy to determine whether acute ischaemia is embolic or thrombotic [4].

Embolism

Peripheral arterial embolism classically presents with a pale, painful, pulseless, paralysed, perishing cold, paraesthetic leg. There may be an obvious

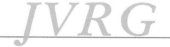

source for the embolus, such as atrial fibrillation or recent myocardial infarction; a history of peripheral vascular disease is unlikely. When clot or atherosclerotic plaque detaches from the heart or great vessels, it usually lodges at a major arterial bifurcation such as the common femoral artery or popliteal arteries. This sudden event occurs without the opportunity for collateral supply to develop and results in severe acute ischaemia. Conventionally, prompt surgical embolectomy is the best way to restore the circulation in this situation.

Acute, severe ischaemia of the leg caused by embolism is rare today; patients often present with a more complex picture. Most patients with atrial fibrillation have co-existing peripheral vascular disease. They may already have formed collateral blood supply, making the ischaemia less severe. Embolectomy is a less certain procedure in patients with existing arterial disease.

Thrombosis

The most common cause of acute leg ischaemia is thrombosis *in situ*. Patients often have pre-existing claudication that suddenly deteriorates as thrombosis supervenes on an atherosclerotic plaque. Patients with claudication may develop critical ischaemia. In some patients this might be combined with altered plasma coagulation. The resulting symptoms are often less severe as collateral blood vessels have had the opportunity to develop. Although the urgency for treatment is seldom as acute, the management is more complex; embolectomy often adds further intimal damage, so complex vascular reconstruction may be necessary.

A treatment protocol according to the severity of ischaemia

Although, treatment may be based on the cause, a more practical way of managing acute leg ischaemia is to take into account the severity of the ischaemia. Acute total ischaemia with the acute "white leg" indicates the threat of muscle necrosis within 12 hours. Less severe ischaemia needs less urgent

management. The Society for Vascular Surgery/International Society of Cardiovascular Surgery [5] has developed a grading system from I - III (A) that is useful for defining patients for clinical trials and publications.

A simpler version stratifies patients into two groups:

- **acute critical ischaemia** - no audible ankle Doppler signal with a neurosensory deficit or

- **acute subcritical ischaemia** - ischaemic pain at rest with audible ankle Doppler signals and no neurosensory deficit

Patients with acute critical ischaemia need urgent therapy on the day of admission, patients with subcritical ischaemia need prompt treatment, but there is often time for investigation and review [6]. A management based on the severity of ischaemia is outlined in Figure 1. This can be used both in major vascular units and in district hospitals where there is not always a vascular surgeon on call [7]. Whilst this protocol has not been tested in a formal trial, it has stood the test of ten years in Gloucester (B).

Options for treatment

Several major trials have attempted to compare surgery with thrombolysis for acute leg ischaemia. The STILE investigators randomised patients with native arterial or bypass graft occlusion to either surgery or intra-arterial thrombolysis with rt-PA or urokinase [8]. The trial was criticised because many patients had chronic ischaemia (occlusions up to 6 months old were included). The 30-day clinical outcomes were similar in both groups, although thrombolysis improved the outcome in patients with ischaemia of less than 14 days duration. This trial was also criticised because one third of the radiologists failed to insert a catheter for thrombolysis successfully.

Following a preliminary trial in New York that showed a favourable advantage for thrombolysis, the TOPAS investigators repeated their protocol in a

Figure 1 Protocol for the treatment of acute leg ischaemia.

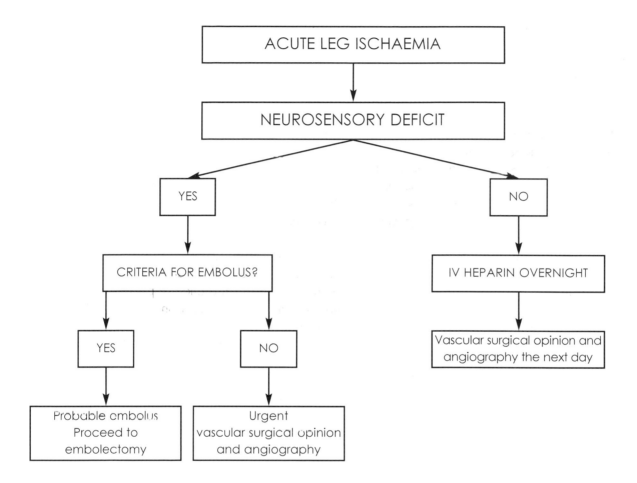

Criteria for an embolus

◆ Sudden onset of painful leg (<24 hours)

◆ Clinically obvious source of embolus, e.g. atrial fibrillation, myocardial infarction

◆ No evidence of peripheral vascular disease (normal pulses other leg)

multicentre, prospective, double blind comparison of thrombolysis and peripheral arterial surgery for severe acute (<14 days) leg ischaemia [9]. An optimal urokinase regimen was used for thrombolysis, and over 500 patients were randomised **(II)**. The study failed to show any difference between thrombolytic therapy and surgery; similar results with regards to 6 month amputation-free survival were demonstrated (72% after thrombolysis versus 75% after surgery).

Perhaps the best conclusion from all the existing research is that acute leg ischaemia should be managed by multi-disciplinary teams including vascular surgeons and radiologists with experience in the optimal techniques of both thrombolysis and vascular reconstruction.

Surgery for acute leg ischaemia

The relatively few patients with the classical presentation of an embolus should have an immediate balloon catheter embolectomy. This can be done under local anaesthetic (LA) in patients with severe cardiorespiratory problems, although intra-operative angiography will be painful. Regional anaesthesia is a possible option but cannot be used if heparin has recently been given, because of the risk of a dural haematoma. An anaesthetist should be present even if the operation is performed under LA, in case the operation needs extending. Intra-operative angiography is required to ensure complete revascularisation, and there should be no reluctance to proceed with intra-operative thrombolysis (see later) or formal vascular reconstruction if indicated [7]. Therefore, full vascular surgical backup must always be available. Post-operatively, these patients require full anticoagulation with a heparin infusion, followed by oral warfarin to prevent further thromboembolic episodes.

Patients with late emboli, or thrombotic or unknown aetiology occlusions should be investigated by angiography or duplex imaging. The severity of ischaemia will determine the urgency of the investigation. Patients with acute critical ischaemia should be treated urgently on admission. These will usually need urgent vascular reconstruction. Patients with stable subacute ischaemia should be anticoagulated and observed for 24 - 48 hours while planning the necessary intervention. It is these patients who are most suited to intervention by thrombolysis **(A)**.

Intra-arterial thrombolysis for acute leg ischaemia

Dissolving thrombi within arteries has been a goal of clinicians since agents became available in the 1950s. Embolectomy often fails because although it clears clot from large arteries, small distal vessels remain occluded. Since 1974, when Dotter first described the use of low dose intra-arterial streptokinase, this technique has become a standard alternative treatment for acute leg ischaemia. Initially, streptokinase 5,000 u/h was used as it was readily available and inexpensive [10]. This was replaced by urokinase and tissue plasminogen activator (t-PA), agents that are more effective, with fewer bleeding and allergic side-effects. In the last couple of years there have been problems with urokinase manufacture, so that t-PA is currently the agent of choice, despite the fact that it has no product licence for peripheral arterial thrombolysis **(C)**.

Which patients are suitable for thrombolysis?

Any patient with a recent arterial or graft occlusion is a potential candidate for thrombolytic therapy. Much recent research has focused on trying to identify patients likely to achieve a good outcome. The duration of ischaemia is important: occlusions over about one month old are less likely to dissolve. The leg must not be so severely ischaemic that muscle necrosis is imminent - lysis usually takes 18-24 hours, so patients with subcritical ischaemia are ideal. Accelerated techniques can be used to speed this up (see below). The randomised trials have suggested that graft occlusions fare better than native vessels [8,9] **(I)**. In contrast, the elderly, women and patients with multiple medical problems tend to have worse outcomes. All these are only relative contraindications to thrombolysis **(B)**. Absolute contraindications include patients at increased risk of bleeding, such as recent surgery, or those who have had a stroke within two months (for full list of absolute and relative contraindications, see reference 10).

Methods of intra-arterial thrombolysis

There are three main methods of intra-arterial thrombolysis, which differ in their indication and speed of action.

Low dose intra-arterial thrombolysis

This is the simplest technique for thrombolysis. A 4 French single lumen catheter is passed via the femoral artery and embedded directly into the artery or graft occlusion. Tissue plasminogen activator is infused at 0.5 - 1 mg/h via a syringe pump. Angiography is done every 6-12 hours to ensure clot lysis is proceeding and the catheter tip resited into remaining thrombus, as necessary. This method is suitable only for patients with subcritical ischaemia, as it often takes 18-24 hours to open the vessel or graft **(II)**.

Accelerated thrombolysis

Several techniques exist that reduce the duration of lysis, often to as little as 4-6 hours. Pulsed spray thrombolysis uses a unique catheter system with multiple side holes that is inserted across the occlusion [11] **(I)**. A dedicated pump infuses a low volume of t-PA into the clot under pressure every few seconds, thus increasing the area of contact with the thrombus. A cheaper alternative is high dose bolus treatment: three 5 mg boluses of t-PA are laced throughout the clot at 10 minute intervals [12] **(I)**. An angiogram after this 30 minutes can be used to predict if the treatment is likely to be effective (significant lysis should have occurred). A high dose infusion of 3.5 mg/h is then continued for four hours. By this time many patients will have completed lysis, if not the infusion rate is reduced to 1mg/h and the treatment continued as low dose therapy. In randomised trials, both pulsed spray and high dose bolus thrombolysis speed up the procedure, though neither has produced clinical results superior to the low dose technique in equivalent patients [11,12] **(II)**.

Intra-operative thrombolysis

There are several situations when this method is useful: after failed embolectomy, thrombosed popliteal aneurysm and trash foot. A catheter is inserted at the occlusion and the inflow clamped. Streptokinase (100,000u) or t-PA (15mg) is given over 30 minutes using an infusion pump. The surgeon can either relax and have a coffee break or perform the proximal anastomosis of a vein bypass. No randomised trials exist in acute leg ischaemia, but consecutive series suggest that about two thirds of infusions improve the distal circulation [13] **(II)**.

Optimal care of patients having thrombolysis

Intra-arterial thrombolysis is a high risk therapy. Complications are frequent, but with good planning, communication and care, they can be minimised. Vascular surgeons and their teams who regularly employ thrombolysis should design a protocol for its use and educate all participants (an example of the Gloucester protocol is available on the JVRG website). Whereas there is no documented evidence regarding the influence of medical and nursing management, the following practical advice can be given.

Consent

All patients with acute leg ischaemia should be made aware of the seriousness of their condition. If thrombolysis is to be used, an experienced team member should counsel the patient and take written consent, explaining the risks, including bleeding, and in particular the 2% risk of stroke **(A)**.

Location

There is no documented advantage in ITU or HDU care for patients receiving thrombolysis, as long as they are managed on wards with experienced nurses who are familiar with vascular patients and the risks of thrombolysis.

Monitoring

Vital signs and condition of the leg should be monitored regularly. The groin puncture site should be checked for bleeding. If there is a low grade ooze, this can be controlled with pressure from a one litre bag of intravenous fluid. Monitoring of coagulation tests has not been shown to be helpful.

Analgesia

Intramuscular analgesia risks bruising. Either oral or intravenous morphine using patient controlled analgesia pump is best if opiate pain relief is required.

Hydration

It is not necessary for a patient to be nil by mouth unless urgent surgery is a significant possibility. Patients may easily become dehydrated (increasing viscosity). Oral fluids should be encouraged and intravenous fluids may be necessary. Urinary catheterisation helps monitor the situation and avoids the need for movement to the commode.

Immobilisation

Patients have to lie flat for many hours. Pressure area care and pressure relieving mattresses improve comfort. Supplemental oxygen can improve the oxygen supply to the leg.

Anticoagulation

Once the catheter is removed, it is necessary to press on the puncture site for about 30 minutes. This may be done in the ward or in x-ray. Anticoagulation with heparin is then necessary for at least 48 hours to counteract the rebound hyperviscosity seen after thrombolytic therapy. Thereafter an individual decision is made whether warfarin, or aspirin and/or clopidogrel is used long term. During the interval after thrombolysis, continued vigilance is necessary (many bleeding complications actually occur at this stage). Regular blood testing should be done to ensure anticoagulation is therapeutic.

Results of intra-arterial thrombolysis

Many open series of patients with acute leg ischaemia treated with thrombolysis have been published. The largest is from the British Thrombolysis Study Group and concerns a consecutive series of over 1000 episodes from 13 centres collated from the NATALI (National Audit of Thrombolysis for Acute Leg Ischaemia) database [14]. The overall results for the collected database were that complete or partial lysis was observed in over two thirds of patients. The 30-day outcome was a limb salvage rate of 72.9 %, an amputation rate of 12.6%, and 12.9% of patients died. The main complications were due to bleeding; minor haemorrhage was common, but 8% had major bleeding that affected the outcome. Stroke is the most feared complication of thrombolysis. Twenty patients developed this complication, though only half of these events were due to intracranial haemorrhage, the rest were thrombotic (I).

Summary

- The large randomised trials suggest that surgery and thrombolysis are both effective treatments for acute leg ischaemia (I).

- Thrombolysis can dissolve thrombus and reveal the underlying cause of vessel occlusion, such as a critical stenosis. Secondary intervention with angioplasty or bypass is often required to achieve long-term patency (I).

- Both interventions carry a high risk of amputation and mortality, related to the severity of the ischaemia and associated co-morbidity. Thrombolysis has an increased risk of major haemorrhage compared to surgery (I).

- A modern vascular unit should have experience of both thrombolysis and advanced vascular reconstruction techniques. Decisions about treatment should be individualised and made in collaboration (A).

- Formal protocols are required for the management of patients with acute leg ischaemia, particularly those undergoing thrombolysis (A).

Further reading

1   Earnshaw JJ, Gregson RHS, Eds. *Practical Peripheral Arterial Thrombolysis*. Butterworth Heinemann Ltd, London, 1994.

References (grade I evidence and grade A recommendations in bold)

1   Campbell WB, Ridler BMF, Szymanska TH on behalf of the Vascular Surgical Society of Great Britain and Ireland. Current management of acute leg ischaemia: results of an audit by the Vascular Surgical Society of Great Britain and Ireland. *Br J Surg* 1998; 85: 1498-1503.

2   Working party on thrombolysis in the management of limb ischemia. Thrombolysis in the management of lower limb peripheral arterial occlusion - a consensus document. *J Am Coll Cardiol* 1998; 81: 207-18.

3   Thompson JF. Treatment of acute leg ischaemia. In: *The Evidence for Vascular Surgery*. Earnshaw JJ, Murie JA, Eds. Tfm publishing limited, Shropshire, 1999; 13: 79-83.

4   Earnshaw JJ. Demography and etiology of acute leg ischemia. *Semin Vasc Surg* 2001; 14: 86-92.

5   **Rutherford RB, Flanigan DP, Gupta SK *et al*. Suggested standards for reports dealing with lower extremity ischemia. *J Vasc Surg* 1986; 4: 80-94.**

6   Earnshaw JJ, Hopkinson BR, Makin GS. Acute critical ischaemia of the limb: a prospective evaluation. *Eur J Vasc Surg* 1990; 4: 365-8.

7   Earnshaw JJ, Gaines PA, Beard JD. Management of acute lower limb ischaemia. In: *Vascular and endovascular surgery*, Beard JD, Gaines PA, Eds, second edition. WB Saunders, London 2001; 7: 149-68.

8   **The STILE Investigators. Results of a prospective randomized trial evaluating surgery versus thrombolysis for ischaemia of the lower extremity. *Ann Surg* 1994; 220: 251-268.**

9   **Ouriel K, Veith FJ, Sasahara AA for the TOPAS investigators. A comparison of recombinant urokinase with vascular surgery as initial treatment for acute arterial occlusion of the legs. *N Engl J Med* 1998; 338: 1105-1111.**

10 Earnshaw JJ. Thrombolytic therapy in the management of acute limb ischaemia. *Br J Surg* 1991; 78: 261-9.

11 **Yusuf SW, Whitaker SC, Gregson RHS, Whenham PW, Hopkinson BR, Makin GS. Prospective randomised comparative study of pulse spray and conventional local thrombolysis. *Eur J Vasc Endovasc Surg* 1995; 10: 136-41.**

12 **Braithwaite BB, Buckenham TM, Galland RB, Heather BP, Earnshaw JJ on behalf of the Thrombolysis Study Group. Prospective randomized trial of high-dose bolus versus low-dose tissue plasminogen activator infusion in the management of acute limb ischaemia. *Br J Surg* 1997; 84: 646-650.**

13 Earnshaw JJ, Beard JD. Intraoperative use of thrombolytic agents. *BMJ* 1993; 307: 638-9.

14 **Braithwaite BD, Whitman B, Foy C on behalf of the Thrombolysis Study Group. Outcome analysis of over 1000 episodes of limb ischaemia treated by peripheral thrombolysis. *Br J Surg* 2001; 88: A618.**

Management of acute leg ischaemia

Chapter 13

Graft surveillance programmes

David K Beattie Specialist Registrar

Mary Ellis Chief Vascular Technologist

Alun H Davies Reader in Surgery and Consultant Surgeon

IMPERIAL COLLEGE SCHOOL OF MEDICINE, CHARING CROSS HOSPITAL, LONDON, UK

Introduction

Graft surveillance programmes based on duplex ultrasound are conceptually attractive. The increasing availability of duplex means that this is now the primary modality for graft surveillance following infrainguinal arterial reconstruction and it is now standard procedure in many vascular units for patients to be entered into a surveillance programme. This chapter reviews some of the available evidence as to the efficacy of graft surveillance and describes the surveillance "pathway".

The evidence for graft surveillance

Current recommendations

Many recommendations regarding graft surveillance have been made in the literature over the past few years. Amongst the most authoritative however were those from the TransAtlantic Inter-Society Consensus on the Management of Peripheral Arterial Disease [1]. The resultant document encompassed a comprehensive review of current evidence and management of all aspects of peripheral vascular disease and made 107 recommendations with respect to such. The recommendations with respect to surveillance following infrainguinal reconstruction with vein were as follows:

Patients undergoing vein bypass graft placement in the lower extremity for the treatment of claudication or limb-threatening ischaemia should be entered into a surveillance programme. This programme should consist of:

◆ Interval history (new symptoms).

◆ Vascular examination of the leg with palpation of inflow, graft and outflow pulses.

◆ Periodic measurement of resting and, if possible, post-exercise ankle:brachial indices.

◆ Duplex scanning of the entire length of the graft, with calculation of the peak systolic velocities and the velocity ratios across all identified lesions.

◆ Surveillance should be performed in the immediate post-operative period and at regular intervals for at least 2 years.

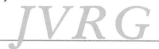

The recommendations in the case of reconstruction with a prosthetic conduit were similar with the exception that duplex scanning of the graft was not recommended. No grading was assigned to these recommendations; the grading that might be inferred is discussed later.

The sequelae of bypass graft failure are clearly potentially severe. Following graft occlusion approximately 80% of those operated upon for critical ischaemia are again at risk of limb loss, and some 90% operated on for claudication experience worse or similar symptoms to those they had pre-operatively [2]. **(II)** Technically, it is usually easier to revise a graft before it fails rather than afterwards. These facts suggest graft surveillance to be of paramount importance, but is there sufficient evidence to suggest that graft surveillance is indeed effective and to support the TASC recommendations?

What must graft surveillance accomplish?

The benefit derived from a graft surveillance programme must be significantly more than the simple identification of graft stenoses, the consequences of which are presumed but still uncertain.

It is beyond reasonable doubt that duplex ultrasound is able to detect haemodynamically significant stenoses, either within the body of a graft, or within the native inflow and outflow vessels. Duplex graft surveillance programmes are based upon a supposition that extrapolates from this however, namely that detected stenoses are responsible for subsequent graft failure and that their correction will hence improve graft patency; there is evidence for this [3,4] **(I)**. The presumption is also made however, that the revision of duplex-detected graft stenoses will improve outcome. If this were to prove not to be the case then the use of duplex surveillance becomes untenable.

Outcome can be measured in many ways, including the effect of surveillance upon limb salvage, upon quality of life and by economic analysis. Graft surveillance programmes can only really be deemed effective, and hence desirable, if positive correlations with respect to all these outcome parameters can be demonstrated. Certainly, a positive effect upon patency rates without an effect upon the other parameters could not support the use of duplex surveillance. Patency should perhaps be considered a soft end-point when assessing the outcome of infrainguinal bypass.

Level I evidence

Level 1 evidence is that derived from meta-analyses of randomised controlled trials (the strongest evidence), from individual randomised controlled trials and, for the purposes of this publication, that from systematic reviews, decision analyses, cost-effectiveness analyses or large observational datasets. This is at slight variance with the accepted US Agency for Health Care Policy and Research Classification [5] in that this requires a randomised controlled trial in order to make a grade A recommendation.

There are only two randomised controlled trials with respect to duplex-based vein graft surveillance. The first was that by Lundell et al in 1995 [3] **(I)**. One hundred and fifty-six grafts, both vein and prosthetic, were randomised to duplex or non-duplex surveillance. Primary-assisted graft patency rates were shown to be better in the duplex group, but the effects upon limb salvage rates were not reported. The authors made several criticisms of their own study, including the small size, the lack of a pre-recruitment biostatistical sample size calculation, and the long delays between duplex scanning and eventual decision-making. Nevertheless, the trial did demonstrate in a randomised manner for the first time, that graft surveillance has a positive effect upon patency rates.

A second randomised trial was that reported by Ihlberg et al in 1998 [6] **(I)**. One hundred and eighty-five grafts were recruited and randomised to clinical examination and ABPI measurement with or without duplex scanning. Primary-assisted and secondary patency rates and limb salvage were actually better in the group randomised not to receive duplex graft surveillance, though not significantly so. The study thus failed to show any benefit at all to routine duplex-based graft surveillance, but did note that such a programme was hard to accomplish within the confines of normal clinical practice. Furthermore, what outcome differences there were appeared during the first post-operative month, prior to surveillance.

The combined evidence from these two randomised trials with respect to the effect of surveillance upon primary patency is shown in Figure 1. Although individually each of these trials provides level I evidence of the effect of surveillance upon patency they are contradictory and hence a meta-analysis of the available randomised controlled trials yields level III evidence only **(III)**.

Given the conflicting level I evidence as to whether duplex surveillance improves vein graft patency, and no evidence to support the concept that it improves limb salvage rates it is not possible to make a grade A recommendation as to the implementation of duplex-based graft surveillance programmes.

Further evidence is derived from a published summation analysis [4] **(I)**. Whilst not strictly providing level I evidence, this analysis was the result of a detailed systematic review of the available literature. A total of 17 published vein graft series were analysed, these encompassing a total of 6649 vein grafts. The results from series where duplex graft surveillance had been employed were compared with the results from series where it had not. Data extraction was hampered by the variety of techniques used to confirm patency, and only six series reported amputation rates. The analysis demonstrated that duplex graft surveillance was associated with an increase in vein graft patency rates following infrainguinal reconstruction, but that no improvement in limb salvage was evident. Again, no recommendation can be made.

Figure 1 Meta-analysis of the two randomised controlled trials showing combined effect of vein graft surveillance on primary-assisted patency rates.

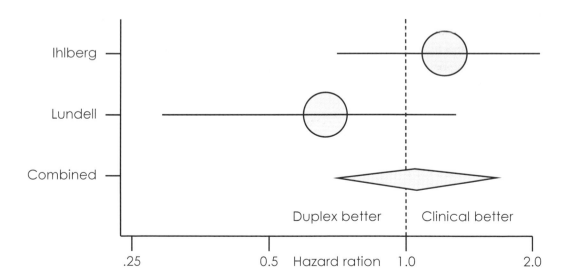

Level II evidence ... or worse

There is considerable further evidence available in the literature, though it is often conflicting. Mills analysed much of this [7] and found a "*substantial body of evidence*" that graft surveillance is clinically useful, cost-effective, and results in improvements in long-term patency and limb salvage rates of 10 to 15%. Only one of the two randomised trials was included in this review, so his conclusion, at least in part, must be drawn from at best, level II evidence.

Duplex may not, however, be sufficiently sensitive in identifying stenoses that lead to graft failure. If so, this means that an unacceptably large number of procedures are performed as a result of abnormal duplex findings, with resultant morbidity and mortality. In one early study only 12% of patients progressed to occlusion whereas it is recognised that up to 30% of grafts may develop a stenosis [8] **(II)**. Furthermore, duplex did not improve stenosis identification as the only stenoses where outcome was altered were those where synchronous symptomatology or the ankle:brachial pressure index had also changed. In another early study however, only 29% of grafts found to be failing on duplex were associated with a fall in the pressure index of greater than 0.15 [9] **(II)**.

In a further study of 275 grafts [10], 24 of 85 grafts that developed a stenosis were treated. A further 28 of 64 that developed an inflow or outflow stenosis were left alone. At a year there were no differences in patency rates for treated and untreated grafts **(II)**. A contemporary study suggests however that stratification of stenoses will detect those grafts most likely to fail [11]. Grafts deemed to be at intermediate risk of failure by virtue of a peak systolic velocity of between 200 and 300 cm/s or a velocity ratio between two and four were no more likely to occlude than those shown to have no stenosis. Most grafts deemed at high risk of failure were electively revised, but seven of nine such grafts that did not undergo repair occluded within 4 months of detection **(II)**. Might the pragmatic approach therefore be to target duplex surveillance only at high-risk grafts?

The generally accepted duplex criteria for the detection of a haemodynamically significant lesion are as follows, these corresponding to a 50% stenosis:

- Peak systolic velocity < 45cm/s.

- Peak systolic velocity > 150cm/s.

- Peak systolic velocity ratio across a stenosis > 2.0.

- ABPI fall > 0.15.

It has been suggested however, that as long as a graft is surveyed every 3 months, intervention can be avoided as long as the peak systolic velocity ratio remains below 3.0 [12]. Further evidence supports this targeted use of duplex surveillance [13]. Dougherty *et al* followed 46 grafts with a duplex defined stenosis and a peak systolic velocity in excess of 3.0. Just 14 of these were revised and only three occluded, all of which showed a velocity ratio prior to occlusion in excess of 7.0. The same group however subsequently compared the outcome for failing grafts as shown by duplex and where revision was undertaken with those where, despite duplex evidence of stenosis, it was not [14]. The outcome was the same for the two groups with respect to both patency rates and to limb salvage.

Should duplex graft surveillance programmes be life-long?

The optimum period for which duplex surveillance of vein grafts should be undertaken has been the subject of one controlled trial, that by Lundell *et al* [3]. Differences in graft patency between the groups randomised to duplex surveillance or clinical and pressure index surveillance were only apparent by the second post-operative year. This suggests that a grade A recommendation can be made such that duplex-based graft surveillance programmes should be continued for more than 1 year, but it must be remembered that the only other level one evidence [6] demonstrated that duplex surveillance does not alter patency rates at all.

Level II evidence is again conflicting, making recommendation at a grade lower than grade A difficult. In one study [15] over a fifth of all vein graft stenoses occurred more than a year after arterial reconstruction. Mills *et al* however [16] suggested that a

Chapter 13

normal early post-operative scan defines a cohort who will not benefit from further intensive duplex surveillance. This was based on a series of 91 grafts that were normal at 3 months, only two of which progressed to stenosis. Additionally, all grafts showing high-grade stenosis had a duplex-detectable abnormality by 6 weeks. Idu *et al* [17] studied 300 grafts and concluded that the duration of surveillance may be restricted to the first 6 months after operation in those who have a normal bypass during that time.

Late graft failure may result from the development of de novo inflow and outflow stenoses and Ihnat *et al* found 7% of grafts to need inflow or outflow reconstruction during long-term follow-up [18]. A retrospective analysis of 159 grafts originating below the femoral artery concluded however that stenoses proximal to the graft do not affect bypass patency and hence do not require repair to prevent graft occlusion [19]. Surveillance of these lesions may thus be unnecessary.

Duplex graft surveillance - economic and quality of life considerations

There has been no significant data published with respect to the effects of duplex surveillance on quality of life and these are eagerly awaited. To make a duplex-based surveillance programme cost-effective it has been suggested that limb salvage rates must be improved by at least 5% [20]. A retrospective appraisal of the costs of lower extremity bypass graft maintenance has been made [21]. Of 155 grafts, a total of 61 needed 86 revisions. Thirty-six percent of all grafts needed revision within one year. The cost of the initial bypass together with the costs of a 5-year graft maintenance programme were similar to those for amputation. Grafts revised for duplex-detected stenoses compared to those revised after failure had better 1-year patency, needed fewer amputations and were cheaper. Overall, the costs of limb salvage were felt to be justifiable compared to amputation. **(II)**

The pathway of care

It is likely that future data will lend stronger support to vein graft surveillance than that currently available

and that the current trend towards enrolling patients in such a programme will accelerate. It seems justifiable therefore to recommend a pathway for the use of vein graft surveillance and to incorporate the TASC guidelines as noted earlier. These guidelines may be amended as more data becomes available and, in particular, as the optimal frequency and duration of surveillance becomes clear. In addition, the criteria for re-intervention are likely to be more accurately defined. In the absence of scientifically validated data to enable construction of the pathway, such a pathway must inevitably be pragmatic. A suggested pathway is shown in Figure 2.

It is important that, prior to discharge, a post-operative quality control check is performed to confirm successful revascularisation and to provide a baseline against which to perform graft surveillance. Prior to discharge the patient should be formally enrolled into the surveillance programme and the importance of this discussed. It is tempting to equate graft surveillance with the performance of duplex ultrasound at regular intervals. It must however be remembered that best practice is to enrol both vein grafts and prosthetic grafts into a surveillance programme and that, for vein grafts, a duplex scan is just one component of the surveillance; an interval history, ABPI measurements and examination being the others. For prosthetic grafts, duplex is not indicated at all, the other components being the mainstay of surveillance. The frequency and duration of surveillance has been discussed above.

Undoubtedly the ideal in graft surveillance is the dedicated one-stop vein graft surveillance clinic where all appropriate imaging can take place prior to an interval history and examination with a surgeon. The vascular laboratory servicing such a clinic should be fully validated. In practice however, few departments have sufficient facilities or patients to enable such clinics to be initiated. Furthermore, the availability of duplex ultrasound is outwith the control of the vascular department and instead rests with a medical physics department or is under the control of the radiology department. It is often the case that these departments have insufficient capacity to provide a comprehensive graft surveillance programme for all patients. Compromises must therefore be reached that take due account of the available local resources.

Figure 2 A suggested duplex-based vein graft surveillance protocol.

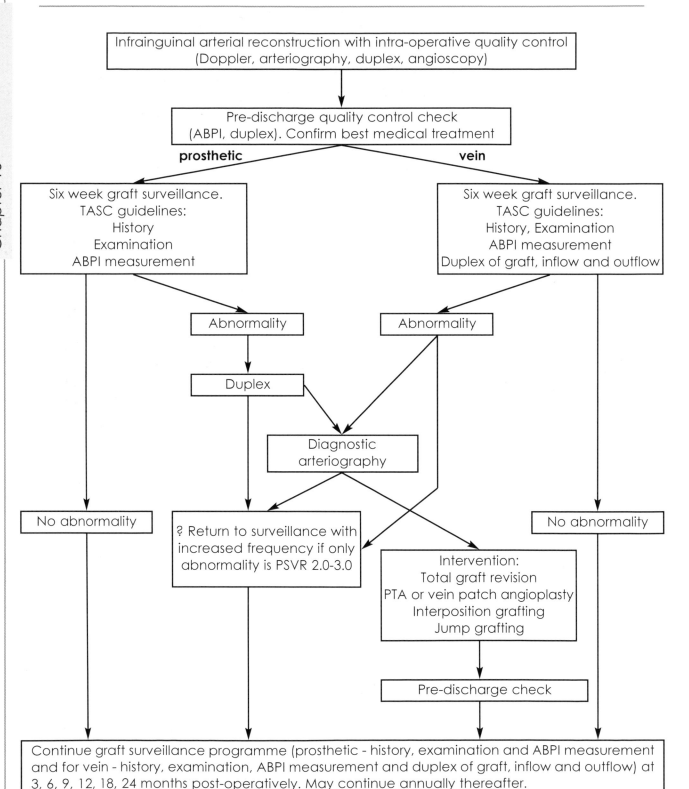

Figure 3 Arteriogram showing a vein graft stenosis developing over a 3-month period during a trial comparing arteriography and duplex for surveillance.

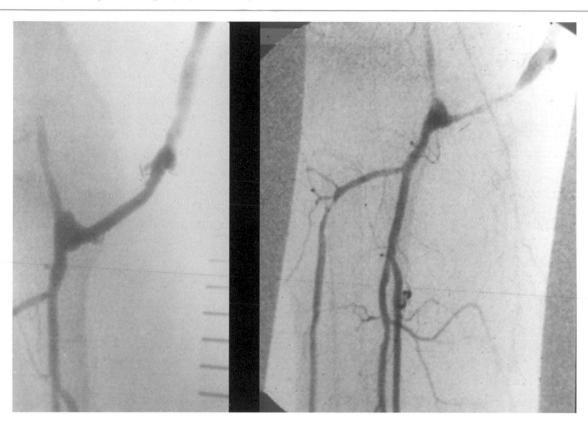

There are potential pitfalls to be avoided. It is the practice in some institutions to delegate the task of graft follow-up entirely to an imaging department such as the medical physics department. This practice is adequate only where facilities exist in that department for history taking and examination. The patient's old records must be available to detect any interval change. It is not acceptable for graft surveillance to take the form of duplex imaging or ABPI measurement alone, with recourse to the physician only when an abnormality is detected. In teaching institutions graft surveillance may be undertaken by a research fellow or similar as part of that individual's research. It is important that, when the researcher leaves and the work is finished, arrangements are made to continue the surveillance.

In most institutions the best compromise will often be to arrange a duplex scan at the time indicated by the surveillance programme, then review the patient in a standard vascular clinic. A protocol for such a review should be in place so that all necessary information is collected at each assesment. These tasks might ideally be performed by a nurse specialist.

The criteria by which a graft may be deemed to be at risk are discussed above. What course of action should be followed where such criteria are satisfied however and the graft is considered to be at risk of failure?

Management of the failing graft

If the sole abnormality detected at graft surveillance is a peak systolic velocity ratio of between 2.0 and 3.0 the graft may be safely kept under close scrutiny [12,13,14]. Most authorities would argue that a ratio in excess of 3.0 is an indication for graft revision.

This raises a number of questions: for example, should graft revision be surgical or endovascular? Is angiography always required prior to re-intervention? Should angiography and percutaneous angioplasty be performed at the same time?

Many vein graft stenoses are best treated by surgery, but duplex data can select those that may be treated by percutaneous transluminal angioplasty (PTA) (Figure 3) [22]. It is suggested that stenoses of less than 2 cm in veins of greater than 3.5 mm diameter may be treated by PTA in cases where the lesion has appeared more than 3 months after surgery. Where such criteria have been applied late intervention rates of just 10% have been recorded [23]. There is however a high incidence of restenosis after PTA of stenoses in the distal third of vein grafts [24]. Several studies have shown equivalent patency rates for surgical revision and PTA for vein graft stenosis [25], but generally these studies have not been randomised, the stenoses suitable for PTA being selected out. In practice therefore, short lesions such as isolated stenoses or webs tend to be treated with PTA or, increasingly, vein patch angioplasty, with more extensive revision or graft replacement being reserved for long stenoses and those grafts exhibiting multiple lesions. Stenoses at or near distal anastomoses are usually treated by jump grafting.

If a stenosis requires surgical intervention on the basis of duplex-derived data, is pre-operative angiography mandatory? Some authorities suggest pre-operative arteriography to be mandatory prior to graft revision in all cases as studies have shown all frequently performed bypass graft configurations to have some discrepancy between duplex and arteriographic findings [26]. Others feel that surgery may be performed based on duplex data alone [27,28]. It is the authors' practice to obtain pre-operative arteriography in the majority of cases prior to graft revision, the exceptions being those cases where, for example, operative intervention has been decided upon in a graft with an isolated well-defined lesion in an otherwise normal vessel. Most surgeons will determine their own policy according to the quality of the duplex service available locally.

Angiography is, of course, mandatory in those patients whose stenosis is to be treated by PTA on the basis of duplex-derived data. Such data should be of sufficient quality to allow an ipsilateral antegrade approach to the lesion with simultaneous angioplasty at the same sitting, without recourse to a preceding diagnostic arteriogram. In the opinion of the author it is untenable to subject a patient to two invasive procedures where such duplex data exists. All patients undergoing angiography for graft stenosis should be prepared and consented for angioplasty, and the risks of such should be fully explained. It is our practice for consent to be taken from each patient by the surgical team on the ward, and again in the radiology department by the radiologist performing the procedure.

Following any graft intervention, be it angioplasty of a short segment or revision of the entire graft, the patient must again be entered into a graft surveillance programme after a suitable post-operative check to confirm successful revascularisation.

There remains much controversy over these issues in the literature and each case should be treated on its own merits. It is best practice therefore for all duplex-detected vein graft stenoses to be reviewed jointly by both the surgeon and the interventional radiologist together. Most departments have radiology meetings at regular intervals to facilitate this, and this type of multi-disciplinary practice undoubtedly points the way to the future.

Summary

- Grade A recommendations require level I evidence and there is very little available with respect to vein graft surveillance.

- The level I evidence that is available is contradictory with respect to the important end-point of patency and the only trial looking at limb salvage found no benefit.

- Grade A recommendations cannot be made with respect to the utility of vein graft surveillance after infrainguinal arterial reconstruction.

- The remainder of the evidence is level II because it is evidence of "best practice," or is level III because it is contradictory.

- As noted earlier, the TASC document [2] recommends that all vein grafts should be entered into graft surveillance programmes according to the protocol outlined earlier. The level of evidence available however, suggests that the grade of this recommendation can only be grade B.

- The TASC recommendations identify three critical issues requiring further investigation:

   "There is a need for documenting the cost-effectiveness of using duplex imaging for vein graft surveillance at all periods."

   "There is a need to establish the optimal frequency and duration of surveillance testing in vein grafts."

   "There is a need for further information to identify what degree of stenosis, as detected by surveillance studies, must be corrected."

- The results of the vein graft surveillance trial [29], a large multicentred trial assessing the benefits of graft surveillance with respect to the end points of patency, limb salvage, quality of life and cost-benefit analysis, are awaited.

Further reading

1   Chant AB, Barros D'Sa AAB, Eds. Graft Maintenance and Graft Failure. In: *Emergency Vascular Practice*. Arnold, London, re-issued 1996.

References (grade I evidence and grade A recommendations in bold)

1   TASC Working Group. Management of peripheral arterial disease. TransAtlantic Inter-Society Consensus. *Eur J Vasc Endovasc Surg* 2000; 19 (suppl A): S217-218.

2   Brewster DC, Lasalle AJ, Robinson JG, Strayhorn EC, Darling RC. Femoropoliteal graft failures: Clinical consequences of success of secondary reconstructions. *Arch Surg* 1983; 118: 1043-7.

3   **Lundell A, Lindblad B, Bergqvist D, Hansen F. Femoropopliteal-crural graft patency is improved by an intensive graft surveillance programme: A prospective randomised study. *J Vasc Surg* 1995; 21: 26-34.**

4   **Golledge J, Beattie DK, Greenhalgh RM, Davies AH. Have the results of infrainguinal bypass improved with the widespread utilisation of postoperative surveillance? *Eur J Vasc Endovasc Surg* 1996; 11: 388-92.**

5   US Department of Health and Human Services. Agency for health care policy and research. The Agency; 1993. Clinical practice guidelines. AHCPR publication No 92-0023 p107.

6   **Ihlberg L, Luther M, Tierala E, Lapantalo M. The utility of duplex scanning in infrainguinal vein graft surveillance: results from a randomised controlled study. *Eur J Vasc Endovasc Surg* 1998; 16: 19-27.**

7   Mills JL. Infrainguinal vein graft surveillance: How and when. *Semin Vasc Surg* 2001; 14: 169-76.

8   Grigg MJ, Nicolaides AN, Wolfe JH. Femorodistal vein bypass graft stenoses. *Br J Surg* 1988; 75: 737-40.

9   Mills JL, Harris EJ, Taylor LM, Beckett WC, Porter JM. The importance of routine surveillance of distal bypass grafts with duplex scanning: a study of 379 reversed vein grafts. *J Vasc Surg* 1990; 12: 379-86.

10   Wilson YG, Davies AH, Currie IC, Morgan M, McGrath C, Baird RN, Lamont PM. Vein graft stenosis; incidence and intervention. *Eur J Vasc Endovasc Surg* 1996; 11: 164-9.

11   Mills JL, Wixon CL, James DC, Devine J, Westerband A, Hughes JD. The natural history of intermediate and critical vein graft stenosis: recommendations for continued surveillance or repair. *J Vasc Surg* 2001; 33: 273-8.

12   Olojugba DH, McCarthy MJ, Naylor AR, Bell PR, London NJ. At what peak velocity ratio should duplex-detected vein graft stenoses be revised? *Eur J Vasc Endovasc Surg* 1998; 15: 258-60.

13   Dougherly MJ, Calligaro KD, DeLaurentis DA. The natural history of "failing" arterial bypass grafts in a duplex surveillance protocol. *Ann Vasc Surg* 1998; 12: 255-9.

14   Dougherty MJ, Calligaro KD, DeLaurentis DA. Revision of failing lower extremity bypass grafts. *Am J Surg* 1998; 176: 126-30.

15   Dunlop P, Hartshorne T, Bolia A, Bell PR, London NJ. The long-term outcome of infrainguinal vein graft surveillance. *Eur J Vasc Endovasc Surg* 1995; 10: 352-5.

16   Mills JL, Bandyk DF, Gahtan V, Esses G. The origin of infrainguinal vein graft stenosis: a prospective randomised trial based on duplex surveillance. *J Vasc Surg* 1995; 21: 16-25.

17   Idu MM, Buth J, Cuypers P, Hop WC, van de Pavoordt ED, Tordoir JM. Economising vein-graft surveillance programmes. *Eur J Vasc Endovasc Surg* 1998; 15:432-8.

18   Ihnat DM, Mills JL, Dawson DL, Hughes JD Hagino RT, De Maioribus CA, Gentile AT, Westerband A. The correlation of early flow disturbances with the development of infrainguinal graft stenosis; a 10-year study of 341 autogenous vein grafts. *J Vasc Surg* 1999; 30: 8-15.

Chapter 13

19   Treiman GS, Ashrafi A, Lawrence PF. Incidentally detected stenoses proximal to grafts originating below the common femoral artery: do they affect graft patency or warrant repair in asymptomatic patients? *J Vasc Surg* 2000; 32: 1180-9.

20   Cheshire NJW, Wolfe JHN. Infrainguinal graft surveillance: a biased overview. *Sem Vasc Surg* 1993; 6: 143-9.

21   Wixon CL, Mills JL, Westerband A, Hughes JD, Ihnat DM. An economic appraisal of lower extremity bypass graft maintenance. *J Vasc Surg* 2000; 32: 1-12.

22   AvinoAJ, Bandyk DF, Gonsalves AJ, Johnson BL, Black TJ, Zwiebel BR, Rahaim MJ, Cantor A. Surgical and endovascular intervention for infrainguinal vein graft stenosis. *J Vasc Surg* 1999; 29: 60-70

23   Gonsalves C, Bandyk DK, Avino AJ, Johnson BL. Duplex features of vein graft stenosis and the success of percutaneous transluminal angioplasty. *J Endovasc Surg* 1999; 6: 66-72.

24   Dunlop P, Varty K, Hartshorne T, Bell PR, Bolia A, London, NJ. Percutaneous transluminal angioplasty of infrainguinal vein graft stenosis: long term outcome. *Br J Surg* 1995; 82: 204-6.

25   Tonnesen KH, Holstein P, Rordam L, Bulow J, Helgstrand U, Dreyer M. Early results of percutaneous transluminal angioplasty of failing below-knee bypass grafts. *Eur J Vasc Endovasc Surg* 1998; 15: 51-56.

26   Landry GJ, Moneta GL, Taylor LM, McLafferty RB, Edwards JM, Yaeger RA, Porter JM. Duplex scanning alone is not sufficient imaging before secondary procedures after lower extremity reversed vein bypass graft. *J Vasc Surg* 1999; 29: 270-80.

27   Lewis DR, McGrath C, Irvine CD, Jones A, Murphy P, Smith FC, Baird RN, Lamont PM. The progression and correction of duplex detected velocity shifts in angiographically normal vein grafts. *Eur J Vasc Endovasc Surg* 1998; 15: 394-7.

28   Idu MM, Buth J, Hop WC, Cuypers P, van de Pavoordt ED, Tordoir JM. Vein graft surveillance: is graft revision without angiography justified and what criteria should be used? *J Vasc Surg* 1998; 27: 399-411.

29   Kirby PL, Brady AR, Thompson SG, Torgerson D, Davies AH. The vein graft surveillance trial: rationale, design and methods. VGST participants. *Eur J Vasc Endovasc Surg* 1999; 18: 469-74.

Chapter 14

Aortic aneurysm screening and surveillance

Elaine Shaw Aneurysm Screening Co-ordinator

Brian Heather Consultant Vascular Surgeon

DEPARTMENT OF VASCULAR SURGERY,
GLOUCESTERSHIRE ROYAL HOSPITAL, GLOUCESTER, UK

Introduction

Aortic aneurysms become increasingly common in men over the age of 65 [1]. Rupture of an abdominal aortic aneurysm (AAA) accounts for approximately 6,000 deaths per year in England and Wales and represents 1.4% of all deaths in this age group [2]. The mortality rate following elective surgical repair of an AAA is approximately 5% [3,4] compared to the overall mortality if an AAA ruptures from 80 - 94% [5,6] **(I)**.

Aortic aneurysms often remain asymptomatic and undetected until they rupture. There is considerable potential to reduce the high mortality rate associated with this condition, by introducing a screening programme to detect aortic aneurysms in a population at risk and to offer elective surgical repair.

Gloucestershire's aneurysm screening programme

In 1990 a screening programme was introduced in Gloucestershire. All 65 year old men were invited to their GP's surgery for an ultrasound scan to screen for an abdominal aortic aneurysm. By targeting this age group it was expected that the majority of aneurysms would be detected prior to rupture. An additional advantage of screening at this age is that most of this group will be retired and able to attend. Gloucestershire has a population of approximately 560,000 and each year nearly 2,700 men are invited for screening.

Capital/running costs

It costs £36,000 per year to run the programme, approximately £12 for each scan performed. The capital outlay to set up the programme totalled £15,000 to purchase a portable ultrasound machine, a lap top computer and a printer.

The annual running costs include salaries for the programme co-ordinator, sessional payments for the radiographers, travelling costs and additional expenditure for stationary and disposables. To offer screening to all of the 65 year old men in the county, it is necessary to run 3 - 4 screening sessions at a GP's surgery each week.

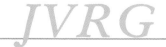

Design of the programme

To achieve high attendance rates, screening is offered at the patient's GP's surgery. Attendance at hospital-based screening programmes has been reported as low as 40% compared to 85% when arranged at a local GP practice [7]. Attending for screening in the more familiar surroundings of the GP's surgery is much more acceptable for the patient as it is less threatening than the ultrasound department of a hospital **(B)**. Some practices use it as an opportunity to perform routine health checks on their patients and to update their records. Of the 87 GP practices in the county, only one declined to take part. Each GP practice is visited once a year in rotation.

The launch of the screening programme co-incided with the new GP contract which had already increased practice workload. It was essential that the screening programme did not also generate too much additional extra work. The Practice Manager produces a list of men eligible for screening by virtue of their date of birth; this is a relatively simple task for the practices as all surgeries in Gloucestershire are computerised. The practices are provided with personalized pre-printed invitation letters, containing the doctor's names and practice address as a heading, the date and time of each patient's appointment and an information sheet which explains the reason for screening. This has meant that the only additional work for the practice is to send out the paperwork to their patients before the screening date (Figure 1).

The practice ensures that a consulting room with a couch and power point is available. The screening sessions are run by the programme co-ordinator (a nurse) and a Senior Radiographer who carries out the ultrasound scan using a portable ultrasound machine.

The benefit of having a nurse at the screening sessions is to ensure that the patient is fully informed about what the screening test is for, the implication of an abnormal result and to answer any questions. An experienced nurse has the ability to put the patient at ease and to help alleviate any anxieties they may have. Whilst the nurse is explaining the procedure, the sonographer can concentrate fully on carrying out the ultrasound examination. This increases the throughput of patients and makes full use of the radiographer's time.

Those patients who do not attend for screening are sent one reminder letter asking them to complete a simple questionnaire which informs the co-ordinator if another appointment is requested. This additional letter has increased attendance by a further 6% since its introduction [8]. When the programme started in 1990, 78% of patients attended for their examination and in 2000 the attendance rate had increased to 87% [9].

Method of diagnosis

Ultrasound imaging is an established tool for accurately assessing the presence and size of aortic aneurysms **(I)**. In the hands of an experienced operator, it is a quick, inexpensive, simple and reliable method of identifying this condition.

The advantage of using suitably trained sonographers is that they are used to working independently. The examination takes about 2 - 3 minutes for each scan and approximately 10 men can be examined per hour.

The examination/potential problems

The abdominal aorta is imaged from the level of the diaphragm to the bifurcation in both longitudinal and transverse planes. It is very important that the correct vessel, i.e. not Inferior Vena Cava (IVC) is identified. In longitudinal section, the coeliac axis and origin of the Superior Mesenteric Artery (SMA) arising anteriorly are markers, not only that the vessel is the aorta but also that it has been visualised to the level of the renal arteries.

Overall visual assessment of the aortic size especially at the level of the bifurcation and in patients with tortuous vessels, is often easier in the transverse plane.

Figure 1 Aortic aneurysm screening:- The Gloucestershire model.

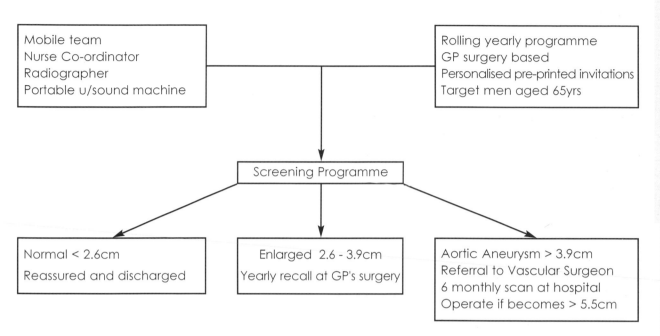

Measurement of aortic diameter is taken ideally, antero-posteriorly on a longitudinal section measuring between the internal surfaces of the true wall.

In large patients, or where overlying bowel gas obscures visualisation of the aorta, it may be necessary to turn the patient into the right decubitus position to image the vessel. It is important that the echoes from the spine are not mistaken for the posterior aortic wall. Fluid filled loops of bowel can mimic a vessel in patients with overlying bowel gas. This mistake should become apparent on the transverse image.

Although in many patients, this is a straightforward examination to perform, it is important to appreciate the need for thorough assessment as well as being aware of potential pitfalls.

The Result

The men are given the result after their examination. An immediate result relieves patient anxiety. A study to assess psychological morbidity associated with AAA screening showed that although the invitation to attend caused some mild anxiety, it was not prolonged, even when an asymptomatic aneurysm was diagnosed [10].

Patients who are found to have aortic aneurysms are referred to one of the four Vascular Surgeons in the county for more frequent ultrasound follow-up, or for consideration of elective repair.

The co-ordinator has agreement from the GPs so that she can make a direct referral to the appropriate surgeon. This again reduces the workload for the GP. The co-ordinator can also take into account individual surgeon's workload and waiting time for surgery. As the co-ordinator is aware which Consultant and

Figure 2 Distribution of aortic diameters.

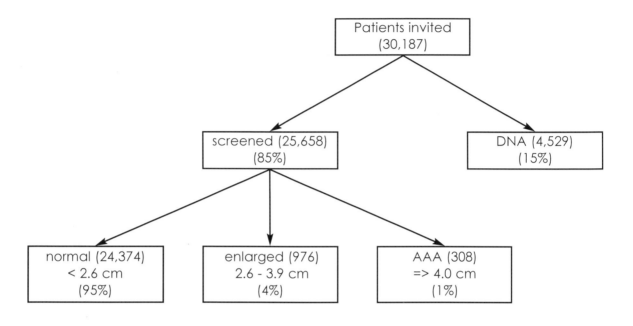

hospital the patient has been referred to, auditing of follow-up and patient outcomes becomes much easier to document.

All patients with an abnormal result are given additional advice on life-style such as giving up smoking, losing weight, having a blood test to check cholesterol levels and having blood pressure checked. An information leaflet to reinforce this information is given to them by the co-ordinator at their appointment. They are also given a telephone number to ring if further advice is needed.

Distribution of aortic diameters

Approximately 95% of men aged 65 have a normal result (aortic diameter below 2.6 cm) and are not recalled. A local follow-up study demonstrated that these men are at a very low risk of development of a significant aneurysm in the future on the basis of a single scan. This is important for the cost-effectiveness of running an aneurysm screening programme, as it eliminates the need for large scale repeat examinations [11].

Approximately 4% of men have an enlarged aorta (aortic diameter 2.6-3.9 cm) and are followed up yearly at their GP's surgery.

A further 1% are found to have an aortic aneurysm (aortic diameter >3.9 cm) and are referred to one of the Vascular Consultants.

Patients with aortic aneurysms of 4.0-5.5 cm are usually followed up with a 6-monthly ultrasound scan or more frequently depending on aneurysm size and rate of growth. Those with aneurysms >5.5 cm, if they are fit, are considered for elective surgical repair as recommended by the UK Small Aneurysm Study [12] **(I)**.

Workload/Results

Over the last 11 years 30,187 men have been invited for screening and 25,658 have attended (85%).

Some 976 enlarged aortas (2.6 - 3.9 cm) have been detected (4%). During follow-up, 277 (28%) have grown to over 3.9 cm and referred to vascular surgery. An additional six patients with enlarged aortas were referred to one of the Vascular Consultants to be considered for surgery as they were found to have an iliac aneurysm measuring over 4 cm.

Some 308 men were found to have an AAA of 4 cm (1.2%) or greater on their initial examination (Figure 2).

By the end of the year 2000, 267 (45%) of the 591 aneurysms detected on the screening programme had undergone elective repair, 257 routinely and ten urgently because of the development of symptoms of pain or tenderness. There were an additional nine screened men who had emergency repair of a ruptured AAA. Of those, two had failed to attend for follow-up, one had previously refused surgery, five had aneurysms less than 5.5 cm and one man ruptured his aneurysm before surgery could be undertaken.

Selective screening

A more cost-effective way to run a screening programme may be to reduce the number of scans necessary by selecting a higher risk group. A recent (unpublished) study examined whether it was possible to reduce the number of men using markers for AAA such as smoking and hypertension.

A total of 1448 consecutive 65 year old men attending for aneurysm screening completed a questionnaire on their smoking habits and history of hypertension. GPs were asked for the information available on each patient's smoking and blood pressure history. Unsurprisingly, the prevalence of AAA was significantly higher both in smokers and patients with hypertension. However, significant numbers of enlarged aortas and aneurysms were detected in the 20% of patients with neither of these risk factors. As a result of this, it was not possible to define a high risk population for screening that produced a worthwhile reduction in screening numbers without an unacceptable fall in detection sensitivity. For example, excluding normotensive patients who had stopped smoking for over 10 years reduced screening numbers by 27% but resulted in failure to detect 19% of aneurysms.

Reducing total community mortality from aortic aneurysms

To evaluate the effectiveness of screening for aortic aneurysms all deaths in the community related to aortic aneurysms were examined. Data were obtained from inpatient records and post mortem results from the counties' two hospitals, together with computerised death certificate records, held by the Health Authority since 1994. This included deaths at home from ruptured AAA, in-hospital deaths from ruptured AAA with or without emergency surgery and all deaths following elective surgery.

There has been an overall two-thirds reduction in deaths in the target population from 1994 - 1998. Screening for asymptomatic abdominal aortic aneurysm results in a significant reduction in numbers of deaths from all aneurysm-related causes in the screened portion of the male population [13] (Figure 3).

Randomised controlled trial

Current Department of Health policy is not to support widespread aneurysm screening until its effectiveness has been fully evaluated. It is therefore essential to prove its efficacy in order to secure funding of further screening programmes. In 1995, Scott *et al* published data from the Chichester area which examined 3,205 men who were offered aneurysm screening compared to a control group without screening. This study showed a small but significant reduction in the incidence of aneurysm rupture together with an overall reduction in the number of aneurysm-related deaths in the screened group [14] (II).

The much larger Multi-centre Aneurysm Screening Study (MASS), currently being performed in the

Chapter 14

Figure 3 Total aneurysm related mortality in Gloucestershire.

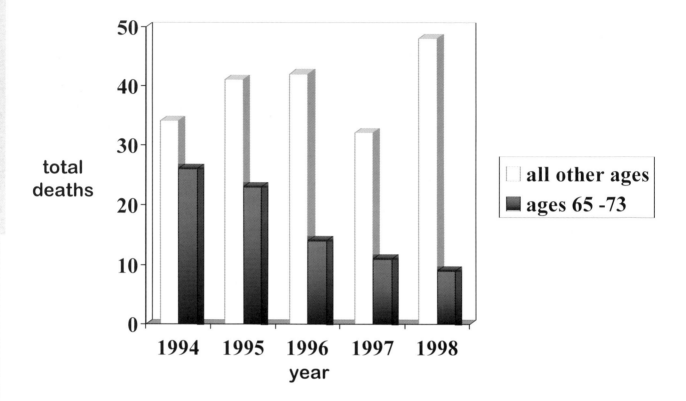

South and East of England will be reporting in 2002/2003 and may pave the way for more widespread screening in the future.

Summary

♦ Aortic aneurysms are more common in males over the age of 65 (I).

♦ Population screening for asymptomatic AAA has the potential to reduce both the risk of rupture and the overall death rate from this condition (I).

♦ GP based screening programmes are more acceptable to the patient and have a much higher attendance rate.

♦ Population screening using ultrasonography is quick, inexpensive and reliable (I).

Further reading

1   Earnshaw JJ, Murie JA, Eds. *The Evidence for Vascular Surgery*. Tfm Publishing Limited, Shropshire, 1999.

References (grade I evidence and grade A recommendations in bold)

1   Fowkes FGR, MacIntyre CCA, Ruckley CV. Increasing incidence of aortic aneurysms in England and Wales. *Br Med J* 1989; 298: 33-5.

2   Office for National Statistics. Mortality Statistics: Cause 1993. London: HMSO, 1995.

3   Veith FJ, Goldsmith J, Leather RP, Hannan EL. The need for quality assurance in vascular surgery. *J Vasc Surg* 1991; 13: 523-6.

4   Akkersdijk GJ, van de Graaf Y, van Bockel JH, de Vries AC, Eikelboom BC. Mortality rates associated with operative treatment of infrarenal abdominal aortic aneurysms in the Netherlands. *Br J Surg* 1994; 81: 706-9.

5   Johansson G, Swendenborg J. Ruptured abdominal aortic aneurysms: a study of incidence and mortality. *Br J Surg* 1986: 73: 101-3.

6   Drott C, Arfvidsson B, Ortenwall P, Lundholm K. Age standardized incidence of ruptured aortic aneurysm in a Swedish population between 1952 and 1988: mortality rate and operative results. *Br J Surg* 1992; 79: 175-9.

7   Collin J, Araujo L, Lindsell D. A Community Screening Programme for Abdominal Aortic Aneurysms. *Eur J Vasc Surg* 1988; 2: 83-86.

8   Gujral S, Shaw E, Earnshaw J, Poskitt K, Heather B. Improving attendance rates for abdominal aortic aneurysm screening. *Ann R Coll Surg Enl* 1997; 79(1): 71.

9   Shaw E. Screening to save lives. The Gloucestershire aneurysm screening project. *Professional Nurse,* December 1992.

10 Lucarotti ME, Heather BP, Shaw E, Poskitt KR. Psychological Morbidity Associated With Abdominal Aortic Aneurysm Screening. *Eur J Vasc Endovasc Surg* 1997; 14, 499-501.

11 Crow P, Shaw E, Earnshaw JJ, Poskitt KR, Whyman MR and Heather BP. A single normal ultrasonographic scan at age 65 years rules out significant aneurysm disease for life in men. *Br J Surg* 2001: 88 (7), 941-944.

12 The UK Small Aneurysm Study Participants. Mortality results for the randomised controlled trial of early selective surgery or ultrasonographic surveillance for small abdominal aortic aneurysms. *Lancet* 1998: 352: 1649-55.

13 Heather BP, Poskitt KR, Earnshaw JJ, Whyman M, Shaw E. Population screening reduces mortality rate from aortic aneurysm in men. *Br J Surg* 2000, 87, 750-753.

14 Scott RAP, Wilson NM, Ashton HA, Kay DN. Influence of screening on the incidence of ruptured abdominal aortic aneurysm: 5-year results of a randomized controlled study. *Br J Surg* 1995, 82, 1066-1070.

Chapter 14

Aortic aneurysm screening and surveillance

Chapter 15

Endovascular AAA repair - *patient selection*

Shiela Dugdill Vascular Nurse Practitioner
Lesley Wilson Vascular Research Sister
Andrew S Brown Specialist Registrar in Vascular Surgery
Mike G Wyatt Consultant Vascular Surgeon

NORTHERN VASCULAR CENTRE, FREEMAN HOSPITAL, NEWCASTLE-UPON-TYNE, UK

Introduction

When determining the correct treatment for any individual condition, clinicians must consider all available options. For many years, the only option for the repair of infra-renal abdominal aortic aneurysm was open operation (see Chapter 22) and this remains the gold standard. Recent advances in both interventional radiology and stent graft technology however, have given surgeons the opportunity to offer endovascular repair (EVR) as an alternative treatment to patients with anatomically suitable aneurysms [1] **(C)**. A suggested clinical care pathway is presented in Table 1.

The wide range of aortic stent grafts available makes it impractical for even the largest vascular units to carry enough devices to suit all patients and it is still the case that most stent grafts are ordered "tailor-made" for each individual. Coupled with the high mortality associated with conversion to open repair, thorough assessment of a patient's suitability for EVR is imperative if we are to realise the benefits of the technique and avoid late device failure.

Indications for endovascular repair

Historically, many surgeons have advised elective repair of aortic aneurysms when they reach a size of 4.0 - 4.5 cm. Recently, however, the UK Small Aneurysm Trial has shown no survival benefit for open repair in patients with asymptomatic aortic aneurysms of less than 5.5 cm in antero-posterior diameter **(A)** [2]. At present there is no good evidence to suggest that the introduction of EVR should result in a change to these criteria [3].

As most stent grafts are ordered on an individual basis the technique is generally not applicable to emergency cases. There are however case reports of the successful treatment of patients with contained rupture [4] and secondary aorto-enteric fistula [5] although the long-term outcome of these patients is unknown. Other situations which have been used as relative indications for EVR include the hostile abdomen [6], horseshoe kidney [7,8], aorto-caval fistula [9], retroperitoneal fibrosis [10] and aortitis [11].

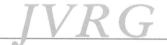

Table 1 Pathway of care for investigation of EVR graft patients.
Patients selected for EVR can be managed pre-operatively according to a clinical care pathway. This pathway for EVR is intended for use by the multi-disciplinary team who are involved on a daily basis with patients in a vascular surgical unit. The pathway is intended as a guide to assessment and treatment and has been developed to reflect evidence-based practice.

Pre admission clinic

Clerk & assess patients
CXR, ECG
Renal scan
Echo
Lung function tests
Blood parameters
Group & Save

MEDICAL

Baseline observations
Ht, Wt, BMI
Urinalysis
Nursing assessment
DVT risk analysis
Pressure sore assessment
Explanation of procedure, Q&A
Health education/promotion
Initiate discharge planning

NURSING

Liaise with physio, OT, discharge co-ordinator
Liaise with x-ray and theatre staff
Book HDU

PAMS

Selection criteria

Specific selection criteria for endovascular aortic aneurysm repair include the following **(C)**:

◆ Patient suitability (heart, chest, kidneys).

◆ Aortic anatomy (size, shape and extent of aneurysmal involvement).

◆ Device considerations (sizing, suitability and availability).

A protocol for patient selection for EVR is illustrated in Figure 1.

Patient suitability

Whilst EVR is often regarded as a minimally invasive procedure, this does not preclude a thorough pre-operative assessment of the patient's general medical state. Many patients with abdominal aortic aneurysms have significant co-morbidity; hypertension (60%), cardiac disease (60%) and respiratory disease (39%) are all prevalent [12] and up to 22.7% of patients may be deemed unfit for open repair on this basis [6]. At present however, there is no good evidence that EVR should be offered to patients who are unfit for a laparotomy.

Figure 1 Protocol for patient selection for EVR.

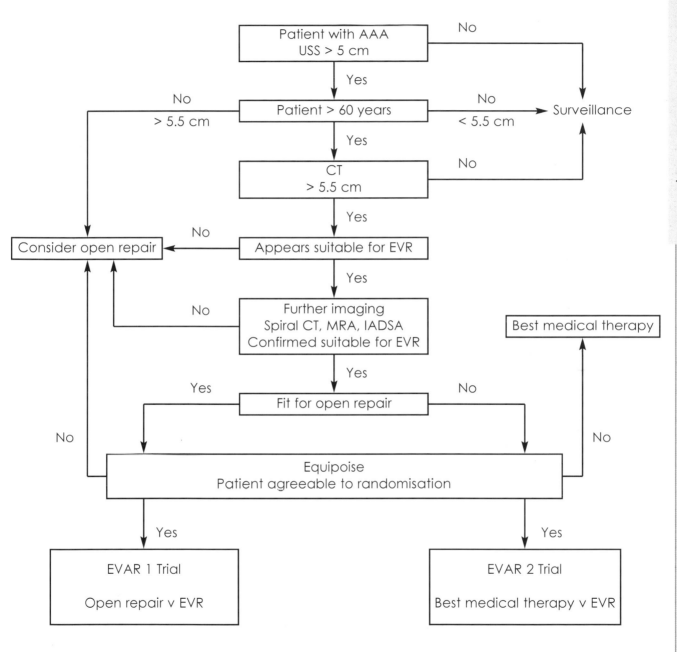

Patients should be worked-up in a similar manner to that for open aortic aneurysm repair. A full past medical history and physical examination should be completed with particular emphasis on the cardiovascular and respiratory systems. A protocol for routine investigations should be agreed with the vascular anaesthetists and might include full blood count, coagulation screen, urea and electrolytes, chest x-ray, pulmonary function tests, electrocardiogram and echocardiography. A renal isotope scan (DTPA) is performed to assess differential renal function, especially when utilising stent grafts which cover the renal arteries.

Further specialised investigations should be tailored to the history of the patient. Stress tests of cardiac function (stress echo and dipyridamole thallium scanning) are reserved for those patients with a history of angina causing functional impairment. Patients found to have significant reversible ischaemia should be referred to a cardiologist for consideration of coronary angiography and coronary revascularisation prior to aneurysm repair.

Much of the above routine can most satisfactorily be carried out at a pre-admission clinic 1 to 2 weeks prior to the procedure. This is close enough that major changes are unlikely to occur in the patient's status but allows time for correction of intercurrent conditions which may be picked up. As these clinics are often held away from the frenetic environment of the ward, it is a useful opportunity to educate the patient on life-style changes as well as providing more information about the procedure.

Aortic anatomy

In order to consider EVR as a treatment option, certain anatomical considerations need to be assessed (Table 2). If a stent graft system is to work it must exclude the aneurysm sac from the systemic circulation by fixing the device within the arterial wall at both proximal and distal ends. Unlike the open repair, where hand-sewn anastomoses provide this attachment, the endovascular stent graft relies on a variety of attachment systems. These include proximal hooks and barbs, radial expansive force and on newer devices, suprarenal fixation [13]. The operator must also consider the route of access, as patients with diseased or tortuous access arteries are often not suitable for endovascular repair.

Specific anatomical considerations prior to endovascular repair include:

- The dimensions of the proximal neck (width and length).

- The extent of aneurysm involvement of the iliac vessels

- Iliac vessel calibre and tortuosity.

Method of assessment

Until recently, many open aneurysm repairs were performed on the basis of ultrasound alone. The nature of EVR however demands a thorough assessment of aneurysm morphology. Conventional CT, with slices taken at 3-5 mm intervals, is able to exclude a number of patients from EVR, for instance because of involvement of the juxta-renal aorta by the aneurysm. Alone however it is insufficient to provide the detailed measurements required for device selection and further imaging is required.

The commonest complementary study is digital subtraction angiography, with a graduated marker placed behind the patient allowing measurements to be made. Precise anatomic information is obtained, especially regarding the presence of occlusive disease in the visceral and iliac arteries, but the extent of aneurysmal disease is frequently under-estimated. In particular the presence of thrombus in the neck of the aneurysm may be overlooked and may only be seen on CT. The images of both modalities must therefore be interpreted together.

Magnetic resonance angiography (MRA) has been used in place of conventional angiography and has a useful role in patients with impaired renal function. Lack of ready availability in many centres, long acquisition times and patient intolerance mean it is unlikely to become a popular method of assessment.

Spiral CT angiography is now becoming more widely available. As well as avoiding an arterial

Table 2 Anatomical considerations for aortic stent graft insertion.

Aneurysm sac	Diameter (AP)	> 5.5cm
Proximal neck	Length	> 15mm
	Width	< 30mm
	Angulation	< 60°
	No thrombus	
Iliac arteries	Internal diameter	> 6mm
	Angulation	< 100°

Chapter 15

puncture, sophisticated software and improved work stations now allow accurate measurement in multiple planes, with sufficient detail for complete evaluation of aneurysm morphology. It seems likely that this will become the single modality of choice in many centres.

Proximal neck

Experience has shown that the aneurysm neck must be within certain limits in terms of length, width and angulation. The current limits that we use are shown in Table 2. Stent grafts inserted into necks shorter than 15mm or with an angulation greater than 60 degrees have a tendency to leak (Type I proximal leak). In addition, the presence of thrombus and proximal neck diameters of greater than 30mm encourage both early and late stent graft migration and result in subsequent proximal endoleak (Type I) formation.

Iliac aneurysmal involvement

With the use of iliac limb extensions for bifurcate grafts, patients with aneurysms involving the iliac arteries can be treated. If this involves stenting across the internal iliac artery, this vessel should be embolised pre-procedure to prevent back bleeding Type II endoleak). Ideally both internal iliac arteries should not be occluded due to the risks of pelvic and colonic ischaemia. Occasionally this is unavoidable and in this instance a staged procedure is performed allowing iliac collateral pelvic and colonic revascularisation prior to aorto-iliac stent grafting.

The distal iliac attachment must be onto as normal artery as is possible, but above the fold of the inguinal ligament. In cases of severe unilateral aneurysmal disease, an aorto-uni-iliac device with a femoro-femoral cross-over would be considered.

Iliac calibre and tortuosity

The systems currently in use have a stent graft packed within an outer sheath, which ranges in size from 18 to 24 french. All devices require an adequate iliac lumen to allow deployment of the system and a minimum diameter of 6 mm is required to allow safe passage of most devices. Any localised stenosis can be angioplastied or stented prior to the procedure in order to facilitate smooth passage of the stent graft within its introducer. Severe angulation of the iliac vessels will preclude endovascular repair, although with the more rigid delivery systems and guide wires moderate angulation can be overcome. If the severe angulation is unilateral then again an aorto-uni-iliac system can be considered.

Device considerations

Several differing system configurations are available when selecting a patient for EVR. Experience with the original tube grafts for aortic-aortic repair has shown that they do not maintain long-term aneurysm exclusion due to problems related to distal fixation [14].

Currently there are two types of device available for the treatment of abdominal aortic aneurysm:

- Bifurcate systems.

- Aorto-uni-iliac systems with femoro-femoral cross-over grafts.

Bifurcate systems have the advantage of maintaining normal patient anatomy. They can be of one piece or modular design and are either fixed in place within the aorta using infrarenal hooks or barbs, centrifugal force or suprarenal bare stent fixators [13].

Aorto-uni-iliac devices can be deployed in a greater proportion of aortic aneurysms (70-80% versus 30-40% for bifurcated grafts), but require occlusion of the contra-lateral iliac system and construction of a cross-over graft [15].

Device choice is usually dependent upon patient anatomy and fitness, availability and personal operator choice. No one device is yet able to fit all aortic aneurysms.

EVAR Trials

Criteria for patient selection are now encompassed by the guidelines governing the EVAR (Endovascular Aneurysm Repair) trial **(C)**. This is a large UK based multi-centre trial funded by the National Health Executive. Suitably trained operators will randomise patients into two distinct limbs of the trial.

- In EVAR 1, fit patients are randomised to either EVR or open repair.

- In EVAR 2, patients deemed unfit for open repair are randomised to EVR + best medical treatment or best medical treatment.

Entry criteria for EVAR are:

- Age at least 60 years.

- Size of aneurysm at least 5.5cm.

- Anatomical suitability for either EVR or open repair (see above).

- Fitness for surgery determined locally according to ASA grading.

The recommended guidelines for assessment of patient fitness for open repair and suitability for EVAR Trial 1 and 2 are as follows.

Cardiac status

Patients should not be recommended for any surgical intervention if they have suffered:

- MI within the last 3 months.

- Onset of angina within the last 3 months.

- Unstable angina at night or at rest.

Normally, patients presenting with the following symptoms would be unsuitable for open repair (EVAR Trial 1):

- Severe valve disease.

- Significant arrhythmia.

- Uncontrolled congestive heart failure.

Respiratory status
(no constraints for EVAR Trial 2)

Open repair (EVAR Trial 1) would not be recommended for patients presenting with the following respiratory symptoms:

- Unable to walk up a flight of stairs without shortness of breath (even if there is some angina of effort).

- $FEV_1 < 1.0$ L.

- $PO_2 < 8.0$ kPa.

- $PCO_2 > 6.5$ kPa.

Renal status

Open repair might not be recommended for patients presenting with serum creatinine levels greater than 200 µmol/litre. These patients may be suitable for EVAR Trial 2.

Each trial will compare EVR against the current best alternative in terms of mortality, durability, safety and cost, as well as generic and patient specific health-related quality of life. Eleven hundred patients will be entered over 4 years, 800 in EVAR 1 and 300 in EVAR 2. Results will give an indication as to the safety, efficacy and durability of new EVR systems as they are introduced.

Until these trials are complete one must rely on the RETA and Eurostar registries to provide data as to the suitability of these devices for the treatment of abdominal aortic aneurysms. This new technology of EVR for the treatment of aortic aneurysms, at present remains of unproven clinical benefit [16].

Risk management

When a patient has completed the work-up and has been selected for EVR, the care pathway described allows for further risk assessment prior to surgery (Table 1). Pre-operative risk management for these patients includes a full nursing assessment, explanation of the procedure, DVT risk analysis, pressure sore assessment, health education and detailed discharge planning.

On the day before surgery all blood and laboratory results are checked, two units of blood cross-matched. The patient is reviewed and examined by the medical staff and the anaesthetist contacted. The patient is orientated to the ward, previous information reinforced and an explanation of expected events and possible complications undertaken.

Informed consent is taken by a senior surgeon and arrangements for the utilisation of theatre and radiological facilities and personnel checked. The attending medical staff should ensure that appropriate antibiotics are prescribed (i.e. single dose of gentamycin 240 mg and metronidazole 500 mg with induction) and prophylactic Tinzaparin prescribed. Anti-embolic stockings are applied (unless contra-indicated) and the patient prepared according to local policy (dentures, wash, shave etc.). A high dependency bed should be booked. This can be on a high dependency unit (HDU) or as part of a specialist vascular ward. The patient is now ready for transportation to theatre accompanied by a nurse from the ward.

Summary

- Endovascular repair (EVR) of abdominal aortic aneurysms is feasible but there is no evidence to suggest that it is preferable to open repair for the treatment of patients with abdominal aortic aneurysms **(III)**.

- Selection for EVR is based on patient, aneurysm and device characteristics. There are no definitive criteria for EVR selection and most centres will apply locally developed policy **(III)**.

- No single device will treat all aneurysms.

- Most patients in the UK are undergoing EVR within the confines of the EVAR Trials 1 and 2. Until these trials report, there is no Grade I evidence to determine which patients if any should be considered for EVR rather than open repair.

Further reading

1   Branchereau A, Jacobs M, Eds. *Surgical and Endovascular Treatment of Aortic Aneurysms*. Futura Publishing Company Inc, Armokk, NY, 2000.

2   Greenhalgh RM, Becquemin JP, Davies A, Harris P, Ivancev K, Mitchell A, Raithel D, Eds. *Vascular and Endovascular Surgical Techniques* (Fourth Edition). WB Saunders, London, 2001.

References (grade I evidence and grade A recommendations in bold)

1   May J, White GH, Hams JP. Devices for aortic aneurysm repair. *Surgical Clinics of North America* 1999; 79: 507-527.

2   **The U.K. small aneurysm trial. Participant mortality results for a randomised controlled trial of early elective surgery or ultrasonographic surveillance for small abdominal aortic aneurysms.** *Lancet* **1998; 352: 1649-1655.**

3   Finlayson SR, Birkmeyer JD, Fillinger MF, Cronenwett JL. Should endovascular surgery lower the threshold for repair fo abdominal aortic aneurysms? *J Vasc Surg* 1999; 29: 973-985.

4   Seelig MH, Berchtold C, Jakob P, Schonleben K. Contained rupture of an infrarenal abdominal aortic aneurysm treated by endoluminal repair. *Eur J Vasc Endovasc Surg* 2000; 19: 202-204.

5   Deshpande A, Lovelock M, Mossop P, Denton M, Vidovich J, Gurry J. Endovascular repair of an aortoenteric fistula in a high-risk patient. *J Endovasc Surg* 1999; 6: 379-384.

6   Fifth report on the Registry For Endovascular Treatment of Aneurysms (RETA). 2001. http://www.vssgbi.org/registries/5thretareport.pdf

7   Loftus IK, Thompson MM, Fishwick G, Boyle JR, Bell PR. Endovascular repair of aortic aneurysms in the presence of a horseshoe kidney. *J Endovasc Surg* 1998; 5: 278-281.

8   Stroosma OB, Kootstra G, Schurink GW. Management of aortic aneurysm in the presence of a horseshoe kidney. *Br J Surg* 2001; 88: 500-509.

9   Lau LL, O'reilly MJ, Johnston LC, Lee B. Endovascular stent-graft repair of primary aortocaval fistula with an abdominal aortoiliac aneurysm. *J Vasc Surg* 2001; 33: 425-428.

10 Boyle JR, Thompson MM, Nasim A, Sayers RD, Holmes M, Bell PR. Endovascular repair of an inflammatory aortic aneurysm. *Eur J Vasc Endovasc Surg* 1997; 13: 328-329.

11 Vasseur MA, Haulon S, Beregi JP, Le Tourneau T, Prat A, Warembourgh H. Endovascular treatment of abdominal aneurysmal aortitis in Behcet's disease. *J Vasc Surg* 1998; 27: 974-976.

12 European Collaborators on Stent-Graft Techniques for Abdominal Aortic Aneurysm Repair. Progress Report, 2001. ftp://ftp.esvs.org/pub/downloads/eurostar_jan_2001.pdf

13 Brown AS, Rose JD, Wyatt MG. What is the case for the bifurcate modular stent-graft for abdominal aneurysms? In: *Indications in vascular and endovascular surgery*. Greenhalgh RM, Ed. WB Saunders, London, 1998

14 May J, White GH, Yu W *et al*. Importance of graft configuration in outcome of endoluminal aortic aneurysm repair: a 5 year analysis by the life table method. *Eur J Vasc Surg* 1988; 15: 406-411.

15 Thompson MM, Boyle JR, Fishwick G, Bell PRF. Aorto-uni-iliac endovascular repair utilising ePTFE and balloon expandable stents: The Leicester experience. In: *Indications in vascular and endovascular surgery*. Greenhalgh RM, Ed. WB Saunders, London, 1998

16 Wyatt MG, Rose JD. Endovascular aneurysm repair: state of the art 2000. In: *The Evidence for Vascular Surgery*. Earnshaw JJ, Murie J, Eds. Tfm Publishing, Shropshire, 1999.

Chapter 16

Endovascular AAA repair - *treatment*

Shiela Dugdill Vascular Nurse Practitioner
Lesley Wilson Vascular Research Sister
Mike G Wyatt Consultant Vascular Surgeon
Michael J Clarke Consultant Vascular Surgeon

NORTHERN VASCULAR CENTRE, FREEMAN HOSPITAL, NEWCASTLE-UPON-TYNE, UK

Introduction

Endovascular abdominal aortic aneurysm repair (EVR) is a minimally invasive technique in which a prosthetic stent graft is introduced endoluminally into the aorta to exclude an aneurysm sac. By avoiding laparotomy and aortic clamping the technique has the potential to reduce peri-operative morbidity and mortality. A search of Medline reveals over 900 articles related to EVR. The majority of these however, report single centre experiences with generally small numbers and one should be careful about reaching firm conclusions on the basis of these. Furthermore, the development of the stent graft devices continues at a rapid pace and many of the published series relate to devices which are no longer available. Two large registries have been collecting data prospectively since 1996. The most recent report from the registry of the European Collaborators on Stent graft Techniques for Abdominal Aortic aneurysm Repair (EUROSTAR) contains data on 3264 stent graft implantations from 98 centres (this includes retrospective data for procedures performed prior to 1996). The Registry for the Endovascular Treatment of Aneurysms (RETA) has now published data on 1000 patients undergoing EVR in centres around the UK.

Two multi-centre randomised controlled trials (EVAR 1 & 2) are now under way to assess the applicability of EVR and these have been described in detail in the previous chapter. It is to be hoped that all centres involved with aortic stenting will participate in these trials. Any patients not entered into the trials should have their data submitted to the RETA or EUROSTAR registries.

Although first described a decade ago [1], the technique has only been widely adopted in the UK in the last 4 or 5 years. Recently though, enthusiasm for EVR has been tempered by reports from both Europe and the USA of late developing device related complications [2,3]. These reports are to a large extent based on the outcome of devices that are no longer available and it is possible (but by no means certain) that the latest generation of stent grafts will overcome some of the earlier problems. Nevertheless, this procedure should still be regarded as developmental. A suggested clinical pathway of care is presented in Table 1.

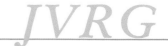

Table 1 Pathway of care

This clinical pathway for endovascular repair of AAA is intended for use by the multi-disciplinary team who are involved on a daily basis with patients in a vascular surgical unit. The pathway is intended as a guide to assessment and treatment and has been developed to reflect evidence-based practice.

Admission Day

Check blood results prior to admission
Review patient
Anaesthetist review

MEDICAL

Orientate to ward
Reinforce previous information, assess understanding
Explain further events/procedures

NURSING

Assess patient
Discuss potential problems
Give relevant information on breathing/mobilisation

PAMS

Pre-operative

Ensure ethical consent given
Ensure induction antibiotics are prescribed
Ensure all test parameters are in medical notes

MEDICAL

NBM 4 hours prior procedure
Antiembolic stockings applied unless contra-indicated
Patient is prepared according to policy
Accompany patient into theatre environment

NURSING

Post-operative

Review patient condition
Check post-operative instructions
Monitor fluid balance
Assess effectiveness of all medications

MEDICAL

Ensure safe environment
Record all observations and fluids
Assess Epidural/PCA pain control
O_2 if required
Observe wound site
Assist with daily activities
Explain all procedures

NURSING

Review by pain service
Commence limb and deep breathing exercises

PAMS

Chapter 16

Table 1 Pathway of care CONTINUED:-

1st Post-operative day

Review patient condition
Check U&E, FBC
Treat accordingly

MEDICAL

Assess analgesia requirements remove PCA/Epidural if necessary
May have diet and fluids as desired
Observe wound site

NURSING

Monitor observations 4hrly
Ensure urinary catheter removed and patient passes urine
Keep informed & updated on condition and length of stay
Commence mobilisation
Assess pain give oral analgesic preparations
Visit from OT & discharge co-ordinator

PAMS

Discussion regarding follow-up with specialist nurse
Stent data correlated

2nd Post-operative day until discharge

Confirm suitability for discharge
Update all medical notes
Write discharge letter & script

MEDICAL

Check wounds
May remove antiembolic stockings once discharged and fully mobile
Arrange district nursing service
Arrange transport for discharge

NURSING

Explain any new medications
Reinforce discharge advice re-lifestyle
Give all documents and medication pertaining to discharge

Ensure patient is able to carry out normal range of activities
Ensure patient aware of the importance of CT follow-up
Given contact number of endovascular team

PAMS

Make follow-up clinic appointment with consultant

Follow-up

4 week clinic appointment and participation with EVAR trial or follow-up into
EUROSTAR Databases

Pre-operative

Admission

The selection and pre-operative work up of patients for EVR has been covered in detail in the preceding chapter. If patients have been fully assessed in a pre-admission clinic they can be brought into hospital on the afternoon prior to surgery. The patient should be reviewed by a member of the medical staff to ensure that there have been no changes to their general health since their visit to the pre-admission clinic. The results of all pre-operative investigations should be available and occasionally it may be necessary to repeat some of these especially if new treatments were started at pre-admission. Modern laboratory techniques have considerably reduced the time taken to obtain cross-matched blood. Whilst some surgeons will still prefer to cross-match patients as if they were undergoing open repair, it is now our policy to cross-match two units of blood prior to the procedure. Pre-operative shaving and showering should be carried out according to local policies. Patients are fasted for 4 hours prior to operation.

Informed consent covers the nature of the procedure and the risks associated with it including a small risk of conversion to open repair. Patients should be informed of the developmental nature of stent graft repair and the need for long-term surveillance as well as the potential for secondary procedures.

Finally, it is often worthwhile to double check that the radiologist and radiographer are available and that the stent graft has arrived from the manufacturer.

Prevention of complications

Deep vein thrombosis prophylaxis is given according to local guidelines. In our institution, Tinzaparin 3500 units s/c is administered at 6 pm the evening prior to surgery and continued daily until discharge. TED stockings can also be applied in patients with no evidence of occlusive lower limb arterial disease. Antibiotic prophylaxis should again be determined by local policy. We use single intra-venous doses of Gentamicin 240 mg and Metronidazole 500 mg on induction of anaesthesia. For those with renal impairment, the Gentamicin is replaced by Teicoplanin 400 mg and Cefuroxime 1.5 g.

The operation

Set-up

A full description of the insertion techniques for the many different stent graft devices currently available is beyond the scope of this chapter but the following are some general points. It is our practice to perform these procedures with a vascular surgeon and an interventional radiologist scrubbed together, with a further surgical assistant. Two scrub nurses are present (one surgical and one radiological) as well as a radiographer. Ideally the procedure is performed in an operating theatre which has been adapted with full angiography facilities including a C-arm and carbon fibre table. This provides the full benefit of the clean theatre environment and access to full surgical facilities should complications occur **(A)**. A significant number of procedures in the UK are performed in the radiology suite however and the incidence of transfer to the operating theatre is low (0.3%) [4].

The majority of endovascular AAA repairs are carried out under general anaesthesia although in patients with severe respiratory disease a regional technique may be considered more appropriate. Some centres have even used local anaesthesia alone [5]. Invasive arterial pressure monitoring and wide bore central venous access are employed as for open aneurysm repair and an indwelling urinary catheter is inserted.

An adjustable radio-opaque marker is placed under the lumbar region of the patient who lies supine on the operating table with the arms at the sides. Immediate conversion to open repair may occur in approximately 3% of cases [4] and so the skin should still be prepped from nipples to knees. The abdomen is draped as for open aneurysm repair and a radiology towel then applied over this.

The device

Bifurcated stent grafts now make up 86 - 90% of devices employed [4,5]. The remainder are predominantly aorto-uni-iliac stents with a femoro-femoral cross-over graft. Very few tube grafts are used. In an attempt to reduce the incidence of distal migration, a number of stent grafts now have an uncovered proximal stent which anchors the device in the supra-renal aorta. This appears to be safe in the short-term [6,7] but careful follow-up is required to determine if there may be a deleterious effect on renal function.

Access

Arterial access is usually achieved via the common femoral arteries. These can be exposed through traditional longitudinal incisions although oblique groin incisions can provide adequate access and in our experience heal more satisfactorily. Retraction of the inguinal ligament allows a silastic Potts' loop to be placed around the distal external iliac artery, just proximal to the inferior epigastric artery origin. A distal loop can then be placed just proximal to the common femoral artery bifurcation. Individual control of the profunda and superficial femoral arteries is not normally necessary.

Occasionally a "hostile" groin is encountered (e.g. following previous infrainguinal bypass). In these circumstances it may be more appropriate to gain arterial access by exposing the external iliac artery through a Rutherford Morrison incision. Excessive tortuosity or narrow calibre of the external iliac artery might also make iliac exposure more attractive. Iliac insertion of the stent graft may however be more awkward on account of the sharp angle created traversing the abdominal wall. Therefore, when determining the entry site, careful consideration should be given to the distal extent of the stent graft to ensure that there is an adequate length of vessel available for deployment.

Deployment

Heparin is administered (5000 units i.v.) and the common femoral artery is punctured. A guide wire

and angiographic catheter are introduced and initial angiography performed to locate the renal arteries. The movement of respiration prevents accurate digital subtraction and breathing must be temporarily arrested by the anaesthetist for each angiographic run. The radio-opaque marker is then positioned in line with the lower margin of the most distal renal artery. The stent graft can now be inserted over a guide wire, a formal arteriotomy usually being unnecessary and deployed as per the manufacturer's recommendations.

Following deployment, completion angiography is performed to confirm satisfactory flow through the graft, patency of the renal arteries and complete exclusion of the aneurysm sac.

Closure

The common femoral artery is closed transversely with interrupted 5/0 Prolene sutures. Drains are not normally required. The subcutaneous layers are closed with Vicryl, and the skin with a subcuticular suture. Finally, the wounds are infiltrated with local anaesthetic. The RETA database reports a median operation time of 150 minutes for bifurcated devices with a median blood loss of 300 mls [4].

Intra-operative complications

Primary endoleaks

Type I (perigraft) endoleaks are seen in approximately 6% of completion angiograms, with similar numbers at the proximal and distal ends [5]. Proximal endoleaks require aggressive management as there is a high (28%) incidence of rupture if left untreated. Ballooning of the proximal end of the graft with a low pressure, high compliance moulding balloon may be sufficient to create an adequate seal. Insertion of a proximal cuff is often successful and in some cases a further stent can be deployed. If endovascular methods prove unsuccessful, laparotomy with proximal banding will exclude 67% of leaks whilst conversion to open repair should be regarded as a last resort. The peri-operative mortality of both these procedures however is in the order of 35% [4].

Distal type I endoleaks are most readily dealt with by ballooning or extension of the limb in to the distal common iliac or external iliac artery (although if the internal iliac is patent, this would first require embolisation). Persisting distal leaks appear to follow a more benign course than their proximal counterparts. Further stenting, embolisation and open repair can all be employed in their treatment, but 36% seal spontaneously within the first 30 days and they do not appear to be associated with rupture [4].

Type II (collateral) endoleaks are seen in up to 7% of cases [5] but a quarter are only seen at 1 month follow-up [4]. They arise most commonly from lumbar vessels, the inferior mesenteric artery or an accessory renal artery. Two thirds of these leaks will seal spontaneously by 30 days and of those persisting beyond the first month, a further third will seal by 1 year. In our practice we have tended to reserve further intervention for patients in whom a persistent type II endoleak is associated with expansion of the aneurysm sac as seen on follow-up CT. In these cases, coil embolisation of branches of the internal iliac artery and percutaneous thrombin injection directly into the sac have both been successfully employed.

Type III (mid-graft) endoleaks are less common (< 3%) [5] and may be seen at junctional areas of a modular graft or from tears in the graft material. Junctional leaks may respond to further ballooning but otherwise are best dealt with by insertion of a further endoluminal stent.

Rarely, a type IV endoleak may occur due to "sweating" of the graft material. This was more common with early devices and these endoleaks will seal spontaneously with time.

Renal artery occlusion

This may occur due to the covered part of the stent graft overlying the renal artery orifice (1.2%) or more commonly an accessory renal artery (2.3%) [5]. In cases where both renal arteries (or the artery to a solitary functioning kidney) are occluded consideration should be given to immediate renal revascularisation. This accounts for about 10% of open conversions [4]. Where a functional kidney remains perfused a conservative approach can be adopted although careful monitoring of renal function is required post-operatively.

Trauma to access vessels

Considering the size of the stent grafts, this complication is surprisingly uncommon. Direct trauma can occur at the entry site to the common femoral artery and the intima is often separated from the media and adventitia. Careful repair with interrupted sutures is usually all that is required although occasionally a formal endarterectomy with or without patch angioplasty may be required. Dissection of an artery is a particular risk in patients with tortuous iliac vessels, especially the external iliac. In some cases this can be corrected by placement of a limb extension stent but, if the external iliac remains occluded, open ilio-femoral bypass or femoro-femoral cross-over grafting will be required. Post-operative thrombosis of the common femoral artery occurs in less than 1% of patients [4].

Embolisation

Considerable amounts of thrombus often exist within the sac of an aortic aneurysm which may be dislodged by manipulation of guide wires and the stent graft within the sac. Significant peripheral embolisation occurs in less than 1% of cases and limb loss was reported in only 2 of 3264 patients [5]. In addition to large vessel emboli, widespread atheromatous embolisation has been reported leading to death from multi-organ failure [8].

Internal iliac artery occlusion

This usually occurs as a planned part of the procedure when it is necessary to extend the limbs of the graft into one or both external iliac arteries but can occur inadvertently. Buttock claudication is reported to occur in 13-50% of cases [9,10,11] with only a minority of patients experiencing a significant improvement over time. Many men with aneurysmal disease have pre-existing erectile dysfunction although this may be worsened following internal iliac occlusion. Severe ischaemic complications such as ischaemic colitis are rare but may occur more frequently when both internal iliac arteries are occluded simultaneously or where there is significant stenosis within the contralateral internal iliac or ipsilateral profunda femoris arteries [12]. When bilateral internal iliac occlusion is planned, it is our practice to sequentially embolise the internal iliac arteries 10 - 14 days apart in order to allow collateral vessel development.

Conversion to open repair

Conversion to open repair occurs in 1.5-3.3% of cases [4,5] and carries with it a 30% mortality rate [4]. Migration of the device or inability to position or advance the delivery system are the most commonly stated indications with conversion for intra-operative rupture only being reported in 0.3% of cases. Similar numbers are seen for persistent endoleak and renal artery damage [4].

Post-operative care

Following recovery from anaesthesia most patients are cared for in an intensive care unit or high dependency unit. Pulse, blood pressure, urine output and peripheral circulation are closely monitored and the wounds inspected regularly. Ileus is not a prominent feature following EVR and no restriction is placed on oral intake which can be commenced immediately. Full blood count, urea and electrolytes are measured the next morning at which stage intravenous fluids are discontinued and all intravenous lines and the urinary catheter removed. The majority of patients are then fit for discharge to the ward where they are encouraged to mobilise early. In the absence of complications, some patients are ready for discharge 3 days post-operatively although the mean length of stay is 6 days [4,5].

CT scanning is performed within the first month following the procedure but is not necessary prior to discharge unless there is a particular concern over the integrity of the repair. Patients are generally fit for discharge 2 to 3 days post-operatively.

Post-operative complications

Overall, complications are reported in 28% of patients undergoing EVR [4]. Technical complications have largely been covered above. The most common wound related complications are bleeding, haematoma and false aneurysm formation (4%) [4,5], whilst wound infection may occur in around 2.5%.

The most serious complications are the associated systemic complications and are reported in 15% of patients. Cardiovascular problems (4%) and renal failure (4%) occur most frequently, but the avoidance of laparotomy may account for the relatively low incidence of respiratory complications (2.1%). Cerebrovascular accidents and confusion are occasionally seen and there are reports of paraplegia due to spinal cord ischaemia [13] and ischaemic sciatic neuropathy [14].

Post-implantation syndrome

This is perhaps not a true complication and indeed is regarded by some as a good sign. A swinging pyrexia and back pain may occur in up to 50% of patients in the first 7 days following stent graft insertion and is thought to be related to thrombosis within the aneurysm sac. Leucocytosis and other features of sepsis are absent and the condition runs a benign course. Discharge need not be delayed if the patient is otherwise clinically well.

Outcome

At 30 days EVR has resulted in successful exclusion of the aneurysm in 81-90% of cases, although 2.4-7.1% of these patients will have required a secondary intervention [4,5]. The overall 30-day mortality in RETA is 5.5%. Nevertheless, patients considered fit for open repair faired better than those who were unfit (3.1% v 14.3%). The 30-day mortality in EUROSTAR is 2.1%.

Follow-up

Perhaps the biggest question hanging over the future of EVR is its long-term durability. In addition to clinical review, careful regular follow-up with CT and plain abdominal x-ray is mandatory. In the EUROSTAR registry, more than half of patients have developed an endoleak by 5 years and 56% have required secondary intervention. Furthermore, there seems to be little sign that the rate of development of late complications is diminishing.

Summary

◆ EVR should be performed by vascular surgeons and interventional radiologists working together as a team. Each have their own individual skills which are essential for accurate stent graft placement **(A)**.

◆ EVR should be performed in a sterile environment with full radiological imaging facilities **(A)**.

◆ Aortic aneurysms can be successfully treated using EVR but there is no evidence that the operative mortality is different from that following open repair **(III)**.

◆ Complications of EVR are common and require awareness by both medical and nursing staff to provide optimum management **(A)**.

Further Reading

1   Branchereau A, Jacobs M, Eds. *Surgical and Endovascular Treatment of Aortic Aneurysms*. Futura Publishing Company, New York, 2000.

2   Waquar Yusuf S, Marin ML, Ivancev K, Hopkison BR, Eds. *Operative Atlas of Endoluminal Aneurysm Surgery*. Isis Medical Media, Oxford, 2000

References

1   Parodi JC, Palmaz JC, Barr H. Transfemoral intraluminal graft implantation for abdominal aortic aneurysms. *Ann Vasc Surg* 1991; 5: 491-499.

2   Harris PL. The highs and lows of endovascular aneurysm repair: the first two years of the Eurostar Registry. *Ann R Coll Surg Engl* 1999; 81: 161-165.

3   Ohki T, Veith FJ, Shaw P *et al*. Increasing incidence of midterm and long-term complications after endovascular graft repair of abdominal aortic aneurysms: a note of caution based on a 9-year experience. *Ann Surg* 2001; 234: 323-334.

4   Fifth report on the Registry For Endovascular Treatment of Aneurysms (RETA). 2001. http://www.vssgbi.org/registries/5thretareport.pdf

5   European Collaborators on Stent-Graft Techniques for Abdominal Aortic Aneurysm Repair. Progress Report, 2001. ftp://ftp.esvs.org/pub/downloads/eurostar_jan_2001.pdf

6   Maclerewicz J, Walker SR, Vincent R, Wastie M, Elmarasy N, Hopkinson BR. Vascular surgical society of great britain and ireland: perioperative renal function following endovascular repair of abdominal aortic aneurysm with suprarenal and infrarenal stents. *Br J Surg* 1999; 86: 696.

7   Bove PG, Long GW, Zelenock GB *et al*. Transrenal fixation of aortic stent-grafts for the treatment of infrarenal aortic aneurysmal disease. *J Vasc Surg* 2000; 32: 697-703.

8   Zempo N, Sakano H, Ikenaga S *et al*. Fatal diffuse atheromatous embolization following endovascular grafting for an abdominal aortic aneurysm: report of a case. *Surg Today* 2001; 31: 269-273.

9   Criado FJ, Wilson EP, Velazquez OC *et al*. Safety of coil embolization of the internal iliac artery in endovascular grafting of abdominal aortic aneurysms. *J Vasc Surg* 2000; 32: 684-688.

10   Lee WA, O'Dorisio J, Wolf YG, Hill BB, Fogarty TJ, Zarins CK. Outcome after unilateral hypogastric artery occlusion during endovascular aneurysm repair. *J Vasc Surg* 2001; 33: 921-926.

11   Wolpert LM, Dittrich KP, Hallisey MJ *et al*. Hypogastric artery embolization in endovascular abdominal aortic aneurysm repair. *J Vasc Surg* 2001; 33: 1193-1198.

12   Yano OJ, Morrissey N, Eisen L *et al*. Intentional internal iliac artery occlusion to facilitate endovascular repair of aortoiliac aneurysms. *J Vasc Surg* 2001; 34: 204-211.

13   Berg P, Kaufmann D, van Marrewijk CJ, Buth J. Spinal cord ischaemia after stent-graft treatment for infra-renal abdominal aortic aneurysms. Analysis of the Eurostar database. *Eur J Vasc Endovasc Surg* 2001; 22: 342-347.

14   Kibria SG, Gough MJ. Ischaemic sciatic neuropathy: a complication of endovascular repair of abdominal aortic aneurysm. *Eur J Vasc Endovasc Surg* 1999; 17: 266-267.

Chapter 17

Endovascular AAA repair - *follow-up*

Rao Vallabhaneni Endovascular Fellow

Geoffrey Gilling-Smith Consultant Vascular Surgeon

REGIONAL VASCULAR UNIT, ROYAL LIVERPOOL UNIVERSITY HOSPITAL, LIVERPOOL, UK

The purpose of follow-up

Patients who have undergone endovascular repair of an aneurysm of the infra-renal abdominal aorta require life-long surveillance in order to ensure that they remain free from the risk of aneurysm rupture and aneurysm related death **(A)**.

Unlike conventional open surgical repair, endovascular repair does not replace the aneurysm with a prosthetic graft. The aim is simply to isolate the aneurysm from the circulation. The aneurysm remains *in situ* and may, therefore, continue to expand and/or rupture should it no longer be properly isolated from systemic arterial pressure and flow.

Late rupture after endovascular repair was first reported by Lumsden in 1995 [1]. Since then several reports have confirmed a small but definite risk of late aneurysm rupture [2,3] **(I)**, [4]. Analysis of the Eurostar database reveals an annual rupture risk of 1% with a cumulative risk of approximately 2.9% 4 years after operation [3] **(II)**. This is probably an under-estimate. Analysis of 161 late deaths of a cohort of 2194 patients showed that ten patients (6.2% of late deaths) suffered sudden unexplained deaths and it is likely that at least some of these deaths were due to late but unrecognised rupture of the aneurysm [5]. It should also be noted that the results reported apply to aneurysms having a median diameter of only 57 mms (range 21-105 mm). A significant number of the aneurysms treated were relatively small and very unlikely to rupture so that the incidence of late rupture in patients with larger aneurysms is probably higher than the relatively conservative 1% reported **(III)**.

It should also be noted that the incidence of late aneurysm rupture does not diminish with duration of follow-up. If anything the trend is the reverse with an increasing risk of rupture as time goes by **(II)**.

What are we looking for?

The rationale for surveillance after endovascular repair is, in general, accepted but there remains uncertainty about the endpoints of surveillance. How can we determine whether or not the aneurysm remains or is again at risk of rupture?

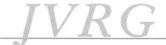

Endoleak

An endoleak is defined as blood flow within the aneurysm sac but outside the stent graft. Endoleaks have been classified according to their site of origin [6,7] (Table 1). Endoleaks may result from failure of the proximal or distal anastomotic seals (Type I), from disconnection of the component parts of a modular stent graft (Type III) or from perforation of the stent graft fabric (Type IV). They may also result from retrograde perfusion of the aneurysm sac via patent lumbar or inferior mesenteric arteries (Type II).

Endoleaks are unequivocal evidence of failure to isolate the aneurysm from the circulation and as such were at first considered evidence of failure of endovascular repair [8]. Later studies, however, revealed continued expansion of the aneurysm in the absence of demonstrable endoleak as well as instances of aneurysm shrinkage in the presence of side-branch reperfusion of the aneurysm sac. The presence or absence of endoleak could not, therefore, be relied upon to determine whether or not the aneurysm was at risk of rupture [9] **(II)**.

Endotension

The realisation that an aneurysm could expand and presumably therefore rupture in the absence of demonstrable endoleak resulted in the concept of endotension which was defined as persistent or recurrent pressurisation of the aneurysm sac after endovascular repair [10,11]. This concept focused attention on the importance of intrasac pressure rather than intrasac flow as the ultimate determinant of the fate of the aneurysm. An aneurysm which remained pressurised would be likely to continue to expand and might rupture whether or not there was flow within the aneurysm sac whereas an aneurysm that was not pressurised would be unlikely to be at risk even if there was evidence of flow within the sac. It should be noted, however, that the consequences of aneurysm rupture would very much depend upon the potential for haemorrhage into and out of the aneurysm sac once rupture had occurred.

Stent graft distortion and migration

Once deployed within the aortic lumen, stent grafts are subject to a variety of forces [12,13]. Haemodynamic forces tend to promote distal displacement of the stent graft and can result in late proximal Type I endoleak if the stent graft is not securely fixed to the aneurysm neck **(II)**. Haemodynamic forces can also result in dislocation of the components of a modular stent graft and if migration occurs can also result in kinking and buckling of the stent graft which, in effect, becomes too long for the aneurysm. Buckling and kinking can also occur if the aneurysm shrinks. Successful isolation and depressurisation of the

Table 1 Classification of endoleaks.

Type of endoleak	Intra-sac flow	Possible intervention
I	Perigraft flow at proximal or distal graft attachment site	Extension cuff Conversion
II	Flow through side branches (e.g. lumbar, IMA)	Coil embolisation, ligation (laparoscopic/open), conservative
III	Fabric tear or modular disconnection	Covered stent/secondary endograft/ conversion
IV	Graft porosity	Conservative

Table 2 Univariate analysis of risk factors for late rupture (Eurostar; n= 2464 median follow-up 11.8 months).

Risk factor	P	Risk Ratio (95% CI)
Proximal type I endoleak	.001	7.59 (2.09 to 27.62)
Type III endoleak	.001	8.95 (2.92 to 27.52)
Stent-graft migration	.001	4.53 (1.24 to 16.66)
Stent-graft kinking	.001	3.13 (1.40 to 11.49)
Type II endoleak*	.415*	
Distal type I endoleak*	.776*	
Stent-graft stenosis*	.646*	
Stent-graft thrombosis*	.503*	

* Statistically not significant.

aneurysm sac often results in circumferential shrinkage and there is now evidence that this can be associated with longitudinal shrinkage [14]. Buckling and kinking can interfere with blood flow to the lower limbs but, perhaps more importantly, tend to increase the haemodynamic force that is applied to the stent graft and increase the risk of migration, dislocation and stent graft fracture **(II)**.

Risk factors for rupture

A recent analysis of the Eurostar database sought to identify the risk factors for rupture. A variety of factors were identified on univariate analysis (Table 2) but multivariate analysis identified migration as the most significant risk factor with a risk ratio of 5.3 [15]. The presence or absence of endotension was not included in this analysis as measures of endotension did not form part of the routine follow-up protocol for these patients. It is interesting to note, however, that endoleak did not feature as a significant risk factor on multivariate analysis. This should not be interpreted as evidence that endoleaks are not dangerous. It is more likely that graft-related endoleaks did not feature as a risk factor simply because when these are recognised they tend to be treated by secondary intervention. The risk of rupture is, therefore, averted. Migration, on the other hand, is often simply observed and it is probable that in many cases, migration results in a late Type I or Type III endoleak and consequent rupture before secondary intervention is considered **(III)**.

There is general agreement that graft-related endoleaks are a significant risk factor for late rupture **(II)**. There is no hard evidence to support this but it would probably now be very difficult to conduct a randomised study to answer this question since most physicians would not consider it ethical to simply observe patients with such endoleaks. The clinical significance of Type II endoleaks, however, remains uncertain. It is probable that some are dangerous while others are not **(III)**.

The laws of physics tell us that an aneurysm which remains pressurised remains at risk of rupture and there is now general agreement that surveillance protocols should include evaluation of the presence or absence of significant intrasac pressure **(B)**.

Other graft-related problems such as migration, distortion and disintegration are also important endpoints as they can herald significant complications.

How do we look for it?

Endoleak

Contrast enhanced CT scanning remains the gold standard for detection of endoleak. (Figure 1 illustrates an algorithm for the post-operative surveillance of endovascular grafts based on CT scanning). There is, however, disagreement as to whether or not single phase CT scanning is sufficient or whether dual or, even, triple phase CT scanning is necessary to reveal endoleaks that might otherwise be missed. It seems clear that dual phase CT scanning is more likely to reveal low flow side branch endoleaks than single phase CT scanning[16] but it may well be that the endoleaks revealed by dual phase CT scanning are not, in fact, clinically significant.

Another problem with CT scanning is that it imposes a significant radiation burden on the patient who will require such scans at intervals throughout the remainder of his/her life. For this reason there has been considerable interest in contrast enhanced ultrasound as an alternative. A prospective study of this performed in Liverpool revealed that contrast enhanced ultrasound failed to identify certain endoleaks revealed on CT scanning [17]. It also revealed that in a number of cases, the scan was, for technical reasons, non-diagnostic. What remains unclear, however, is whether or not the endoleaks revealed only on CT scanning were clinically significant. Since it is likely that an experienced observer can diagnose most high-flow graft-related endoleaks if a state-of-the-art ultrasound machine is available, it may be that Duplex scanning could be employed as first line of investigation with CT scanning reserved only for those patients in whom

Duplex scanning was considered non-diagnostic or for those in whom there was other evidence to suggest continued pressurisation of the aneurysm sac. Such an approach would reduce the overall radiation burden but remains to be validated.

Endotension

It is possible to measure intrasac pressure directly by needle puncture of the aneurysm. This is invasive, however, and there is a theoretical risk of introducing infection. For these reasons, direct sac puncture is not, in general, considered acceptable for routine surveillance.

Several groups are working to develop remote monitoring of intrasac pressure by means of a pressure transducer introduced into the aneurysm sac at the time of endovascular repair and accessed remotely at intervals during follow-up. At the time of writing, however, such technology is not available and the presence or absence of endotension must be deduced indirectly by observation of change in the size of the aneurysm. It is generally believed that if an aneurysm is pressurised it will continue to expand. Conversely an aneurysm which is shrinking is probably not pressurised **(III)**.

Changes in the size of an aneurysm can be determined by observation of serial CT scans, measuring either the widest diameter or the volume of the aneurysm. There is now some evidence to suggest that measurement of volume may be more accurate than measurement of diameter [18]. The problem with the latter technique is that a change in the shape of the aneurysm may result in a change in diameter which is not, in fact, indicative of expansion or shrinkage. It is also difficult to ensure that the same diameter is measured on subsequent CT films. Measurement of volume is, however, more complex and time consuming. In our view, therefore, measurement of aneurysm diameter is probably sufficient for routine surveillance with measurement of volume being reserved for patients in whom there is uncertainty or evidence that the aneurysm may be enlarging **(B)**.

Figure 1 Algorithm for the post-operative surveillance of endovascular grafts based on CT scanning.

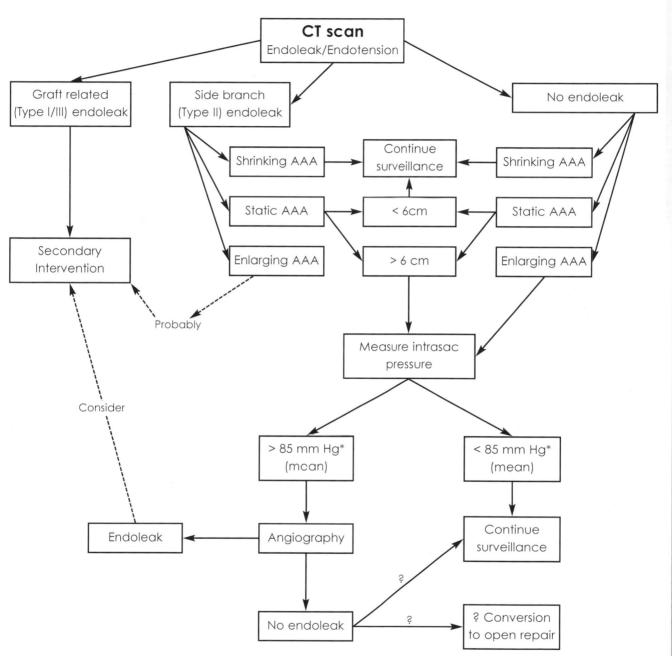

* This is an arbitrary figure based on no hard evidence.

Chapter 17

Structural integrity of the graft

Plain radiography of the abdomen in at least two planes remains the most reliable method for evaluating the integrity of the stent graft. (Figure 2 illustrates an algorithm for the post-operative surveillance of endovascular grafts based on plain abdominal x-rays). Wire-form fractures and separation of stent graft constituents can usually be seen clearly. By reference to adjacent bony landmarks it is also possible to determine whether or not the stent graft is migrating and whether or not there is threatened disconnection of the component parts of a modular device **(II)**. Migration should, however, also be assessed on CT scanning, relating the position of the stent to the origins of the renal arteries on successive CT slices **(B)**.

Frequency of follow-up examination

Patients need to be examined frequently enough to detect the threat of late rupture before it occurs. The longer the interval between successive examinations, the greater the risk that a late graft related endoleak will occur and result in rupture before it is identified. On the other hand, surveillance examinations impose a considerable burden on both patients and physicians. Although patients can, in general, be persuaded to accept the need for surveillance examinations, continued acceptance of this obligation is unlikely if patients are subject to very frequent examinations. Each examination will, in addition, generate CT and other images which need to be reviewed and evaluated. As the number of patients treated in any individual centre increases, so the burden of surveillance also increases.

Currently we recommend surveillance examinations at 1, 3, 6, 12, 18 and 24 months after intervention. Thereafter we examine patients annually but we increase the frequency of examination in cases where there is concern **(A/B)**. Each surveillance examination should include clinical examination (evaluation of peripheral arterial tree), two plane radiography of the abdomen and single phase contrast enhaced CT scan. Duplex scanning may be performed in addition but cannot yet replace CT scanning.

Indications for secondary intervention

Endoleak

There is general agreement (but no hard evidence) that the finding of a graft-related endoleak on surveillance is an indication for early secondary intervention. Anecdotal reports attest to the risk of early rupture following the development of proximal, distal or mid-graft endoleak **(III)**.

We do not believe that a Type II endoleak is an indication for secondary intervention unless it is associated with clear evidence that the aneurysm remains pressurised and at risk of rupture. Thus, we only intervene if the endoleak is associated with expansion of the aneurysm or, occasionally, if it is associated with a large aneurysm that is not expanding but that is not shrinking either and in which direct sac puncture has confirmed significant intrasac pressure **(C)**.

Endotension

Evidence that the aneurysm is pressurised mandates further investigation to determine and if possible treat the cause. If the aneurysm is expanding and there is no evidence of endoleak on CT scanning, we perform angiography to try and establish whether or not an endoleak is present. This requires selective injection into both internal iliac arteries to opacify any patent lumbar arteries that may communicate with the aneurysm sac as well as retrograde injection into the common iliac arteries to establish whether or not there is communication with the aneurysm sac alongside the distal (iliac) anastomotic sites **(B)**.

Where no cause can be identified, it must be assumed that pressure is being transmitted through thrombus sealing an endoleak or through the interstices of the graft itself. Although rupture of an aneurysm in which there is no flow may be considered a relatively benign event, continued enlargement is in our view likely to result in enlargement of the aneurysm neck and late migration with consequent secondary proximal endoleak. For this reason we will, in general, consider the arguments for and against

Figure 2 Algorithm for the post-operative surveillance of endovascular grafts based on plain abdominal X-rays.

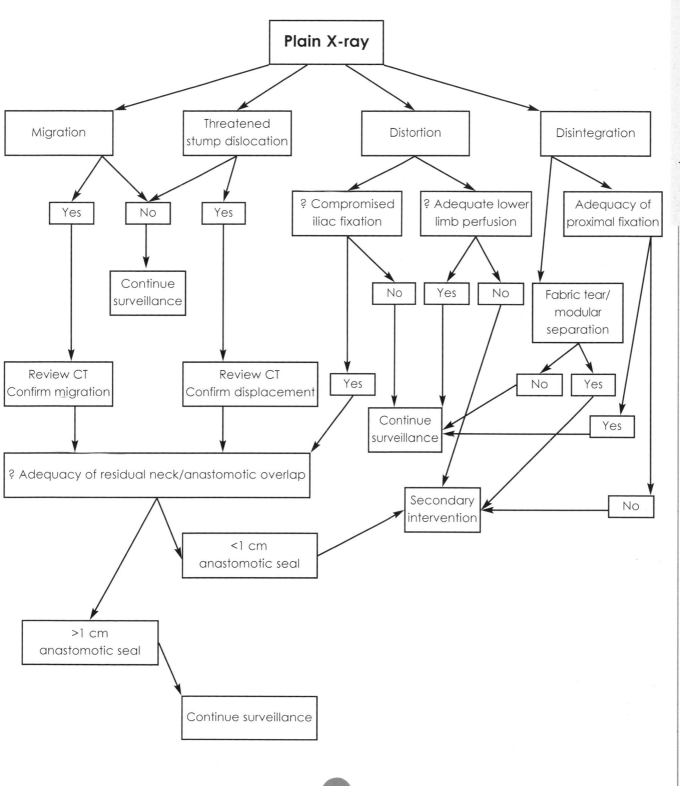

conversion to open repair, the decision being based largely on the perceived balance of risk (**B**).

Migration

Evidence of migration either at the proximal attachment site or at the site of attachment between component parts of a modular graft (threatened dislocation) is, in our view, an indication for early intervention (**A/B**). The available evidence suggests that a policy of observation may well result in endoleak, rupture and death before the patient is next examined (**II**).

Graft distortion and disintegration

Graft distortion is not, in itself, an indication for secondary intervention although it is often associated with migration and/or a reduction in blood flow to the lower limbs. Thus, the finding of graft distortion should prompt a careful examination of available images to determine whether or not there is migration. This should be combined with clinical and non-invasive vascular laboratory evaluation of the patient to assess whether or not lower limb circulation is threatened. Unfortunately, distortion is not easily corrected. If the graft limb is migrating up from its common iliac "attachment site", the limb may be extended to provide increased security. A localised kink can occasionally be straightened by the insertion of a small stent but, in general, severe graft distortion and evidence of migration requires conversion to open repair (**B**).

Evidence of stent graft disintegration and wireform fractures should also prompt a careful evaluation of available images. Loss of structural integrity may be associated with migration while wireform fractures may result in perforation of the graft fabric and late Type III endoleak.

Summary

- There is a small but significant number of patients who remain at risk from aneurysm rupture and death following endovascular repair (**I**).

- Patients who have undergone endovascular aneurysm repair require lifelong surveillance to determine whether or not they remain or are again at risk from aneurysm rupture (**A**).

- The aim of surveillance should be to ensure that the patient remains free of endoleak, that the aneurysm is no longer pressurised and that the stent graft is not migrating, distorting or fragmenting. Surveillance examinations should also include an evaluation of lower limb perfusion (**B**).

- The presence or absence of endoleak is best determined by contrast enhanced CT scanning (**II**).

- Angiography should be reserved for patients in whom there is uncertainty or evidence of endotension in the absence of demonstrable endoleak on the CT scan (**B**).

- The presence or absence of persistent or recurrent pressurisation of the aneurysm sac is best determined by evaluation of change in aneurysm size on successive CT scans (**B**).

- Comparison of successive diameter measurements is probably adequate for routine surveillance with measurement of changes in volume being reserved for cases in which there is uncertainty (**B**).

- Direct measurement of intrasac pressure should only be considered in cases where a large aneurysm fails to shrink and it is suspected that this is because it remains pressurised (**B**).

- Plain radiography should be performed to look for evidence of stent graft migration, distortion or disintegration (**A**).

- Clinical and non-invasive vascular laboratory examinations are necessary to evaluate lower limb perfusion (**B**).

References (grade I evidence and grade A recommendations in bold)

1   Lumsden AB, Allen RC, Chaikof EL, Resnikoff M, Moritz MW, Gerhard H, Castronuovo JJ Jr. Delayed rupture of aortic aneurysms following endovascular stent grafting. *Am J Surg* 1995; 170(2): 174-8.

2   **Zarins CK, White RA, Moll FL, Crabtree T, Bloch DA, Hodgson KJ, Fillinger MF, Fogarty TJ The AneuRx stent graft: four-year results and worldwide experience 2000.** *J Vasc Surg* **2001; 33(2 Suppl): S135-45.**

3   **Harris PL, Vallabhaneni SR, Desgranges P, Becquemin JP, van Marrewijk C and Laheij RJ. Incidence and risk factors of late rupture, conversion, and death after endovascular repair of infrarenal aortic aneurysms: the EUROSTAR experience. European Collaborators on Stent/graft techniques for aortic aneurysm repair.** *J Vasc Surg* **2000; 32(4): 739-49.**

4   Ohki T, Veith FJ, Shaw P, Lipsitz E, Suggs WD, Wain RA, Bade M, Mehta M, Cayne N, Cynamon J, Valldares J, McKay J. Increasing incidence of midterm and long-term complications after endovascular graft repair of abdominal aortic aneurysms: a note of caution based on a 9-year experience. *Ann Surg* 2001; 234(3): 323-34.

5   Vallabhaneni SR, Harris PL, Gilling-Smith GL, Laheij R. Aneurysm-related mortality during late follow-up after endovascular aneurysm repair of infrarenal aorta. *Br J Surg* 2001; 88(4): 598.

6   White GH, May J, Waugh RC, Yu W. MS Type I and Type II endoleaks: a more useful classification for reporting results of endoluminal AAA repair. *J Endovasc Surg* 1998; 5: 189-193.

7   White GH, May J, Waugh RC, Chaufour X, Yu W. Type III and type IV endoleak: toward a complete definition of blood flow in the sac after endoluminal AAA repair. *J Endovasc Surg* 1998; 5(4): 305-9.

8   Cuypers P, Buth J, Harris PL, Gevers E, Lahey R. Realistic expectations for patients with stent-graft treatment of abdominal aortic aneurysms. Results of a European multicentre registry. *Eur J Vasc Endovasc Surg* 1999; 17(6): 507-16.

9   Gilling-Smith GL, Martin J, Sudhindran S, Gould DA, McWilliams RG, Bakran A, Brennan JA, Harris PL. Freedom from endoleak after endovascular aneurysm repair does not equal treatment success. *Eur J Vasc Endovasc Surg* 2000; 19(4): 421-5.

10   Gilling-Smith G, Brennan J, Harris P, Bakran A, Gould D, McWilliams R. Endotension after endovascular aneurysm repair: definition, classification, and strategies for surveillance and intervention. *J Endovasc Surg.* 1999; 6(4): 305-7.

11   White GH, May J, Petrasek P, Waugh R, Stephen M, Harris J.Endotension: an explanation for continued AAA growth after successful endoluminal repair. *J Endovasc Surg* 1999; 6(4): 308-15.

12   Liffman K, Lawrence-Brown MM, Semmens JB, Bui A, Rudman M, Hartley DE. Analytical modelling and numerical simulation of forces in an endoluminal graft. *J Endovasc Ther* 2001; 8(4): 358-71.

13   Mohan IV, van Marriewijk, Laheij RJF, How TV and Harris PL on behalf of the Eurostar collaborators. Factors and forces influencing stent-graft migration. *Eur J Vasc Endovasc Surg* (in press).

14   Harris P, Brennan J, Martin J, Gould D, Bakran A, Gilling-Smith G, Buth J, Gevers E, White D. Longitudinal aneurysm shrinkage following endovascular aortic aneurysm repair: a source of intermediate and late complications. *J Endovasc Surg* 1999; 6(1): 11-6.

15   Vallabhaneni SR, Harris PL. Lessons learnt from the EUROSTAR registry on endovascular repair of abdominal aortic aneurysm repair. *Eur J Radiol* 2001; 39(1): 34-41.

16   Golzarian J, Dussaussois L, Abada HT, Gevenois PA, Van Gansbeke D, Ferreira J, Struyven J. Helical CT of aorta after endoluminal stent-graft therapy: value of biphasic acquisition. *Am J Roentgenol* 1999; 172(6): 1690-1.

17   McWilliams RG, Martin J, White D, Gould DA, Rowlands PC, Haycox A, Brennan J, Gilling-Smith GL and Harris PL. Detection of endoleak with enhanced ultrasound: comparison with biphasic CT. *J Endovasc Ther* (in press).

18   Wever JJ, Blankensteijn JD, Th M Mali WP, Eikelboom BC. Maximal aneurysm diameter follow-up is inadequate after endovascular abdominal aortic aneurysm repair. *Eur J Vasc Endovasc Surg* 2000; 20(2): 177-82.

Endovascular AAA repair - *follow-up*

Chapter 18

Investigation of TIA and stroke

Ross Naylor

Consultant Vascular Surgeon & Honorary Reader in Surgery

DEPARTMENT OF SURGERY, LEICESTER ROYAL INFIRMARY, LEICESTER, UK

Introduction

A number of level I randomised trials have contributed towards rationalising the management of stroke and TIA[1,2]. As with previous chapters, the level of evidence will be detailed. However, the European Carotid Surgery Trial (ECST) and the North American Symptomatic Carotid Endarterectomy Trial (NASCET) have also published secondary analyses (SA) from their databases. Because there is no classification for this type of evidence, they have also been graded level I.

The chapter is based on the sequence of questions faced by the family doctor and/or hospital clinician who is seeing a patient with suspected TIA or stroke.

- Did this patient suffer a TIA or stroke?

- Did the TIA/stroke affect the carotid territory?

- To whom should patients be referred?

- Do some patients warrant expedited referral and investigation?

- Which risk factors require investigation?

- What constitutes optimal medical therapy?

- Does the patient have an ipsilateral carotid stenosis?

- Is there a need for functional CT/MR imaging?

- Which patients should be considered for carotid endarterectomy?

Did this patient suffer a stroke or TIA?

Stroke is a loss of focal cerebral function (occasionally global), lasting for > 24 hours and which has a vascular cause (haemorrhage/ischaemia). A transient ischaemic attack (TIA) has a similar definition, but a time domain < 24 hours. Patients presenting with non-hemispheric symptoms; isolated dizziness, isolated diplopia, isolated vertigo, presyncope and blackout should not be considered to have suffered a TIA unless the symptoms definitely co-

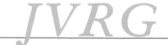

exist with others typical of a carotid or vertebrobasilar event. Alternative aetiologies (labyrinthine disorders, arrhythmias etc) should be sought. Isolated non-hemispheric symptoms are *not* indicative of TIA/stroke and these patients should not be considered for carotid endarterectomy **(A)**.

Did the TIA/stroke affect the carotid territory?

It can be quite difficult, on clinical grounds alone, to reliably determine the vascular territory. The carotid territory is involved in about 70% of ischaemic strokes, while 20% are vertebro-basilar. The territory is difficult to determine in 10% because of overlap of the vascular boundary zones. "Classical" carotid territory symptoms include hemisensory/motor signs, monocular blindness (amaurosis fugax) and higher cortical dysfunction (dysphasia, visuospatial neglect etc). Vertebro-basilar symptoms include bilateral sensory/motor signs, bilateral blindness, dysarthria, homonymous hemianopia, nystagmus, problems with gait, balance and stance and a tendency to veer to one side while walking.

Any patient with a history suggestive of a carotid or vertebrobasilar event should be referred for investigation unless co-morbidity, senility and/or reduced life expectancy warrant a more conservative approach. Even if an operation is not recommended, all will benefit from optimisation of medical therapy **(A)**. Figure 1 outlines the investigation and management of a patient with a suspected stroke or TIA.

To whom should patients be referred?

It is the responsibility of hospital/health administration to ensure access to a cerebrovascular clinic. Unfortunately, provision of such a service varies throughout the UK. The importance of rapid access is borne out by the observation that 5% of medically treated NASCET patients [3] who presented with a stroke, thereafter suffered a further stroke within 30 days **(I)**. In an ideal world, it would be preferable for

TIA/stroke patients to be seen in multi-disciplinary clinics. Unfortunately, a shortage of stroke physicians/neurologists currently makes this impossible.

In the absence of a multi-disciplinary clinic, the patient should be referred to a rapid-access service run by a physician/vascular surgeon interested in cerebral vascular disease who; (i) offers out-patient review within four, preferably two, weeks of referral, (ii) has rapid access to Duplex ultrasound or MR angiography, (iii) will take responsibility for investigating and treating risk factors and (iv) has the facility for discussing complex/atypical cases with neurological colleagues **(B)**. The decision to refer should not be based on the presence of a bruit. Up to 60% of patients with a 90-99% stenosis will not have a carotid bruit **(A)**. Biological, as opposed to chronological age, should determine whether referral is appropriate. Patients aged over 75 years have the highest incidence of stroke **(I)** and can gain significant benefit from carotid surgery **(A)**.

Do some patients warrant expedited referral and investigation?

All patients should be seen as soon as possible, but some require more urgent assessment. It is not possible to predict stenosis severity from either the mode of presentation or the presence/absence of a bruit. The only exception is the rare patient whose symptoms are triggered by exercise, hot baths etc. in whom a critical stenosis should be suspected.

Secondary analyses [4] from the ECST and NASCET **(I)** suggest that an increased stroke risk in medically treated patients can be anticipated from clinical parameters (Table 1). Recognition of one or more of these should alert the clinician to a higher priority for referral, especially if the patient is known to have severe carotid disease. Crescendo TIAs (repeated TIAs within 2 weeks) and progressive worsening of an acute neurological deficit (progressive stroke) are associated with a higher risk of stroke than discrete, non-recurrent neurological events.

Figure 1 Algorithm for the investigation and management of a patient with a suspected stroke/TIA.

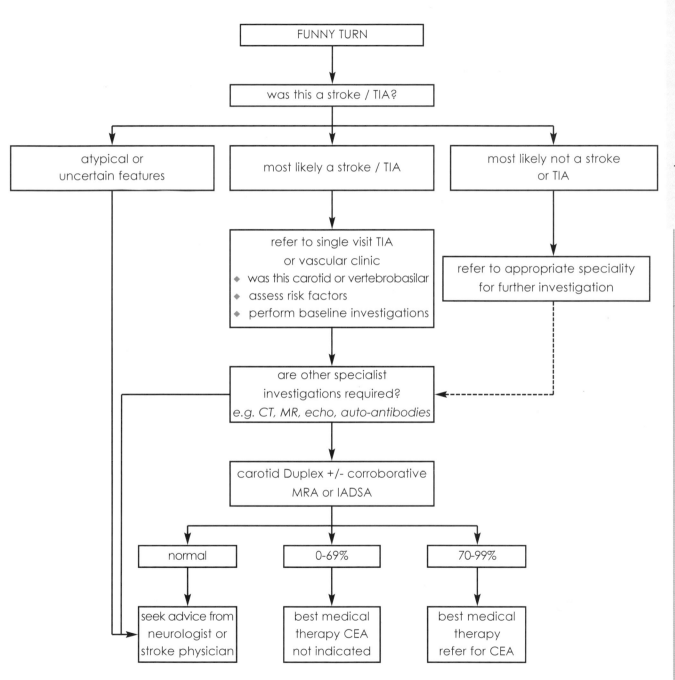

Table 1 Predictors of increased risk of late stroke in medically treated patients with a 70-99% stenosis (*).

clinical factors

Male versus female gender

Hemispheric versus ocular symptoms

Recurrent events for longer than 6 months

Symptoms within the last 2 months

Cortical versus lacunar stroke

Increased number of concurrent risk factors

Increasing age

after imaging

Irregular or ulcerated plaques

Incremental degrees of stenosis above 70% (especially 90-95%)

Severe stenosis with contralateral occlusion

Tandem intracranial disease

No recruitment of intracranial collaterals

*(based on subgroup analyses from ECST and NASCET (ref [4])).

Expedited referral and investigation should be considered in higher risk patients, particularly when one or more of the following co-exist: male sex, hemispheric events, recurrent events, symptoms within 2 months or symptoms for more than 6 months **(A)**. Patients with crescendo TIAs or progressive stroke should be considered neurological emergencies and admitted for investigation **(B)**.

Which risk factors require investigation?

Non-modifiable risk factors for ischaemic stroke include increasing age, male gender and black race. Modifiable risk factors include hypertension, ischaemic heart disease, previous TIA, hyperlipidaemia, smoking and diabetes **(I)**. There is a perception amongst stroke physicians that, if left to their own devices, surgeons will often ignore risk factor management and simply focus their efforts on identifying those suitable for carotid endarterectomy (CEA).

All patients should undergo baseline studies including full blood count, plasma viscosity/erythrocyte sedimentation rate, urea and electrolytes, blood sugar, lipids, chest x-ray and ECG. Second line investigations (immunology, echocardiography, etc.) should be reserved for selected patients and require the input of specialist colleagues **(B)**. Responsibility for ensuring appropriate investigation and best medical therapy should not be delegated to the most junior member of the team **(B)**.

What constitutes optimal medical therapy?

Anti-platelet therapy

A recent meta-analysis [5] showed that aspirin (a cyclo-oxygenase pathway inhibitor) reduced the risk of stroke by 15% in patients with cerebral vascular disease (I). In those with "vascular disease", aspirin [6] conferred a 22% reduction in non-fatal stroke and myocardial infarction and any vascular death (I). A large randomised trial [7] has confirmed that low dose aspirin is associated with a lower incidence of peri-operative stroke/death following CEA and reduces the incidence of side effects (I). Dipyridamole (a weak ADP antagonist) alone does not reduce the risk of stroke. Combination with aspirin [8] confers a 23% risk reduction, although 25% suffer side-effects requiring dipyridamole withdrawal (I). Clopidogrel (ADP inhibitor) has not been evaluated in patients with symptomatic cerebral vascular disease. The CAPRIE study (any vascular patient) observed a small but significant benefit in favour of clopidogrel (0.5% absolute risk reduction, 8.7% relative risk reduction) as compared with aspirin [9] in reducing any late vascular event (I). Clopidogrel is significantly more expensive than aspirin, it trebles the bleeding time [10], while combination with aspirin increases the bleeding time by a factor of five (II).

In summary, aspirin remains the first line antiplatelet agent (A). Low dose aspirin (75-300mg) confers a lower operative risk and reduced side effect profile as compared with higher doses (600-1200mg) (A). Aspirin should not be withdrawn prior to carotid surgery (A). The second line agent is clopidogrel. Surgeons should be aware that increased peri-operative bleeding may be encountered in patients on chronic clopidogrel therapy, especially if in combination with aspirin (C).

Treatment of hypertension

Hypertension is the main risk factor for stroke, but implementation of therapeutic guidelines is generally poor. Few trials have examined hypertension therapy in patients with cerebral vascular disease. A meta-analysis of 48,000 patients from randomised hypertension studies [11] showed that a 5mmHg reduction in diastolic pressure reduced late stroke by 38% (I). Unfortunately, evidence suggests that 40% of known hypertensives destined to suffer a stroke will not be on any treatment prior to suffering the stroke. In addition, only 50% of treated patients will have a documented diastolic pressure < 90mmHg [12]. Controversy persists regarding criteria for treatment. The current recommended threshold is < 140/90mmHg. Uncontrolled hypertension conferred an increased risk of operative stroke in ECST [13] (I).

Control of hypertension is the cornerstone of stroke prevention (A). The aim should be to achieve a blood pressure of < 140/90mmHg, but this may be relaxed slightly in the presence of increasing age (B). No patient should undergo carotid endarterectomy with uncontrolled hypertension (A).

Treatment of hyperlipidaemia

Interpretation of the role of lipid lowering therapy in stroke prevention is confounded by the fact that (i) few randomised trials specifically include patients with cerebral vascular disease and (ii) a meta-analysis of the randomised trials [14] has shown no significant benefit, partly because low cholesterol levels were associated with an increased risk of haemorrhagic stroke while high cholesterol levels were associated with an increased risk of ischaemic stroke! (I). A subsequent meta-analysis [15] has shown that statin therapy conferred a 25% reduction in the risk of ischaemic stroke, but only in those with ischaemic heart disease (I).

Until further trials are published, statin therapy is specifically indicated in TIA/stroke patients with elevated total cholesterol levels and a history of ischaemic heart disease (A).

Cessation of smoking

No randomised trials have been performed! Meta-analyses of cohort and epidemiological studies [16] suggest that stroke risk is doubled in patients who continue to smoke (II).

All TIA/stroke patients should be encouraged to stop smoking **(A)**.

Diabetes mellitus

There is no evidence from randomised trials [17] that tight glycaemic control reduces the risk of stroke **(I)**. However, the UK Prospective Diabetes Study Group [18] showed that type II diabetics randomised to strict anti-hypertensive control had a 44% reduction in late stroke as compared to similar diabetic patients with higher blood pressure thresholds **(I)**.

Type II diabetic, hypertensive patients require strict blood pressure control **(A)**.

Atrial fibrillation

About 20% of strokes are due to non-valvular atrial fibrillation and warfarin therapy confers a 70% risk reduction [19,20]. High risk patients for stroke (6% p.a.) include (i) any age with a history of TIA/stroke, rheumatic heart disease, ischaemic heart disease, impaired left ventricular function and (ii) those aged > 75 years with hypertension or diabetes. Medium risk (2% risk p.a.) comprises (i) those aged < 65 years with a history of diabetes, hypertension, peripheral vascular disease and ischaemic heart disease (group a) or (ii) those aged 65-75 years with no risk factors (group b). Low risk patients (1% p.a.) include patients < 65 years with no risk factors **(I)**.

High risk and group (a) medium risk patients should be considered for warfarinisation (target INR = < 3.0). Medium risk (group b) and low risk patients should be treated with aspirin **(A)**.

Does this patient have an ipsilateral carotid stenosis?

Contrast angiography was a pre-requisite for participation in ECST and NASCET. The main disadvantages, however, are the 1-2% procedural stroke risk [21] and the time delay in making management decisions. Since 1991, there have been major advances in non-invasive imaging (colour duplex ultrasound and MR angiography (MRA)) and an increasing number of experienced centres have now developed validated criteria to diagnose severe carotid disease and select patients for carotid endarterectomy (CEA) without recourse to angiography. The decision to base management decisions on non-invasive imaging has aroused considerable debate. One of the problems being that if one assumes angiography to be the "gold standard", duplex and MRA can only ever come second.

Before any centre considers abandoning routine angiography, a number of criteria must be met **(B)**. The radiologist/technician must be experienced in carotid imaging, diagnostic criteria must be validated against angiography or resected specimens and the workload must be sufficient to maintain expertise. Inter-machine validation studies must be repeated following purchase of new equipment and newly trained technologists must be closely monitored. The single most important factor is the ultrasound operator. There is, however, no evidence that a radiologist is better than a similarly experienced vascular technologist. MRA is a proven alternative to duplex and angiography, provided similar validation studies have been performed. The main problem is the waiting time involved in most UK centres.

For those reliant upon non-invasive assessment, intra-arterial digital subtraction angiography (IADSA) should still be performed in any patient with equivocal duplex/MRA findings. In the case of duplex, this primarily relates to (i) excessive bifurcation calcification, (ii) inability to image above or below the plaque, (iii) high resistant ICA waveform suggestive of severe distal disease and (iv) damped inflow signal suggestive of proximal CCA disease.

In contrast, clinicians who insist on angiography prior to CEA must include the 1-2% angiographic stroke risk in discussion of the overall operative risk. No patient should undergo angiography if the patient is not thereafter also willing to consent to CEA **(A)**. Radiologists undertaking IADSA must minimise the risks of stroke. These include (i) the use of small amounts of non-ionic contrast material, (ii)

Chapter 18

experienced practitioners, (iii) small bore catheters and (v) well hydrated patients [22].

Because of the risks of procedural stroke, angiography should never be used to screen for carotid artery disease **(A)**. Colour duplex ultrasound or MRA are the preferred methods for non-invasive assessment. Both should be performed as quickly as possible (preferably at single visit clinics) though the choice will inevitably reflect local expertise and speed of access **(B)**. Before abandoning a policy of routine angiography, advocates of Duplex or MRA must undertake validation studies against angiography or the resected plaque. The former is preferable so as to derive criteria for diagnosing less severe disease **(B)**. Advocates of routine non-invasive assessment must have defined criteria for referring selected patients for IADSA **(B)**. Centres insisting on pre-operative angiography must add the angiographic stroke risk to the operative risk when discussing the risks and rationales of CEA with their patients **(A)**.

Which patients should be considered for carotid endarterectomy?

Patients with a TIA or minor stroke within 6 months who have a 70-99% stenosis of the ipsilateral internal carotid artery gain a six to tenfold reduction in the risk of late stroke (Table 2) following CEA, compared to best medical therapy alone **(I)**. Patients with 0-69% stenoses derive no clear benefit from CEA. The only exception might be the very rare patient with a moderate stenosis who suffers repeated TIAs/minor strokes despite optimal medical therapy. Any such patient requires the corroborative input of a stroke physician/neurologist. Expedited CEA should be considered in patients exhibiting one or more of the high-risk clinical and investigative factors summarised in Table 1 **(I)**.

The question of extending the six-month threshold in selected patients has been considered following publication of the final results from ECST and NASCET. Both studies [4] showed that the annual risk of stroke was persistently high for the first 12 months after randomisation in symptomatic patients with 80-99% stenoses **(I)**. Accordingly, it may now be

reasonable to extend the threshold to 12 months in selected patients, particularly if they exhibit other factors predictive of increased stroke risk (Table 1) **(B)**.

Is there a need for functional CT/MR imaging?

This has always been a controversial subject. Pre-operative CT scanning was mandatory in the ECST and NASCET to exclude intracranial haemorrhage and unexpected intracranial pathology (tumour, arteriovenous malformation). This attitude changed with increasing awareness that the yield from scanning in TIA patients was < 2% and could otherwise delay referral for surgery in high risk patients **(III)**. There is compelling evidence to advocate routine CT scanning in all stroke patients within 14 days of onset so as to exclude those with haemorrhage **(A)**. In an ideal world, all TIA patients should still undergo CT or MR provided it does not delay referral for surgery **(II)**. Unfortunately this is not usually the case.

CT/MR imaging should be performed within 2 weeks of a stroke to differentiate between ischaemia and haemorrhage **(B)**. Advocates of routine CT/MRI imaging in TIA patients must ensure that this does not incur a significant delay (< 2 weeks from consultation) **(C)**. For those without rapid access to CT/MRI (currently the majority in the UK), clear criteria must be established for imaging unusual or atypical cases **(B)**.

Summary

- All patients with carotid territory symptoms should be referred for investigation unless significant co-morbidity or senility warrants a conservative approach. Referral should not be based on the presence/absence of a bruit **(A)**.

- Non-invasive assessment (Duplex, MRA) should be performed on all patients. Centres requiring angiography prior to surgery must include the risk of stroke in any discussion of the operative risk **(A)**.

Table 2 Long-term risk of ipsilateral stroke *(including peri-operative stroke or death)(*)*.

stenosis (%)	surgical risk (%)	medical risk (%)	ARR (%)	RRR (%)	NNT	strokes prevented per 1000 CEAs
ECST						
<30%	9.8 at 5y	3.9 at 5y	-5.9	n/a	n/a	n/a
30-49%	10.2 at 5y	8.2 at 5y	-2.0	n/a	n/a	n/a
50-69%	15.0 at 5y	12.1 at 5y	-2.9	n/a	n/a	n/a
70-99%	10.5 at 5y	19.0 at 5y	+8.5	45	12	83 at 5y
NASCET						
30-49%	14.9 at 5y	18.7 at 5y	+3.8	20	26	38 at 5y
50-69%	15.7 at 3y	22.2 at 3y	+6.5	29	15	67 at 3y
70-99%	8.9 at 3y	28.3 at 3y	+19.4	69	5	200 at 3y

ARR = absolute risk reduction

RRR = relative risk reduction

NNT = number of CEAs to prevent one ipsilateral stroke

n/a = not applicable

* Reproduced with permission from Naylor A.R. (ref [4])

- All risk factors should be optimised where possible. This duty should not be delegated to the most junior member of the team **(A)**.

- Patients presenting with stroke should have a CT within 2 weeks to exclude haemorrhage. If CT or MR scans are required in TIA patients, this should not unnecessarily delay referral for surgery where appropriate **(B)**.

- High risk patients for stroke (in its natural history) include male patients, those presenting with stroke, hemispheric signs, recurrent events for > 6 months, 90-95% stenoses, contralateral occlusion, multiple risk factors, most recent event within 4 weeks, irregular plaque surface morphology **(A)**.

- Lower risk patients for stroke (in its natural history) include female patients, discrete ocular symptoms, those with string sign, 70-79% stenoses **(A)**.

- Surgeons must quote their own operative risk and this should include the risk of cranial nerve injury **(A)**.

Further reading

1. Moore WS. *Surgery for Cerebrovascular Disease*. WB Saunders, 2000.

2. Naylor AR, Mackey WC. *Carotid Artery Surgery: A Problem Based Approach*. WB Saunders, 2000.

References (grade I evidence and grade A recommendations in bold)

1. **European Carotid Surgery Trialists' Collaborative Group. Randomised trial of endarterectomy for recently symptomatic carotid stenosis: Final results of the MRC European Carotid Surgery Trial (ECST).** *Lancet* **1998; 351: 1379-1387.**

2. **Barnett HJM, Taylor DW, Eliasziw *et al*. Benefit of carotid endarterectomy in patients with symptomatic moderate or severe stenosis.** *N Engl J Med* **1998; 339: 1415-1425.**

3. **Gasecki AP, Ferguson GG, Eliasziw M *et al*. Early endarterectomy for severe carotid artery stenosis after a non-disabling stroke: Results of the NASCET Trial.** *J Vasc Surg* **1994; 20: 288-295.**

4. Naylor AR, Rothwell PM, Bell PRF. Overview of the principal results and secondary analyses from the European and North American randomised trials of carotid endarterectomy. *Eur J Vasc Endovasc Surg* (IN PRESS).

5. **Johnson ES, Lanes SF, Wentworth CE *et al*. A meta-regression analysis of the dose-response effect of aspirin on stroke.** *Arch Int Med* **1999; 159: 12448-1253.**

6. **Antiplatelet Triallists Collaboration. Collaborative overview of randomised trials of anti-platelet therapy - 1: Prevention of death, myocardial infarction and stroke by prolonged antiplatelet therapy in various categories of patients.** *Brit Med J* **1994; 308; 81-106.**

7. **Taylor DW, Barnett HJM, Haynes RB *et al*. Low dose and high dose acetylsalicylic acid for patients undergoing carotid endarterectomy: a randomised trial.** *Lancet* **1999; 353: 2179-2184.**

8. **Wilterdink JL, Easton JD. Dipyridamole plus aspirin in cerebrovascular disease.** *Arch Neurol* **1999; 56: 1087-1092.**

9. **CAPRIE Steering Committee. A randomised blinded trial of Clopidogrel versus Aspirin in patients at risk of ischaemic events. (CAPRIE)** *Lancet* **1996; 348: 1329-39.**

10. Payne D, Hayes PD, Bell PRF, Goodall AH, Naylor AR. Combined effects of aspirin and the novel antiplatelet agent clopidogrel on platelet function in vivo and in vitro. *J Vasc Surg* (IN PRESS).

11. **Collins R, MacMahon S. Blood pressure, antihypertensive drug treatment and the risks of stroke and coronary heart disease.** *Br Med Bull* **1994; 50: 272-298.**

12. Kalra L, Perez I, Melbourn A. Stroke risk management: changes in mainstream practice. *Stroke* 1998; 29: 53-7.

13. **Rothwell PM, Warlow CP. Prediction of benefit from carotid endarterectomy in individual patients: A risk modelling study.** *Lancet* **1999; 353: 2105-2110.**

14. **Qizilbash N, Lewington S, Duffy S *et al*. Cholesterol, diastolic blood pressure and stroke: 13,000 strokes in 450,000 people in 45 prospective cohorts.** *Lancet* **1995; 346; 1647-1653.**

15. **DiMascio R, Marchioli R, Tognoni G. Cholesterol reduction and stroke ocurrence: An overview of randomized clinical trials.** *Cerebrovascular Dis* **2000; 10: 85-92.**

16. **Shinton R, Beevers G. Meta-analysis of relation between cigarette smoking and stroke.** *Brit Med J* **1989; 298; 789-794.**

17. **UK Prospective Diabetes Study Group. Effect of intensive blood glucose control with metformin on complications in overweight patients with type II diabetes.** *Lancet* **1998; 352: 854-865.**

18. **UK Prospective Diabetes Study Group. Tight blood pressure control and risk of macrovascular and microvascular complications in type II diabetics.** *Brit Med J* **1998; 317; 2035-2038**

19. **Goldstein LB, Adams R, Becker K, Furberg CD, Gorelick PB, Hademenos G *et al*. Primary prevention of ischaemic stroke: A statement for Healthcare Professionals from the Stroke Council of the American Heart Association.** *Stroke* **2001; 32: 280-299.**

20. **Gubitz G, Sandercock PAG, Lip GYH. What are the effects of anticoagulant and antiplatelet treatment in people with atrial fibrillation? In:** *Clinical Evidence.* **BMJ Publishing Group and American College of Physicians - American Society of Internal Medicine, London, December 1999. pp122-126.**

21. **Hankey GJ, Warlow CP, Sellar RJ. Cerebral angiographic risk in mild cerebrovascular disease.** *Stroke* **1990; 21: 209-222.**

22. Scottish Intercollegiate Guidelines Network (SIGN). Management of patients with stroke (II) Management of carotid stenosis and carotid endarterectomy, 1997.

Investigation of TIA and stroke

Chapter 19

The diagnosis of deep venous thrombosis

Kok-tee Khaw Consultant Radiologist

DEPARTMENT OF RADIOLOGY, ST GEORGE'S HOSPITAL, LONDON, UK

Introduction

Significant changes have occurred in the diagnosis of deep venous thrombosis (DVT) in recent years. Venography has been replaced as the first-line test of choice by duplex ultrasonography, but there is at present still no universal consensus as to the most cost-efficient and accurate practice for the diagnosis of acute symptomatic DVT. Full duplex sonography is time-consuming and requires skill and training, and recent studies have attempted to determine if more limited tests can safely be used. Methods used for diagnosis will be dictated by availability of facilities and clinical practices in individual centres, but to optimise patient management a diagnostic strategy should be adopted that will ensure that the diagnosis of clinically relevant DVT is confirmed or excluded as accurately and quickly as possible after initial presentation.

Clinical evaluation and risk probability assessment

Objective testing for diagnosis of DVT is necessary as clinical evaluation is unreliable, with sensitivities and specificities as low as 60% and 20% respectively [1]. Accuracy of clinical evaluation can be increased with the use of models for risk probability assessment (RPA). These use specific combinations of symptoms, physical signs and risk factors which can stratify patients into low, moderate or high risk groups (Table 1). They are simple to use and have shown considerable potential for increasing the predictive value and decreasing the number of objective tests required [1-3].

Venography

Venography is now recognised to have many disadvantages. It is still used extensively and preferred by some clinicians because of accuracy, familiarity with the method and routine evaluation of calf veins. However, it is invasive, uncomfortable and expensive in comparison to non-invasive techniques, and requires the use of ionising radiation and contrast media. It should not be used for follow-up studies. Contrast induced thrombosis is an uncommon but well-recognised complication, and technical failure to opacify all the deep veins may occur in up to 15% of patients [4]. Studies have also shown inter- and intra-

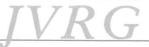

Table 1 Risk probability score sheet for assessment of DVT.

Risk Probability Assessment:		Score
History:	Paralysis/paresis/plaster immobilisation of lower limbs	+1
	Bedridden >3 days, major surgery in <4/52, airline flight > 4hrs	+1
	Active cancer - Rx in previous 6/12 or on palliative treatment	+1
O/E:	Entire leg swollen	+1
	Calf swollen >3 cm than other leg (10 cm below tibial tuberosity)	+1
	Tenderness along deep veins	+1
	Pitting oedema worse in symptomatic leg	+1
	Collateral superficial veins (non-varicose)	+1
	Alternative diagnosis more likely than DVT	-2

Score:	HIGH	≥3
	MODERATE	1-2
	LOW	≤0

observer variability of up to 30% for the presence of thrombus, with greatest discordance for distal involvement [5,6]. It is because of its invasive nature that venography is now used mainly as an adjunct to non-invasive tests when these are equivocal, or when special clarification of a diagnostic problem is required. Its routine use for the diagnosis of DVT should be discouraged when alternative non-invasive methods such as sonography are available.

Physiological methods

These tests reflect the haemodynamic effects of venous obstruction. They include simple continuous-wave hand-held Doppler and various types of plethysmography such as impedance, air and photo-plethysmography. Extrinsic venous compression is applied with cuffs. Local physiological response is measured by assessing changes such as electrical impedance, or light reflected from the dermal venous plexus, as a reflection of venous capacitance, emptying and refilling. Impedance plethysmography is the most extensively documented and used of these methods.

Studies have shown reasonably high sensitivities and specificities for these methods [7-9] and they require relatively little training to perform. They are consistently less accurate than venography or ultrasonography, with a comparatively high false positive or equivocal rate, and are unsatisfactory in the diagnosis of asymptomatic DVT [10]. They also show much lower predictive values for distal as opposed to proximal DVT. They do however provide physiological information that is not available from more direct imaging methods such as venography and ultrasonography, and when initially abnormal, are useful for assessing resolution of obstructive changes due to recanalisation or collateral formation. Plethysmographic methods are still commonly used in the initial diagnosis of DVT in centres with access to a dedicated vascular laboratory or when more definitive diagnostic tests are not freely available.

Biochemical assays

D-dimer is a product formed by the interaction of fibrin and plasmin, and elevated D-dimer levels are associated with the presence of DVT [11-13]. However, increased levels are also seen in many different pathologies such as infection and malignancy. They therefore have a high sensitivity but low specificity in the diagnosis of DVT with negative predictive values of up to 98% and positive predictive values as low as 50% for proximal vein and 8.2% for distal vein thrombus [11,12,15]. Another recognised cause of variability in results is the wide variety of different assays available [7,14]. D-dimer estimation is thus best used as part of an overall diagnostic strategy for DVT in conjunction with other tests. The combination of D-dimer testing and RPA alone increases positive and negative predictive value for DVT significantly, and the addition of another objective test such as plethysmography or ultrasonography increases them further [2,3,9,12]. It must be noted that a negative D-dimer test makes DVT very unlikely but does not exclude it entirely, so that high-risk patients require further imaging or serial follow-up [16].

Duplex ultrasonography

Colour duplex ultrasonography (CDU) is now considered the method of choice in the imaging of acute symptomatic DVT. It is non-invasive and inexpensive and provides detailed anatomic and flow information. It is greatly preferred to venography by patients. It can differentiate extrinsic compression from thrombus, identify collaterals and venous recanalisation in chronic venous disease and diagnose other causes of calf swelling such as ruptured Baker's cysts, thrombophlebitis or haematomas. Thrombophlebitis should not be ignored because thrombus in the saphenous veins at or near the junctions can extend into the deep venous systems and may require anticoagulation [17]. CDU is also extremely accurate. It is the best test for above-knee DVT and compares favourably with venography for below knee thrombus [18,19]. Factors that limit its more widespread usage are availability, the operator-dependent nature of duplex and the time required to perform a complete lower limb examination. Technical difficulty in duplex assessment and decreased sensitivity and specificity in the detection of distal thrombus may be caused by the number of calf veins, their small calibre and relatively low flow. An experienced operator can perform an above-knee vein examination in a few minutes but may require another 15-20 minutes to assess all calf veins fully. This has been one of the major factors leading to the evaluation of whether simpler forms of examination can satisfactorily be used to identify clinically relevant DVT.

Is it necessary to evaluate calf veins?

Management of infrapopliteal thrombus and whether calf veins should be routinely imaged remain one of the most contentious issues in deep vein thrombosis, and opinions vary according to clinician and centre. Reasons for treating calf vein thrombus are the potential risk of extension and pulmonary embolus (PE), the risk of post-phlebitic syndrome, and the possibility of recurrent thromboembolic disease.

The risk of PE is probably of most importance. Conventional wisdom holds that patients with infrapopliteal DVT should be anticoagulated because of the risk of pulmonary embolus, and indeed approximately 20% of below-knee DVT may extend proximally and propagate, and about 10% of these patients will have PE. However, the potential risk of PE in untreated patients with below-knee DVT is only 2% [20]. Many other clinicians feel that this order of risk does not warrant anticoagulation in isolated below-knee DVT with the attendant potential complications of treatment, costs and difficulties to patients. Serial investigation will detect those patients who develop proximal extension who are then at higher risk. Routine calf vein imaging is also time-consuming and expensive and a recent study by Kim *et al* has indicated that it is not cost-effective [21].

The potential long-term risk of post-phlebitic syndrome is another reason often quoted for treatment of infrapopliteal DVT. The role of isolated calf thrombus in the causation of post-phlebitic syndrome, remains uncertain. The pathophysiology of development of significant residual obstruction or valvular reflux after DVT is complex, and the main risk of development of post-phlebitic symptoms relates to above-knee DVT and in particular ilio-femoral thrombus. Venographic studies have been quoted by Rutherford [22] as showing that the majority (up to 95%) of popliteal or tibial thromboses recanalise completely. Recanalisation of thrombus involving the femoral segment is less frequent at about 50%, and although partial resolution may occur, less than 20% of iliofemoral DVT recanalise completely. Opinions vary as to whether serious post-phlebitic complications are frequent or uncommon with isolated calf thrombus [22-24]. The role of anticoagulation in the prevention of this condition is also still uncertain [22].

There is also a low frequency of recurrent thromboembolic disease (<2% serially tested patients) in isolated calf vein DVT if proximal extension does not occur [25].

Compression ultrasound - a simpler test

The clinical considerations above, and difficulties in providing full duplex ultrasonography as a screening test for DVT, has led to consideration of whether more limited tests can be used effectively for diagnosis and treatment.

The normal vein has phasic flow, fills with colour and collapses completely on compression. The single most useful ultrasound parameter for vein normality is complete compressibility. Many studies have now been performed assessing the ability of limited compression ultrasound scans (CUS) to diagnose femoropopliteal DVT [26-28] (II). This is because thrombus isolated to a single short segment (e.g. mid-superficial femoral vein) is extremely rare affecting 0 - 2.4% of DVT documented with venography or ultrasound in symptomatic patients [29,30]. If the common femoral and popliteal veins are fully compressible, clinically significant acute above-knee DVT can be excluded. The technique is simple, fast and requires little operator training and skill.

These studies suggest that simpler, limited compression scans will diagnose 99% of symptomatic femoropopliteal DVT. However, if CUS is the sole method used for evaluation, data indicate that serial rescanning is required to exclude thrombus extension. In earlier studies up to 5 rescans could be performed with 15-25% repeat scans positive [26,27]. A more recent multicentre outcome study involving 1702 patients extended compression to include the distal popliteal vein (3-point compression) with only one repeat scan a week later [28] (II). In a 6 month follow-up only 0.7% patients in whom both scans were normal presented with thrombosis or embolism and 0.1% died of PE. The pick-up rate from the second scan was also very low at only 3% (12/412) of the total number of abnormal scans and <1% (12/1300) of all patients rescanned. Simple CUS is therefore a very safe and accurate test for the diagnosis of clinically relevant DVT (B). As serial scanning is expensive and inconvenient, CUS is best used in combination with risk probability assessment and/or D-dimers to optimise pick-up rate and decrease the need for follow-up scans [8,13,31].

Asymptomatic patients

It is important to note that CUS is most suited to assessment of the acute symptomatic patient without previous venous problems. The sensitivity of ultrasound when blinded to venography was only

62% in a trial of asymptomatic patients [32]. Sensitivities for impedance plethysmography fall from the 87-100% range in symptomatic patients to as low as 13% for asymptomatic patients [31,33]. Caution should be exercised in patients who are asymptomatic or have a previous history of DVT, venous insufficiency or high risk factors, and if CUS is negative or equivocal in these patients, further serial scanning, full duplex or venography must be considered.

Other methods of imaging

Radioisotope scintigraphy

(125)I-labelled fibrinogen is sensitive in the detection of developing thrombus. It was used frequently in post-operative patients but is unable to detect established thrombus and unsuitable for the diagnosis of clinically suspected acute symptomatic DVT [34,35]. It is now of historical interest only owing to the availability of better tests and the risk of blood-borne infection. Other methods have included injection of autologous Tc-labelled red blood cells [36] and indium-111-labelled platelets [37]; it is improbable that these will gain common usage when more accurate non-invasive methods are available.

Contrast-enhanced CT scanning

CT is not used as a primary modality for investigation of DVT as it involves radiation and administration of contrast, although pelvic and abdominal venous thrombosis is readily diagnosed. It is capable of diagnosing lower extremity DVT, however. In a recent study, spiral CT pulmonary angiography for suspected pulmonary embolism was extended to include imaging of the lower limb in the venous phase during the same scanning episode. Exact correlation with ultrasound findings for femoropopliteal DVT was found in 19/71 patients scanned [38].

Magnetic resonance imaging

Magnetic resonance imaging has not been widely used for venous imaging but shows considerable potential. Earlier studies have demonstrated flow-related changes in occluded or partially occluded veins with varying techniques (spin-echo, gradient-echo or time-of-flight). Comparisons of MRI, venography and duplex have found sensitivities and specificities of up to 100% for detection of proximal thrombus and 97% for distal thrombus [39,40]. Intraluminal thrombus has been directly visualised by Moody et al [41] using a 3-D blood and fat suppressed sequence which relies on the formation of methaemoglobin. Changes in the signal over time may indicate the chronicity of the thrombus. MRI will undoubtedly play a larger part in the imaging of vascular disease as availability and experience increase.

St George's experience and diagnostic imaging algorithm

Limited 3-point colour compression ultrasound for diagnosis of acute DVT was introduced in our centre in mid-1998. A same-day service is provided by the radiology department for patients presenting to the casualty or out-patients departments. Patients who present outside working hours are given a therapeutic dose of low molecular weight heparin (LMWH) and scanned the next morning. Second scans were initially performed on all patients, but the introduction of risk probability assessment and D-dimer estimation has decreased the number performed. Scans are performed by all personnel in the department as the technique is simple. Scans by staff new to the method are checked by more senior personnel for 2-3 months. Even inexperienced personnel appear able to confidently exclude or diagnose definite above-knee DVT after performing 5-10 scans although experienced colleagues will find fewer scans equivocal. Preliminary audit has confirmed that it is an accurate and safe method of diagnosis with less than 1% of patients with negative scans re-presenting with venous thromboembolic disease within 6 months. This is comparable to the previous studies quoted and comparable to negative venography [4]. One important consequence of introducing such a policy is that although the scans are simple to perform, demand has increased significantly. The number of requests for imaging has tripled since 1996 and continues to rise with a significant drop in the percentage of positive scans (Figure 1).

Figure 1 Figures are shown projected to the end of 2000. Prior to 1996 mainly venography was performed. In 1997 duplex imaging was introduced as first line for diagnosis of DVT and in 1998 immediate access compression USS with follow-up scanning was commenced. The number of positive diagnoses doubled in 1997 from previous years but since then has remained static while the numbers of scans requested continues to rise.

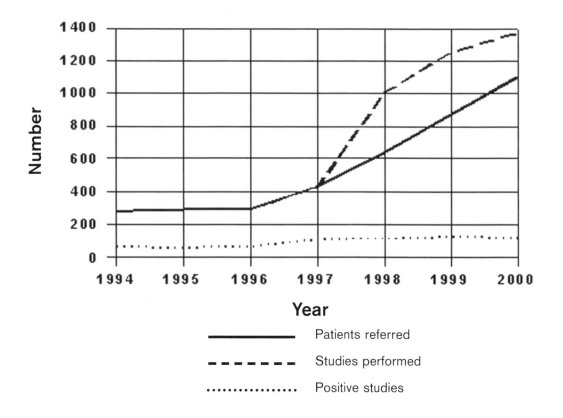

DVT IMAGING 1994-2000

The diagnostic algorithm that is used at present is shown in Figure 2.

Conclusion

The diagnostic strategy adopted in individual centres will depend on the diagnostic facilities available and the clinical practices of the clinicians involved. The demand for diagnostic tests means that full duplex ultrasonography for all patients cannot be achieved in the majority of centres, but data indicate that simpler methods are a viable option. Varying non-invasive methods such as plethysmography and simple compression ultrasound can be used but compression ultrasound is the most safe and accurate. Ideally serial scans should be performed in all patients with an initial negative scan, but this places an unacceptable workload on many departments and in practice is often not possible. To obtain maximal positive and negative predictive value and to decrease the number of unnecessary imaging requests, the objective test of choice should be combined with RPA and D-dimer estimation. Patients with low RPA and negative D-dimers who do not have follow-up scans should be advised to return for review if symptoms fail to resolve or worsen. Full colour duplex sonography by a skilled operator and venography should continue to be real options for patients with equivocal initial diagnoses and who are at high risk. For maximum benefit and cost-effectiveness in the management of DVT, if resources allow, consideration should be given

Figure 2 Screening protocol for patients presenting with possible acute symptomatic DVT.

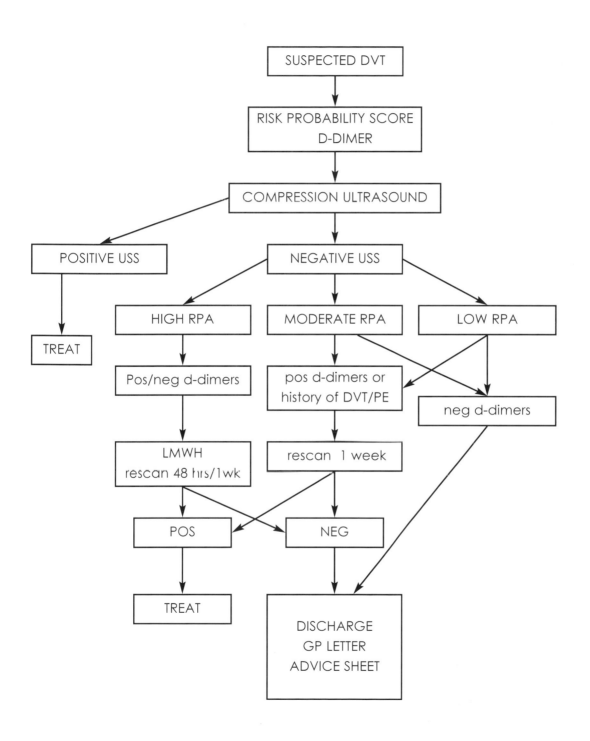

to establishing specific multi-disciplinary units for management of venous thrombosis with staff (e.g. specialist nurse-clinicians) who are trained in assessment and management of these patients when they present.

Summary

♦ A combination of simple tests such as compression ultrasound, risk probability assessment and D-dimer testing can be used to diagnose clinically significant acute symptomatic DVT **(I)**.

♦ Clinical evaluation with risk probability assessment will stratify patients into low, moderate and high risk groups **(I)**.

♦ If compression ultrasound is negative, moderate and low-risk patients with negative D-dimers can be discharged. Rescans should be performed on patients with positive D-dimers, and high-risk patients with negative D-dimers **(A)**.

♦ Full colour duplex or venography should continue to be an option on high risk patients, those with equivocal compression scans, or who have persisting symptoms **(B)**.

Further reading

1 Browse NL, Burnand KG, Lea Thomas M. *Diseases of the Veins: Pathology. Diagnosis and Treatment.* Edward Arnold (Hodder Stoughton), London UK, 1998.

2 Zwiebel WJ. *Introduction to Vascular Sonography (4th Edition).* WB Saunders, Philadelphia, 2000.

References

1 Anand SS, Wells PS, Hunt D *et al*. Does this patient have deep vein thrombosis? *JAMA* 1998; 279: 1094-1099.

2 Wells PS, Hirsh J, Anderson DR. Accuracy of clinical assessment of deep vein thrombosis. *Lancet* 1995; 345: 1326-1330.

3 Wells PS, Anderson DR, Bormanis J *et al*. Value of assessment of pre-test probability of deep vein thrombosis in clinical management. *Lancet* 1997; 350: 1795-1798.

4 Leclerc J, Illescas F, Jarzem P. Diagnosis of Deep Vein Thrombosis, Leclerc J (editor). In: *Venous Thromboembolic Disorders.* Lea and Febiger, 1991; 176-228.

5 Kalodiki E, Nicolaides AN, Al-Kutoubi A *et al*. How "gold" is the standard? Interobservers' variation on venograms. *International Angiology* 1998; 17: 83-88.

6 Wille-Jorgensen P, Borris L, Jorgensen LN . Phlebography as the gold standard in thromboprophylactic studies? A multicentre interobserver variation study. *Acta Radiol* 1992; 33: 24-28.

7 Comerota AJ, Katz ML, Grossi RJ *et al*. The comparative value of non-invasive testing for diagnosis and surveillance of deep vein thrombosis. *J Vasc Surg* 1998; 7: 40-49.

8 Kearon C, Julian JA, Newman TE, Ginsberg JS. Noninvasive diagnosis of deep venous thrombosis. *Ann Intern Med* 1998; 128: 663-677.

9 Thomas PRS, Butler CM, Bowman J *et al*. Light reflection rheography: an effective non-invasive technique for screening patients with suspected deep vein thrombosis. *Br J Surg* 1991; 78: 207-209.

10 Agnelli G, Cosmi B, Radicchia S *et al*. Features of thrombi and diagnostic accuracy of impedance plethysmography in symptomatic and asymptomatic deep vein thrombosis. *Thrombosis and Haemostasis* 1993; 70: 266-269.

11 Brill-Edwards P, Lee A. D-dimer testing in the diagnosis of acute venous thromboembolism. *Thrombosis and Haemostasis* 1999; 82: 688-694.

12 Aschwanden M, Labs KH, Jenneret C at al. The value of rapid D-dimer testing combined with structured clinical evaluation for the diagnosis of deep vein thrombosis. *J Vasc Surg* 1999; 30: 929-935.

13 Bernardi E, Prandoni P, Lensing A *et al*. D-dimer testing as an adjunct to ultrasonography in patients with clinically suspected deep vein thrombosis: prospective cohort study. *BMJ* 1998; 317: 1037-1040.

14 Dale S, Gogstad GO, Brosstad F *et al*. Comparison of three D-dimer assays for the diagnosis of DVT: ELISA, latex and an immunofiltration assay (Byco Card D-dimer). *Thrombosis and Haemostasis* 1994; 71, 270-274.

15 Wells PS, Brill-Edwards P, Stevens P *et al*. A novel and rapid whole-blood assay for D-dimer in patients with clinically suspected deep vein thrombosis. *Circulation* 1995; 91: 2184-2187.

16 Farrell S, Hayes T, Shaw M. A negative SimpliRED D-dimer assay result does not exclude the diagnosis of deep vein thrombosis or pulmonary embolus in emergency department patients. *Ann Emerg Med* 2000; 35: 121-125.

17 Chengelis DL, Bendick PJ, Glover JL *et al*. Progression of superficial venous thrombosis to deep vein thrombosis. *J Vasc Surg* 1996: 24: 745-749.

18   Rosen MP, McArdle C. Controversies in the use of lower extremity sonography in the diagnosis of acute deep vein thrombosis and a proposal for a unified approach: Seminars in CT, US and MR 1997; 18: 362-368.

19   Mattos MA, Londrey GL, Leutz DW *et al.* Colour flow duplex scanning for the surveillance and diagnosis of acute deep vein thrombosis. *J Vasc Surg* 1992; 15: 366-375.

20   Moser KM, LeMoine JR. Is embolic risk conditioned by location of deep venous thrombosis? *Ann Intern Med* 1981; 94: 439-444.

21   Kim HZ, Kuntz KM, Cronan JJ. Optimal management strategy for use of compression ultrasound for management of deep venous thrombosis in symptomatic patients; a cost-effectiveness analysis. *Acad Radiol* 2000; 7: 67-76.

22   Rutherford RB. Pathogenesis and pathophysiology of the post-phlebitic syndrome. *Sem Vasc Surg* 1996; 9: 21-25.

23   Browse NL, Clemenson G, Thomas ML. Is the post-phlebitic leg always post-phlebitic? Relation between phlebographic appearances of deep vein thrombosis and late sequelae. *BMJ* 1980; 2: 1167-1170.

24   Moneta GL, Nehler MR, Chitwood RW, Porter JM. The natural history, pathophysiology and non-operative treatment of chronic venous insufficiency. In: *Vascular Surgery*, Rutherford RB, Ed. WB Saunders, 1995; 1837-1850.

25   Leclerc J. Natural history of venous thromboembolism. In: *Venous Thromboembolic Disorders*, Leclerc J, Ed. Lee and Febiger, 1991; 166-175.

26   Pezzullo JA, Perkins AB, Cronan JJ. Symptomatic deep vein thrombosis; diagnosis with limited compression US. *Rad* 1996; 198: 67-70.

27   Frederick MG, Hertzberg BS, Kliewer MA *et al.* Can the examination for lower extremity DVT be abbreviated? A prospective study of 755 examinations. *Rad* 1996; 199: 45-47.

28   Cogo A, Lensing AW, Koupman MM, et al. Compression Ultrasonography for diagnostic management of patients with clinically suspected DVT: prospective multicentre cohort study. *BMJ* 1998; 316, 17-20.

29   Cogo A, Lensing AW, Prandoni P *et al.* Distribution of thrombosis in patients with symptomatic deep vein thrombosis. *Arch Intern Med* 1993; 153: 2777-2780.

30   Markel A, Manzo RA, Bergelin RO *et al.* Pattern and distribution of thrombi in acute venous thrombosis. *Arch Surg* 1992; 127: 305-312.

31   Lynch TG, Dalsing MC, Ouriel K *et al.* Developments in diagnosis and classification of venous disorders: non-invasive diagnosis. *Cardiovasc Surg* 1999; 7: 160-178.

32   Agnelli G, Radicchia S, Nenci GG. Diagnosis of deep vein thrombosis in asymptomatic high-risk patients. *Haemostasis* 1995; 25: 40-48.

33   Cruickshank MK Levine MN Hirsh J *et al.* An evaluation of impedance plethysmography and 125I fibrinogen leg scanning in patients following hip surgery. *Thrombosis and Haemostasis*, 1989; 62: 830-834.

34   Lensing AWA Hirsh J. 125I fibrinogen leg scanning: reassessment of its role for the diagnosis of venous thrombosis in post-operative patients. *Thrombosis and Haemostasis*, 1993; 69: 2-7.

35   Weinmann EE, Slazman EW. Deep vein thrombosis. *New Engl J Med*, 1994; 331: 1630-1641.

36   Leclerc JR, Wolfson C, Arzoumanian A *et al.* Tc-99m red blood cell venography in patients with clinically suspected deep vein thrombosis : a prospective study. *J Nuc Med* 1988; 29: 1498-1506.

37   Ezekowitz M, Pope CF, Sostman HD. Indium111 platelet scintigraphy for the diagnosis of acute venous thrombosis. *Circulation* 1986; 73: 668-674.

38   Loud PA, Katz DS, Klippinstein DL *et al.* Combined CT venography and pulmonary angiography in suspected thromboembolic disease: diagnostic accuracy for deep venous evaluation. *AJR* 2000; 174: 61-65.

39   Carpenter JP, Holland GA, Baum RA, Owen RS. Magnetic resonance venography for the detection of deep venous thrombosis: comparison with contrast venography and duplex Dopper ultrasonography. *J Vasc Surg* 1993; 18: 734-741.

40   Evans AJ, Sostman HD, Knelson MH *et al.* Detection of deep venous thrombosis: prospective comparison of MR imaging with contrast venography. *AJR* 1993; 16: 131-139.

41   Moody AR, Pollock JG, O'Connor AR, Bagnall M. Lower limb deep venous thrombosis: direct MR imaging of the thrombus. *Radiology* 1998; 20: 349-355.

The diagnosis of deep venous thrombosis

Chapter 20

Infrainguinal bypass

Shirley A Murray Clinical Research Nurse

Judith G McClements Vascular Ward Sister

Paul HB Blair Consultant Vascular Surgeon

REGIONAL VASCULAR UNIT, ROYAL VICTORIA HOSPITAL, BELFAST, NORTHERN IRELAND

Introduction

Although infrainguinal bypass surgery for patients with claudication continues to be performed, effective risk factor modification and exercise clinics have led to a much more conservative management of claudicants. This chapter outlines the pathway of care for those patients with critical ischaemia requiring infrainguinal bypass surgery. Space does not permit a comprehensive discussion and therefore only selected areas have been included.

The clinical definition of critical limb ischaemia (CLI) may vary slightly but, in general, it is defined as "severe rest pain or the presence of ulceration or gangrene with a low ankle artery pressure (< 40-60mmHg)" [1] **(I)**. The report of a national survey of the Vascular Surgical Society of Great Britain and Ireland, published in 1995 revealed that the condition is common, affecting 1 in 2500 of the population on an annual basis. This represents a major burden on hospital services with mean mortality and amputation rates of 13.5 and 21.5% respectively [2] **(II)**. Patients with CLI are often elderly and have co-morbid medical problems: up to 30% may present with diabetes in addition to significant cardio-respiratory disease **(II)**. These patients are often admitted as emergencies or directly from the out-patient clinic and represent a major challenge to the vascular team, as they require urgent assessment and treatment, if limb salvage is to be achieved.

General assessment

A thorough history should identify risk factors and co-morbid medical conditions in addition to life-style risks. Limb examination should include signs of ischaemia, absent pulses, poor skin nutrition, loss of hair and cool temperature. There may be pallor on foot elevation, redness due to injured dilated superficial capillaries and reduced toe and foot movement. Confirmation of the degree of ischaemia should be undertaken by a non-invasive means to confirm the diagnosis of critical ischaemia. It is important to be aware of the patient's life-style and expectations.

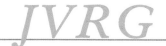

Although outcomes of care are frequently less predictable in patients with CLI, identification of specific nursing requirements, the patients' home circumstances and provisional discharge planning need to be considered at an early stage in the pathway. Patients with CLI often have a morbid fear of amputation and these fears should be addressed [3]. Particular care should be paid to pain control, nutrition, hydration, pressure care area and specific ulcer treatment **(A)**.

Nutrition

The importance of nutrition in hospital patients was highlighted in the 1992 publication of the Kings Fund Centre. This report provided evidence that illness was frequently associated with malnutrition and that appropriate nutritional support conferred significant clinical benefits [4] **(I)**. The potential financial savings in the UK NHS, resulting from appropriate use of the nutritional support, were estimated to be £266 million. Failure to recognise and treat malnutrition in hospital patients may be due to lack of training and knowledge of medical nursing staff, lack of interest and failure to regard nutrition as important and the lack of organisation of nutritional services within a hospital linking relevant disciplines. Disease related malnutrition is associated with impairment in functional capacity, immune function and wound healing and is associated with an increased incidence of complications and poor clinical outcomes [5] **(I)**.

Due to their reduced mobility, co-morbid medical problems and social circumstances, a vascular patient may present in a pre-existing malnourished state. The problem is then compounded by drowsiness induced by opiate analgesia and intermittent fasting prior to certain diagnostic and therapeutic procedures. These patients are therefore at significant risk of problems with wound healing and the development of pressure ulcers in addition to reduced healing capacity of their presenting lower limb ulceration. It has been demonstrated that very simple measures such as supplementation of a normal hospital diet with oral sip feeds may have a significant benefit [6]. Potential nutritional problems should therefore be recognised as early as possible using a nutritional assessment tool and appropriate steps taken during the pre- and post-operative period **(A)**. Early involvement of the dietician and multi-disciplinary nutrition team may be required.

Pain control

Pain control is dealt with in the chapters on acute and chronic pain. It is important to assess and monitor a patient's analgesia requirement carefully. Excessive drowsiness can occur, leading to poor hydration and reduced nutritional intake.

Pressure area care

Guidelines concerning pressure ulcer risk assessment and prevention have recently been produced by the National Institute for Clinical Excellence [7] **(A)**. A patient's potential to develop pressure ulcers may be influenced by a variety of intrinsic risk factors, which should be considered when performing a risk assessment. The risk assessment should take place within 6 hours of the patient's admission, preferably using a chosen risk assessment tool with appropriate formal documentation. The risk factors are summarised in Table 1.

Potential extrinsic factors that may be involved in tissue damage include pressure, shearing and friction and attempts should be made to remove or diminish these factors. Skin inspection should occur regularly, particularly of the most vulnerable areas i.e. heels, sacrum and ischial tuberosities **(A)**. Healthcare professionals should be aware of the following signs, which may indicate incipient pressure ulcer development; persistent erythema, non-blanching hyperaemia, blisters, discoloration, localised oedema and/or induration. In those patients with darkly pigmented skin, purplish bluish localised areas of skin may occur.

Water-filled gloves; synthetic and genuine sheepskin; and doughnut-type devices should not be used. Patients deemed at risk of pressure ulceration should be repositioned with the frequency determined by the results of skin inspection and with due consideration for the patient's medical condition and

Table 1 Intrinsic risk factors associated with the development of pressure ulcers.

- Reduced mobility or immobility

- Sensory impairment

- Acute illness

- Level of consciousness

- Extremes of age

- Vascular disease

- Severe chronic or terminal illness

- Previous history of pressure damage

- Malnutrition and dehydration

comfort **(A)**. Where appropriate, pressure-relieving devices should be considered. Static overlays, mattresses and cushions may be employed to conform to the patient's shape and redistribute weight over a larger surface. Alternating pressure mattresses use inflation and deflation of sealed cells while high air loss therapy uses warm air circulated through a bed of ceramic beads. NICE are currently updating the guidelines in this area.

Thromboprophylaxis

The majority of patients with critical limb ischaemia are bed or chair bound. DVT prophylaxis in the form of low molecular weight heparin should be given pre- and post-operatively in addition to low-dose aspirin. The morning dose of heparin should be omitted on the day of surgery to avoid the risk of dural haematoma associated with epidural anaesthesia. Although rare, heparin induced thrombocytopenia can occur and platelet counts should be monitored according to standard protocols in patients receiving long-term therapeutic doses of low molecular weight heparin **(C)**.

Local management of ischaemic ulceration

Dressings

Patients with critical limb ischaemia often present with dry necrosis and only simple dressings are therefore required. In general the primary aim is to revascularise the limb, followed by debridement or some degree of minor amputation if required. The application of expensive wound dressings seems of little value until the factors that are responsible for delayed wound healing have been identified and addressed. The ideal dressing should maintain a moist wound environment by maintaining thermal insulation, be highly absorbable and permeable to bacteria, free of contaminants, non-adherent and non-toxic [8] **(II)**. A brief overview of dressings that create optimum wound environment is given below:

- **Alginates** made from seaweed can be composed of galuronic and mannuronic acid, are best used in moderate to highly exudating wounds.

- **Hydrocolloids** consist of a mixture of pectins, gelatines carboxymethylcellulose and elastomers.

They create an environment that encourages autolysis and are particularly useful for sloughy or necrotic wounds. The dressing should be large enough to cover the wound with an overlap of at least 2 cms. Hydrocolloid dressings are waterproof, facilitating bathing or showering.

◆ **Hydrogels** can be used as a sheet or in a gel form. The gels are extremely moist facilitating autolysis in necrotic wounds, although maceration and excoriation of the surrounding skin may occur due to leakage of the gel and exudate. A protective barrier film should be employed if this occurs [9] **(C)**.

Larval therapy

Although they have been used for many centuries, there has been a recent revival in larval therapy. They are particularly useful for debridement of necrotic wounds in patients for whom surgical debridement may not be the best option. They are applied when 2-3 mms long, and if the conditions are favourable they rapidly increase in size to 8-10 mms in length when removed. They use powerful proteolytic enzymes to break down and liquefy necrotic tissue. They should be applied to the wound as soon as possible, after delivery, if this is not possible they should be stored in a cool, dark place at a temperature of 8-10°. After a period of 48-72 hours, the larvae should be removed and disposed of by incineration [10] **(C)**.

Although sterile larvae have been produced commercially for some years, some patients find the concept unacceptable and should not be pressurised into accepting larvae therapy.

Assessment for intervention

The ultimate aim of successful infrainguinal bypass surgery should be a pain-free patient with a functional limb. Prospective studies have shown that following successful infrainguinal arterial reconstruction, patients with critical ischaemia do obtain immediate and lasting improvement in health related quality of life [11]. Activities of daily living and pain scores have been shown to improve significantly after successful reconstruction

and primary amputation, although mobility was only improved by successful reconstruction [12] **(II)**. Figure 1 outlines an algorithm for the management of a patient with CLI.

Primary amputation should be considered where there is necrosis and destruction of significant weight bearing areas of the foot (see chapter on amputation). A fixed flexion deformity of the limb or limited life expectancy due to terminal illness or grave co-morbid medical conditions should also be considered as indications for primary amputation **(B)**. The worst case scenario is the frail elderly patient who undergoes an unsuccessful vascular reconstruction and ultimately comes to amputation several weeks after their admission. It has been estimated that median inpatient and rehabilitation costs in such a patient may be in excess of £17,000 as opposed to £4320 for a successful distal bypass [13]. Although successful reconstructive surgery is the ultimate goal it should be appreciated that problems occurring as a result of delayed wound healing, episodes of recurrent ischaemia and the need for repeat operations can occur despite initial successful bypass surgery. In a retrospective series of 112 patients, repeat operations to maintain graft patency, treat wound complications or treat recurrent or contra-lateral ischaemia were required in 61 patients. The surgical ideal of an uncomplicated procedure with long-term symptom relief, maintenance of functional status and no recurrence or repeat operations was only achieved in 16 of 112 patients [14]. A large retrospective study of patients treated in the Veterans Affairs system has attempted to identify risk factors associated with post-operative mortality in patients undergoing femorodistal bypass. Patients who died were older and four times more likely to have had a recent MI, twice as likely to have had heart failure and four times as likely to have been on dialysis at the time of surgery [15]. Age in itself does not appear to preclude successful bypass surgery as the results of lower extremity reconstruction in octogenarians would appear to be comparable to those reported for younger patients [16] **(II)**.

Patients with end stage renal disease constitute a particularly difficult group with regard to infrainguinal bypass surgery. A recent review of these patients has reported a 2-year survival rate of 49%, peri-operative

Figure 1 Algorithm for the management of a patient with chronic critical limb ischaemia (CLI).

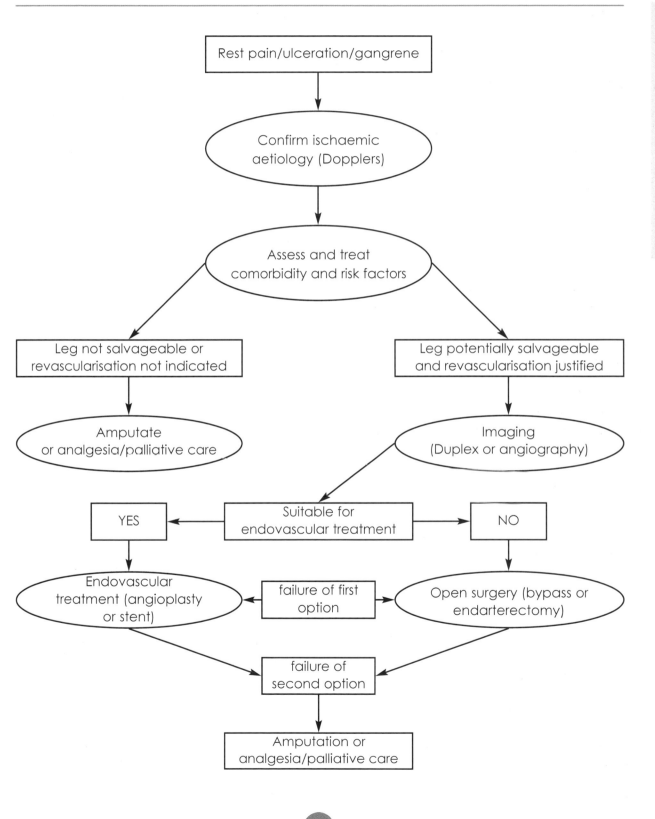

mortality rate of 9%, early graft thrombosis rate of 14% and a 14% amputation rate in the presence of a functioning graft [17] **(II)**. A recent retrospective review of dialysis dependent patients undergoing infra-inguinal bypass surgery has reported more encouraging results with a peri-operative mortality of 1.3% and a 4-year survival, primary, and secondary patency rates of 51%, 60% and 86% respectively. Of 78 patients with end stage renal disease undergoing bypass surgery, 16 required amputation, 9 in whom the graft was still patent. The only absolute predictor of limb loss, despite a patent graft, appeared to be the presence of a healed ulcer more than 4 cms in diameter [18]. Although not documented in the literature, patients with rheumatoid arthritis often fair badly in terms of delayed wound healing following bypass surgery **(III)**.

The management of a chair or bed bound patient can be particularly difficult. Pre-operative independence and mobility have been shown to predict post-operative independence and mobility after bypass surgery for critical limb ischaemia. Of 25 survivors who were not living independently before surgery, only 1 achieved independent living 6 months post-operatively. Undertaking extensive revascularisation in the hope of achieving independence in a previously dependent patient is unlikely [19].

Obtaining informed consent requires discussion with the patient and the patient's family, and should bear the above points in mind **(C)**. An information leaflet explaining the risks and benefits of surgery helps this process (see website).

Time does not usually permit a lengthy formal cardio-respiratory assessment of these patients. Frequently, sufficient information can be gleaned from adequate history and examination, chest x-ray, ECG and routine blood investigations. Blood gases, respiratory function tests and measurement of left ventricular function may be useful but the ability to perform distal bypass surgery under epidural anaesthesia allows most patients to proceed to surgery. Transfusion is not usually required and group and save is usually sufficient unless there is pre-existing anaemia.

Specific investigations

Imaging techniques are discussed in the chapter on day-case angiography. The choice of pre-operative imaging technique depends on local resources and experience. The majority of patients will require angiography, which remains the commonest pre-operative imaging technique. The x-ray request should mention the diagnosis of critical ischaemia and stress the importance of obtaining images of the distal foot vessels. CO_2 angiography should be considered for patients with renal impairment although frequently only the proximal vessels may be imaged satisfactorily. The films can be supplemented with MR angiogram of the calf and foot vessels. Gadolinium enhanced MR angiography can produce images of an extremely high quality comparable to conventional digital subtraction views, although this facility may not be available in all hospitals. Completely non-invasive assessment by duplex arteriography has been reported from several units. Employing duplex arteriography to direct infrainguinal bypass surgery has provided similar patency limb salvage rates compared with contrast arteriography [20]. The procedure, however, requires a highly skilled technician and is time consuming. Duplex evaluation can be useful when contrast angiography does not reveal any pedal vessel. This may be as a result of very poor proximal flow and a distal vessel suitable for distal anastomosis may be detected by this technique **(C)**.

Treatment options

It is not uncommon to identify several levels of disease in patients with critical limb ischaemia. Aorto-iliac disease should be treated first by endovascular and/or surgical means, depending on the extent of the disease and patient fitness. Consideration should be given to an endovascular technique since the combination of a surgical inflow procedure and concomitant distal bypass increases the operating time and constitutes an increased risk to the patient. Alternatively axillo-femoral or femoro-femoral cross over surgery may be required. Occasionally if the profunda artery is of good calibre and the patient has minimal tissue loss, then no further procedure may be required. However, if significant ulceration or gangrene exists, a more distal bypass will usually be required **(C)** (Figure 2).

Figure 2 Possible infrainguinal revascularisation options in a patient with CLI. Angioplasty (a) should be considered but may need to be extensive with the risk of re-occlusion. A femoropopliteal bypass (b) may fail to reperfuse the foot unless at least one tibial artery is patent. Extensive tissue loss often requires a tibial bypass (c), especially in diabetics.

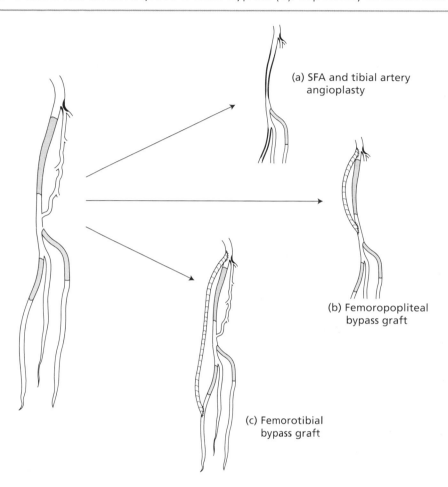

(a) SFA and tibial artery angioplasty

(b) Femoropopliteal bypass graft

(c) Femorotibial bypass graft

Reprinted from 'Vascular and Endovascular Surgery', 2nd Edition, Beard JD and Gaines PA (eds), by permission of the publisher, WB Saunders, © 2001.

Some patients may be suitable for infrainguinal endovascular intervention. Although the results are not as durable as bypass surgery, the short-term effects may facilitate ulcer healing with re-occlusion not necessarily resulting in clinical deterioration [21]. Endovascular techniques should be considered in patients unfit for surgery and promising results have been reported with sub-intimal angioplasty by a few centres [22] **(II)**.

Operating room care

Infrainguinal bypass surgery for critical limb ischaemia can be a lengthy procedure and appropriate care of the patient in the operating theatre is important. Hypothermia, hypoxia and blood loss are poorly tolerated therefore appropriate monitoring and support measures should be employed.

Anaesthetised patients are subject to prolonged pressure on dependent body parts due to gravity compressing the patient's skin and muscle between the bones and the operating table. Prolonged pressure has the potential to damage skin integrity while anaesthetic agents contribute by lowering blood pressure and reducing tissue perfusion. Pooling from prep solutions, skin shearing and friction during positioning and indeed the use of positioning devices themselves may increase the risk of pressure ulcer development [23]. An extensive review of the importance of the operating theatre in the development of pressure ulcers has recently been published [24] **(I)**. Twenty-two articles were reviewed. The most common statistically significant risk factor appeared to be time on the operating table mattress. Several studies identified the standard operating theatre mattress to be a significant risk factor in prolonged operations. Placing the patients directly on a warming blanket has also been criticised because of the correlation with pressure ulcer formation. Most studies suggested that a dry visco-elastic polymer pad or gel pad reduced pressure better than foam overlays and standard operating room mattresses. Static air mattresses appear to offer the most protection, however, they require further assessment with regard to maintaining the position of the surgical patient. The reviewed research suggested that every pre-operative assessment should include an evaluation of skin integrity and pressure ulcer risk factors. A nursing plan should be formulated and implemented based on the type and length of the surgical procedure, patient position, positioning devices to be used and identified patient risk factors **(A)**.

Choice of conduit

The majority of patients with critical limb ischaemia require bypass surgery to infrageniculate vessels. Where possible autologous saphenous vein should be used as it has the best patency and is less likely to cause problems with infection [25] **(A)**. Pre-operative duplex ultrasound mapping can help with identification of adequate vein and may facilitate marking of the vein pre-operatively [26,27]. Several studies have shown that there does not appear to be a significant difference in patency between *in situ* and reversed saphenous vein graft for femoropopliteal and femorodistal bypass procedures [28-32] **(I)**. Some centres have suggested the *in situ* technique is preferable when the vein is of

small calibre, however, the technique appears to have an increased requirement for secondary procedures.

When the ipsilateral saphenous vein is not available then alternative sites for vein harvest may be explored such as the contralateral long saphenous, short saphenous, superficial femoral, basilic or cephalic veins. Although it seems reasonable to use the best available saphenous vein from either leg, some surgeons prefer to avoid using the contralateral long saphenous vein as 20% of patients with critical limb ischaemia may require intervention in the contralateral limb [33]. Arm veins have been shown to be durable grafts and have been employed successfully in preference to the contralateral long saphenous vein [34] but they require careful handling and are more prone to aneurysmal dilatation [35]. When autologous vein is in short supply, splice vein reconstructions consisting of saphenous and basilic and cephalic veins can be employed. This is a time consuming procedure although patency rates similar to conventional vein graft techniques have been reported [36]. If vein length is short, profunda may be used as a suitable inflow vessel. Vein grafts performed to an isolated popliteal segment are unlikely to heal tissue ulceration or gangrene. An alternative is to perform a prosthetic femoropopliteal bypass with a vein extension to the crural vessel [37]. Similarly some centres have suggested intra-operation balloon angioplasty of the superficial femoral artery, followed by popliteal to distal bypass graft [38] **(III)**.

If autologous vein is not available or its removal is not desirable for reasons stated above, a prosthetic graft may be employed. Patency rates for prosthetic grafts to distal limb vessels are poor and as a result a variety of adjunctive techniques have been suggested. Construction of distal arteriovenous fistulas has been claimed to improve patency rates [37]. However, a recent prospective randomised trial failed to show a significant clinical advantage with the distal arteriovenous fistula [40] **(I)**. Interestingly this trial incorporated an interposition vein cuff at the distal anastomosis in all patients. The use of a vein cuff at the distal anastomosis has been shown to significantly improve patency rates for infra-popliteal grafts at 2 years [41] **(I)**. It therefore seems reasonable to employ a vein cuff at the distal anastomosis with a crural vessel if a synthetic graft is being employed **(B)**.

Technical considerations

Distal bypass surgery can be technically demanding and obsessive attention to detail is required. Procedures can be lengthy, ideally at least two experienced operators should take part to facilitate synchronous vein harvesting and proximal and distal vessel dissection. The distal vessel must be approached carefully to avoid damage and should be carefully inspected to facilitate an appropriate distal anastomotic site. Clamps and sloops may damage the distal vessel and intra-luminal occlusion devices or operating under tourniquet control may have some advantages. The distal anastomosis should be performed using some form of magnification with 7/0 polypropylene sutures. Care should be given to graft tunnelling to prevent kinking or twisting of the graft. It is important that whatever form of bypass is constructed, some form of intra-operative assessment should be performed on completion. Angiography, duplex ultrasonography or vascular endoscopy have all been employed. The optimal method of confirming technical adequacy is not clear. Surgical debridement of gangrenous lesions should be performed at the end of arterial reconstruction. Small dry necrotic lesions may be left for a secondary procedure as revascularisation may improve the situation dramatically. The operative wound should also be closed carefully, avoiding tension. A clear indication to the recovery room staff should be given regarding the presence or absence of pulses so that early graft closure may be detected **(C)**.

Systemic anticoagulation with intravenous heparin (5,000 units) is required during the procedure. A single dose of a broad-spectrum antibiotic (e.g. Augmentin) should be given intra-operatively.

Post-operative care

Perfusion of the distal limb should be inspected regularly to detect early signs of ischaemia. In particular records should be kept of the limb colour, temperature, capillary return, presence or absence of pulses and degree of pain. In some patients reperfusion can occasionally lead to a compartment syndrome requiring fasciotomy. Severe muscle pain or tenderness should be reported early. Vital signs should be recorded including heart rate, blood pressure, temperature, respiratory rate and oxygen saturation. Hypotension and dehydration should be avoided to reduce the risk of graft closure. Careful fluid balance is required in these patients who frequently have concomitant coronary heart disease **(B)**. If graft closure is detected early (within a few hours) some vein grafts can be salvaged in the operating theatre.

Wound care

Most surgical wounds heal relatively quickly by primary intention. A simple non-adherent dressing applied in theatre can be left for up to 48 hours and frequently no further dressings may be applied. If the dressing becomes blood stained or heavily soiled it should be replaced. In general, the less a wound is disturbed the better but it must be inspected once within the first 24-48 hours and thereafter if the patient complains of pain or discomfort **(C)**. It is not unusual to notice some degree of inflammation, swelling and redness 2-3 days post-operatively.

Mobility

Regular evaluation of the patient's pain control is particularly important in the post-operative period to allow early mobilisation. Epidural anaesthesia has a great advantage here as the infusion can be continued post-operatively (see acute pain chapter). Following distal bypass procedures, patients are usually nursed in bed for at least 24 hours and then are carefully mobilised to a chair within 48 hours. Mobilisation may then proceed depending on the patient's general health. Reperfusion oedema is a common problem following bypass surgery and it is important that patients elevate their feet while sitting out of bed. Wound healing in the foot may be compromised by peripheral oedema. Class I (TED) stockings can reduce the degree of oedema, however, they are probably best avoided in the initial few days until the graft beds down as they can cause compression of a superficially placed vein graft **(C)**.

Discharge planning

Plans for discharge will have been considered pre-operatively and should be reviewed early in the post-operative period with the multi-disciplinary team, especially the physiotherapist, social worker and occupational therapist. It is important to define the patient's social circumstances, their ability to perform activities of daily living and short or long-term care needs following discharge. Patients with CLI, like claudicants, require risk factor modification and life-style advice (see chapter on risk factor modification). A leaflet containing post-operative and health education advice, as well as a contact phone number should be supplied at discharge.

Adjuvant medical therapy following bypass surgery is usually employed in an attempt to improve graft patency and also to reduce morbidity and mortality from myocardial infarction and stroke (B). Some studies suggest aspirin in combination with dipyrimamole or ticlopidine improves graft patency [42], however only aspirin in prosthetic grafts and ticlodipine in vein grafts have been shown in well designed, double-blind, randomised controlled trials to reduce the risk of occlusion in infrainguinal bypass grafts [43] (A). Research for larger studies in the Netherlands has suggested no overall difference in treatment between oral anticoagulation and aspirin [44] (II). However, the risk of adverse effects from warfarin and the need for INR monitoring should be considered. The issue of graft surveillance is discussed in the relevant chapter.

Summary

♦ Critical limb ischaemia is a common condition with significant associated morbidity and mortality (I).

♦ Optimal care includes particular attention to nutrition, pain relief, pressure area and specific ulcer care (A).

♦ Patients presenting with critical limb ischaemia need careful assessment of their associated co-morbidities and risk factors (A).

♦ Reconstruction should be considered in terms of overall patient fitness and quality of life (B).

♦ Primary amputation may be the best option for some patients (II).

♦ Vein grafts achieve the best results for infrainguinal bypass (A).

♦ Alternative endovascular and prosthetic bypass procedures should be considered in unfit patients or when autologous vein is unavailable (B).

♦ Discharge planning should begin as soon as possible and include secondary prevention measures (A).

Further reading

1   Beard JD, Gaines PA. Treatment of chronic lower limb ischaemia. In: *Vascular and Endovascular Surgery*. 2nd Ed. WB Saunders, London, 2001.

2   Miller M, Glover D, Eds. *Wound Management theory and practice*. The Friary Press, Dorchester, Dorset. 1999.

References (grade I evidence and grade A recommendations in bold)

1   **Tyrrell MR, Wolfe JHN. Critical leg ischaemia: an appraisal of clinical definitions. *Br J Surg* 1993; 80: 177-80.**

2   Critical limb ischaemia: management and outcome. Report of a national survey. The Vascular Surgical Society of Great Britain and Ireland. *Eur J Vasc Endovasc Surg* 1995; 10:103-13.

3   Goodall S. Peripheral vascular disease. *Nursing Standard* 2000; 14: 48-52.

4   **Lennard-Jones JE, Ed. A positive approach to nutrition as treatment. London King's Fund Centre 1992. Available from the King's Fund Centre, 126 Albert St, London, NW1 7NF.**

5   **Green CJ. Existence, causes and consequences of disease-related malnutrition in the hospital and the community, and clinical and financial benefits of nutritional intervention. *Clinical Nutrition* 1999: 18 (supplement 2) 1-28.**

6 Delmi M, Rapin CH. Bengoa JM, Delmas PD. Dietary supplementation in elderly patients with fractured neck of femurs. *Lancet* 1990; 335: 1013-1016.

7 **National Institute for Clinical Excellence (2001). Inherited clinical guidelines B: Pressure ulcer risk assessment and prevention. NICE, London, April 2001.**

8 Turner TD. Which dressing and why? *Nursing Times* 1982 (Supplement) 78 (29): 1-5.

9 Hampton S. Choosing the right dressing. In: *Wound management theory and practice*. Miller M, Glover D, Eds. The Friary Press, Dorchester, Dorset, UK,1999; 116-128.

10 Jones M, Andrews A. Larval Therapy. In: *Wound management theory and practice*. Miller M, Glover D, Eds. The Friary Press, Dorchester, Dorset, UK, 1999.

11 Chetter I, Spark JI, Scott PJA, Kent PJ, Bevridge DC, Kester RC. Prospective analysis of quality of life in patients following infrainguinal reconstruction for chronic critical ischaemia. *Br J Surg* 1998; 85: 951-955.

12 Johnson BF, Singh S, Evans L, Drury R, Datta D, Beard JD. A prospective study of the effect of limb threatening ischaemia and its surgical treatment on the quality of life. *Eur J Vasc Endovasc Surg* 1997; 13: 306-314.

13 Panayiotopoulos AP, Tyrrell MR, Ready JF, Taylor PR. Outcome and cost analysis after femorocrural and femoropedal grafting for critical limb ischaemia. *Br J Surg* 1997; 84: 207-12.

14 Nicoloft AD, Taylor LM, McCafferty RB, Moneta GL, Porter JM. Patient recovery after infrainguinal bypass grafting for limb salvage. *J Vasc Surg* 1998; 27: 256-66.

15 Feinglass J, Pearce WH, Martin GJ, Gibbs J, Compar D, Sovensen M, Khuvi S, Daley J, Henderson WG. Post operative and amputation-free survival outcomes after femorodistal bypass grafting surgery: Findings from the Department of Veterans Affairs. National Surgical Quality Improvement Programme. *J Vasc Surg* 2001; 34 (2).

16 Pomposelli FB, Arora S, Gibbons GW, Frykberg R, Smakourshi P, Campbell DR, Freeman DV, Loterfo FW. Lower extremity arterial reconstruction in the very elderly: Successful outcome preserves not only the limb but also residential status and ambulatory function. *J Vasc Surg* 1998; 28(2).

17 Dorgan PS, Shepard AD, Nypauer TJ. Critical limb ischaemia in patients with end stage renal disease: do long term results justify an aggressive surgical approach? In: *Perspectives in vascular surgery*. Gloviczki P, Ed. Vol 12:1. Thieme Pub, New York: 81-92.

18 Lantis JC, Conte MS, Belkin M, Whittemore AD, Mannick JA, Donaldson MC. Infrainguinal bypass grafting in patients with end stage renal disease: Improving outcomes? *J Vasc Surg* 2001; 34: 1171-1177.

19 Abou-Zaman AM. Lee RW, Moneta GL, Taylor LM, Porter JM. Functional outcome after infrainguinal bypass for limb salvage. *J Vasc Surg* 1997; 25: 287-97.

20 Proia RR, Walsh DB, Nelson PR, Connors TP, Powerr RJ, Zwolak RM, Fillinger MR, Cronemmett JL. Early results of infragenicular revascularisation based solely on duplex arteriography. *J Vasc Surg* 2001; 34: 1165-1170.

21 London NJM, Varty K, Sayers RD *et al*. Percutaneous transluminal angioplasty for lower limb critical ischaemia. *Br J Surg* 1995; 82: 1217-1221.

22 Nydahl S, Hatshorne T, Bell PRF, Bolia A. Subintimal angioplasty of infrapopliteal occlusions in critically ischaemic legs. *Eur J Vasc Endovasc Surg* 1997; 14: 212-216.

23 Scott SM, Mayhew PA, Harris EA. Pressure ulcer development in the operating room: Nursing implications. *AORN Journal* 1992; 56: 242-250.

24 **Armstrong D. An intra-operative review of pressure relief in surgical patients. *AORN Journal* 2001; 73: 645-674.**

25 **Beard JD, Gaines PA. Treatment of lower limb ischaemia. In: *Vascular and Endovascular Surgery,* 2nd Ed. Beard JD, Gaines PA, Eds. WB Saunders, London, 2001.**

26 Lemmer JH Jr, Meng RL, Corson JD, Miller E. Division of Cardiothoracic Surgery, University of Iowa Hospital and Clinics, Iowa City 52242. Preoperative saphenous vein mapping for coronary artery bypass. *Journal of Cardiac Surgery* 1988; 3(3): 237-40.

27 Kupinski AM, Evans SM, Khan AM, Zorn TJ, Darling RC 3rd, Chang BB, Leather RP, Shah DM. Karmody Vascular Laboratory, Department of Surgery, Albany Medical College, New York 12208. Ultrasonic characterization of the saphenous vein. *Cardiovascular Surgery* 1993; 1(5): 513-7.

28 **Harris PL, How TV, Jones DR. Prospectively randomised clinical trial to compare *in situ* and reversed saphenous vein grafts for femoropopliteal bypass. *Br J Surg* 1978; 74: 252-255.**

29 **Moody AP, Edwards PR, Harris PL. *Insitu* versus reversed femoropopliteal vein grafts: long-term follow-up of a prospective randomised trial. *Br J Surg* 1992; 79: 750-753.**

30 **Wengerter KR, Veith FJ, Gupta SK, Goldsmith J, Farrell E, Harris P L, Moore D, Shanik G. Prospective randomised multicentre comparison of *insitu* and reversed vein infrapopliteal bypasses. *J Vasc Surg* 1991; 13: 189-199.**

31 **Lawson JA, Tangelder MJD, Algra A, Eikelboom BC on behalf of the Dutch BOA Study Group. The myth of the *insitu* graft: superiority in infrainguinal bypass surgery? *Eur J Vasc Endovasc Surg* 1999; 18: 149-157.**

32 **Harris PL, Veith FJ, Shanik GD, Nott P, Wengerter KR, Moore DJ. Prospective randomised of *in situ* and reversed infrapopliteal vein grafts. *Br J Surg* 1993; 80: 173-176.**

33   Tarry WC, Walsh DB, Birkmeyer NJO, Fillinger MR, Zwolak RM, Cronenwett JL. Fate of the contralateral leg after infrainguinal bypass. *J Vasc Surg* 1998; 27: 1039-48.

34   Holzenbein TJ, Pomposelli F B, Miller A *et al*. Results of a policy with arm veins used as the first alternative to an unavailable ipsilateral greater saphenous vein for infrainguinal bypass. *J Vasc Surg* 1996; 23: 130-40.

35   Shulman ML, Badhey MRI. Late results and angiographic evaluation of arm veins as long bypass grafts. *Surgery* 1982; 96: 1032-41.

36   Eugster T, Stierli P, Fischer G, Gurke L. Long-term results of infrainguinal arterial reconstruction with spliced veins are equal to results with non spliced veins. *Eur J Vasc Endovasc Surg* 2001; 22: 152-156.

37   McCarthy WJ, Pearce WH, Flinn WR, McGee GS, Wang R, Yao J S. Long-term evaluation of composite sequential bypass for limb threatening ischaemia. *J Vasc Surg* 1992; 15(5).

38   Schneider PA, Caps MT, Ogaws DY, Hayman ES. Intraoperative superficial femoral artery balloon angioplasty and popliteal to distal bypass graft: An option for combined open and endovascular treatment of diabetic gangrene. *J Vasc Surg* 2000; 33: 955-962.

39   Dardik H, Berry Sm, Dardik A, Wolodiger, Pecoraro J, Ibrahim IM, Kahn M, Sussman B. Infrapopliteal prosthetic graft patency by use of the distal adjunctive arteriovenous fistula. *J Vasc Surg* 1991; 13(5).

40   Hamsho A, Nott D, Harris PL. Prospective randomised trial of distal arteriovenous fistula as an adjunct to femoro-popliteal PTFE bypass. *Eur J Vasc Endovasc Surg* 1999; 17: 197-201.

41   Stonebridge PA, Prescott RJ, Buckley CV. Randomised trial comparing infrainguinal PTFE bypass grafting with and without vein interposition cuff at the distal anastomosis. *J Vasc Surg* 1997; 26: 543-50.

42   Girolami B, Bernardi E, Priris MH, tenCate JW, Prandoni P, Simioni P, Andreozzi GM, Girolami A, Buller HR. Antiplatelet therapy and other interventions after revascularisation procedures in patients with peripheral arterial disease: A meta-analysis. *Eur J Vasc Endovasc Surg* 2000; 19: 370-380.

43   Watson HR, Belcher G, Horrocks M. Adjuvant medical therapy in peripheral bypass surgery. *Br J Surg* 1999; 86: 981-991.

44   Tangelder MJD, Algra A, Lawson JA, Eikelboom BC. Systematic review of randomised controlled trials of aspirin and oral anticoagulation in the prevention of graft occlusion and ischaemic events after infrainguinal bypass surgery. *J Vasc Surg* 1999; 30: 701-9.

Chapter 21

Lower limb amputation and rehabilitation

Joan A Potterton Vascular Nurse

Robert B Galland Consultant Vascular Surgeon

DEPARTMENT OF SURGERY, ROYAL BERKSHIRE HOSPITAL, READING, UK

Introduction

Amputation may be the best or only option for some patients with critical leg ischaemia. This may be because revascularisation appears impracticable or unjustified, or because it has not succeeded. Primary amputation should not be regarded as "failure" of treatment, but viewed positively by patients as well as clinicians. The aim of amputation is to relieve pain, remove dead or severely ischaemic or infected tissue whilst maintaining function and quality of life.

Approximately 5,000 lower limb amputations are performed in the United Kingdom each year [1]. About 90% of these are as a result of peripheral vascular disease. Men account for 66% with a mean age of 72 years [2]. Female amputees are on average five years older. They often have elderly husbands or are widowed and therefore rely on others for their care [3]. Unfortunately, prognosis for patients who have an amputation as a result of peripheral vascular disease is poor. Many have coexistent cardiac, respiratory or neurological disease. This is reflected in the high operative mortality of patients undergoing major amputation. Hospital statistics in the United Kingdom suggest a 30-day operative mortality of at least 10% [4].

About half of those patients undergoing major amputation will have died within three years of their amputation [5] (I).

Although mobility is important for many patients, other factors such as pain relief and returning home to family and friends also contribute to quality of life [6]. Some 56% of patients will be fitted with a limb [2]. Although 85% of these patients are still walking to varying degrees at one year, only 31% are doing so at five years (I). Conversely the number of patients who are totally dependent on a wheelchair rises from 13% at one year to 39% at five years. A study of major amputations carried out in the South East Thames Region found that only 5% of amputees were totally free of a wheelchair i.e. Mobility Grade 5, (Table 1) [7]. With time against amputees, it is vital that their rehabilitation and discharge from hospital are well planned so that they can enjoy the best quality of life possible during their remaining years. Rehabilitation and discharge of patients undergoing amputation is often poorly planned and fragmented. There are few groups of patients who require the care of so many disciplines of health care (Figure 1). Coordination of the multi-disciplinary team is key to improving care of these patients. On a busy acute surgical ward nursing

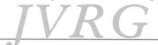

Table 1 Mobility grading.

0   Bedridden (cannot transfer from wheelchair)

1   Wheelchair mobility

2   Limited household ambulation

3   Unlimited household ambulation

4   Limited community ambulation

5   Unlimited community ambulation

staff are rarely in a position to make this a priority. The role of a vascular nurse specialist on the other hand should be focused on improving quality of care of all vascular patients and may include implementing and coordinating care programs to meet this need. There is increasing economic demand to reduce length of stay of all patients. Amputees, although a small group of patients, put a significant demand on the acute vascular/surgical ward. The post-operative duration of hospital stay varies greatly but some patients remain in hospital for many months.

The need for a care pathway

The potential value of an integrated care pathway (ICP) is illustrated in an audit recently completed in our unit. Data were collected for two periods, each of

Figure 1 Multi-disciplinary team caring for the amputee.

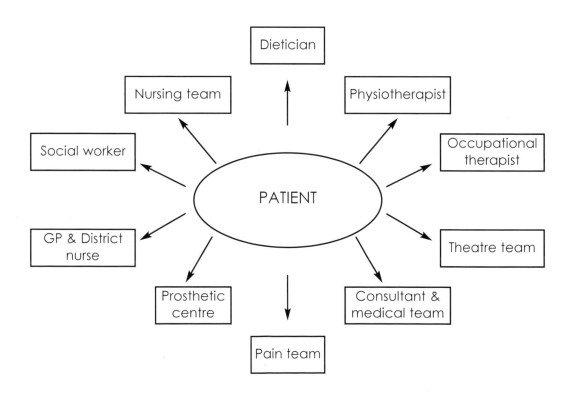

Figure 2 Scattergram showing post-operative stay of amputees before and after appointment of a vascular nurse. Bars represent medians.

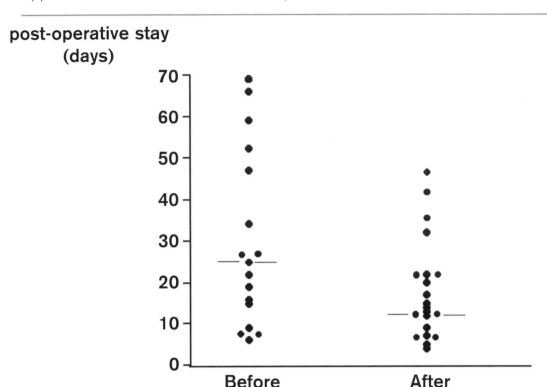

post-operative stay
(days)

8 months before and after appointment of a vascular nurse. All vascular amputees on the acute surgical ward were included. Amputees on medical wards were excluded, as the aim was to look specifically at length of stay on the surgical ward. Data were collected as part of a continuing audit supplemented by information from theatre registers and the Patient Management System (PMS) to find discharge dates. Length of stay was calculated from day of operation to day of discharge. In the first period (1st June 1999 to 31st January 2000) there were 17 patients. Amputations performed were above knee, ten, below knee, five and through knee, two. There were 11 men and six women. Median length of stay was 25 days (range 6 - 69 days) (Figure 2).

Discharge was often delayed because of social problems. Planning rehabilitation often didn't happen until several days after operation. A meeting with the occupational therapy department revealed that they were often unaware of the presence of an amputee on the ward until the physiotherapist requested a wheelchair several days after operation. The occupational therapy department felt that they could improve their service to the patient if they were aware of the patient's admission at an earlier stage.

Amputation for vascular disease is performed to relieve pain and save life. A decision to carry out the amputation is often made while the patient is still in hospital after a failed attempt at revascularisation. Under these circumstances advanced planning is not possible. However for a number of patients the decision to amputate is made in the out-patient clinic.

In an attempt to improve care of these patients the vascular clinical nurse specialist introduced several changes:

♦ Where possible the vascular clinical nurse specialist sees patients in the out-patient department to provide support, answer questions and start care planning.

◆ Vascular nurse makes referrals to occupational therapist (OT) and social worker as soon as decision to amputate is made.

◆ OT carries out a home access visit as early as possible, preferably before the patient comes into hospital.

◆ OT orders wheelchair before operation.

◆ Better use of community hospitals with early referral made for rehabilitation.

◆ Multi-disciplinary team meetings are held weekly, coordinated by the vascular nurse. Goals are set for rehabilitation and discharge. The meetings are sometimes used as a case conference with patient, relatives and social worker.

Following implementation of these changes, 21 amputations were carried out in the period - 1st February 2000 to 30th September 2000. There were 19 men and two women with 11 below knee amputations and ten above knee amputations. The post-operative length of hospital stay was reduced to a median of 13 days (range 4-46 days). This was statistically significant P = 0.044 (Mann Whitney U test) (Figure 2).

These results were encouraging but it was recognized that in the absence of the vascular nurse, for example during holiday time, this level of care might not happen for every patient. We needed to find a means of standardizing care. Integrated care pathways are an established means of providing this for a given diagnosis.

Evidence for a care pathway

There is little evidence for the use of ICPs in the care of amputees. Several circumstances have been identified as being conducive to success of ICPs [8]. These include the following:

◆ Small teams.

◆ Defined predictable groups.

◆ Containable setting.

◆ A high volume of cases.

◆ Established guidelines for best practice.

As amputees fit very few of these criteria there has perhaps been an understandable inertia in their use. After fractured neck of femur, integrated care pathway for stroke is the one most commonly used [8]. There are several common denominators between patients with stroke and amputees. There are many generally reported benefits arising from use of care pathways, including enhancement of multi-disciplinary working and collaboration, active patient involvement in planning care, a unified patient record and a significant reduction in length of hospital stay, all of which satisfy clinical governance.

Mikulaninec [10] identified that patients were staying longer in hospital following major amputation than accepted national figures. A care pathway was introduced to address this issue. A reduction in hospital stay of 2 days was achieved **(II)**. The ability to reduce hospital stay was confirmed in another study [11]. In addition, that study, of amputees being managed by a multi-disciplinary plan of rehabilitation care, showed that more patients were referred for limb fitting and there was a decreased need for post-hospital physiotherapy **(II)**. Schaldach [12] described a survey of 184 patients comprising three consecutive phases. In the first phase patients received routine hospital care, patients in the second phase received a rehabilitation consult. Neither group used a care pathway. In the third phase they were subjected to a rehabilitation-focused ICP. There was an overall reduction in hospital stay from 11 to 8 days with a low rate of readmission. In addition there was a slight increase in the number of patients discharged to their own home in the third phase. This was achieved with a significant reduction in cost to the patient **(II)**.

Our experience in developing the care pathway

Traditionally nurses have been the professionals most likely to initiate and coordinate care pathways. In order for them to succeed, motivation and commitment of all members of the multi-disciplinary team are required. Most hospitals that are committed to using care pathways employ a care pathway facilitator. The latter brings experience gained from other ICPs and is also the person best equipped to train other staff. Staff training in the use of new ICPs is identified as crucial to their success [8]. The care pathway facilitator is also involved with audit after the initial pilot.

Our first task was to organize a multi-disciplinary meeting, which was well attended. It is vital at this early stage that all members of the team are involved and take ownership of the pathway. Various members of the group took responsibility for elements of the ICP and a draft pathway was defined for the next meeting. The second meeting lasted 2 hours, which was unacceptably long, so it was decided that the group should split into smaller units. The occupational therapist and physiotherapist took responsibility for the rehabilitation section. The anaesthetist, pain nurse and theatre nurse worked together on the section on epidural pain relief and care during operation and recovery. The out-patient nurse, ward nurse, pre-operative clerking nurse, vascular nurse and vascular surgeon took responsibility for the sections on pre and post-operative care and discharge planning. The facilitator attended all meetings and correlated the various elements to produce another draft. Many problems were encountered along the way. People often found it difficult to find time to attend meetings and staff changes made it difficult to maintain continuity. The occupational therapist changed four times in 6 months and the physiotherapist twice. When key people are lost from the group the fundamental element of ownership and commitment is lost. It has taken over a year to develop the care pathway. At the time of writing the final draft has been approved and is ready to be piloted.

Elements of the pathway

It has been identified that for the majority of elderly amputees, mobility will often depend on a wheelchair [3]. Therefore adaptation of the home so that it is wheelchair-accessible is probably the most important aspect of rehabilitation. Although it is our policy to refer all amputees for limb fitting, the overall aim of the

care pathway was to improve the quality of the patient's life by ensuring that timely referrals for home adaptations were made. The pathway was also aimed at reducing length of hospital stay. This meant for many patients a further period of rehabilitation at a community hospital was needed. An achievable discharge date of 10 days after the operation was agreed. From our own small study and the few studies where ICPs were used in the care of amputees it is clear that early planning is crucial. It was therefore decided that the care pathway should start in the out-patient department wherever possible. An out-patient nurse makes appropriate referrals at this stage. If possible the vascular nurse sees the patient in out-patients to offer emotional support, provide information and establish a rapport with the patient and relatives. The patient is given an information leaflet to reinforce verbal information given. The pre-operative clerking nurse also plays a major role by confirming that referral to occupational therapy has been made and making further referrals to social services and community hospitals. We recognize that in some cases it may not be possible for the patient to attend the pre-operative clerking clinic in advance due to poor mobility and their inevitable poor general medical condition. In a study of 300 vascular patients, 91% of those with varicose veins attend pre-operative clerking clinic whereas only 24% of those being admitted for major arterial surgery attended [13]. The latter were either not fit enough to attend or had no means of transport. In these cases our patients will be clerked in the pre-operative clerking clinic on the day of admission.

The ward nurse makes referrals for those patients who are already in hospital. A full physiotherapy assessment is carried out pre-operatively to establish functional status so that realistic rehabilitation goals can be set. Post-operatively, elements of the pathway include nursing interventions such as pain relief, pressure area care, nutrition and hygiene. Physiotherapy is planned along a continuum of goals with progress documented. Referral for limb fitting and out-patient physiotherapy is made by the ward physiotherapist. Discharge planning is reviewed daily, confirming that all necessary referrals have been made and a discharge date set. Development of good relationships with subacute units such as community hospitals is fundamental in achieving the planned discharge date. Accurate documentation of variables in the pathway is necessary for auditing purposes. If a clear reason for the variance is given, this information can be used to reshape the pathway after the initial pilot. It is useful to identify elements of the pathway that don't work or may not be necessary. Inevitably there will be some patients who do not fit the ICP, for example patients needing renal dialysis. A summary of our ICP is shown in Table 2.

Selection of amputation level

The ideal level of amputation depends upon vascularity, rehabilitation potential and prosthetic considerations. The potential for rehabilitation and likely goals can only be set by a full and holistic assessment of the patient to include other illnesses and disabilities, cognitive state and motivation, likely discharge destination and life-style, as well as the patient's own aspirations and wishes.

In general terms more proximal the level of amputation, the more difficult it will be for the patient to achieve independent walking. Therefore more distal the amputation site, the better the rehabilitation potential for walking, as these provide longer stump length and preserve more joints and hence more control of the prosthesis. Preservation of the knee joint has enormous advantages in terms of mobility. 80% of the trans-tibial amputees achieved unlimited housebound mobility or better compared to 40% of the above knee amputees in one study [14] (II).

Many surgeons now favour the skew flap technique compared to the traditional Burgess long posterior flap for transtibial amputation. A randomised trial has shown no difference in healing between the skew flap and traditional Burgess long posterior flap but the time to limb-fitting and early mobility was shorter in the skew-flap group due to a less bulbous stump [15] (I). The Gritti-Stokes knee-level amputation seems a useful option for patients where a transtibial amputation will not heal and who are deemed incapable of walking. The longer stump assists transfers, sitting balance, maintains muscle attachment and proprioception. Limitations in prosthetic fitting make this level unpopular with prosthetists, although good ambulation can be achieved [16]. Healing is better than the conventional through-knee amputation [17] (I).

Transcutaneous oximetry ($TcPo_2$), photoplethysmography, laser Doppler velocimetry, thermography and isotope clearance rates have all been shown to correlate with subsequent stump healing. However, whilst all these methods seem superior to Doppler ankle pressures [18], a systematic review concluded that the sensitivities and specificities were inadequate to recommend their clinical use [19] (I). Figure 3 outlines an algorithm for the selection of amputation level.

Stump management

Tight or elasticated bandages should not be used in vascular amputees as they can generate unacceptable pressures and cause tissue breakdown.[20] (B). Rigid dressings of Plaster of Paris are not generally used in the vascular amputees in the UK. Adhesive clear plastic film type of dressing applied post-operatively can be very useful as this allows easier and regular wound inspections. This type of dressing may maintain shape and certainly makes life easier for the physiotherapists to inspect wounds before and after application of early walking aids. Once the wound is healed or healing satisfactorily then elasticated and graduated pressure stump shrinker socks like Juzo® are applied to the stump at about 2-3 weeks post-operatively to control post-operative oedema. Stump boards should be fitted to the wheelchairs of patients with transtibial amputations to reduce dependent oedema and knee contracture. Appropriate and specialist footwear such as a PRAFO boot protects the other leg from damage by the wheelchair.

Pain management

Controlling stump and phantom pain seems vital for the patient to participate successfully in a rehabilitation programme. Measures include appropriate regular analgesics, and drugs like Amitriptyline, Gabapentin, Carbamazepine, as well as physical treatment modalities like transcutaneous nerve stimulators, acupuncture and Capsaicin cream. There is some evidence that complete pain relief for

Table 2 Summary of the care pathway.

Components	Personnel responsible	Action	Timing
Discharge planning	Out-patient nurse	Make referral to OT Physiotherapist Vascular nurse Pain team	At out-patient clinic, when the decision to amputate is made.
	Occupational therapist (OT) Pre-operative clerking nurse	Carry out pre-operative home visit and order wheelchair. Confirm referrals made by OPD nurse. Make referral to social worker and community hospital.	Before the patient is admitted. During pre-operative clerking clinic.
	Ward nurse Vascular nurse	Confirm discharge plans. See patient to provide support and answer questions. Coordinate discharge plans and weekly multi-disciplinary team meetings.	On admission. Pre-operatively in out-patients or on admission. Weekly.
Patient assessment	Pre-operative clerking nurse	Medical assessment questions. Relevant blood tests, ECG, Chest x-ray.	During pre-operative clerking clinic.
	House surgeon Ward nurse	Medical assessment. Nursing assessment of activities of daily living. Nutritional risk assessment. Pressure sore risk assessment.	On admission.
	Physiotherapist	Assessment of functional status.	On admission.
Pain relief	Pain nurse	Pre-operative assessment. Discusses post-operative pain relief options. Advises on pre-operative pain relief.	On admission.
	Anaesthetist	Assesses general condition and rationalises pain relief. Gives epidural if appropriate.	
	Recovery nurse	Ensures adequate pain relief prior to discharge from recovery. Aim for pain score <5.	Immediately after operation.
	Ward nurse	Assesses pain. Aims for pain score of <5.	Twice per shift or hourly if epidural insitu
Rehabilitation	Physiotherapist	Assesses chest and treat if necessary. Assesses sitting balance. Teaches exercises.	Day one after operation.
		Teaches transfer methods and practices safe transfers. Sets mobility goals using a continuum of care. Wheelchair assessment.	Day two after operation.
		Physiotherapy in the gym to start walking practice. Referral to out-patient physiotherapy. Referral for limb fitting.	Day three after operation. Day six onwards
	Occupational therapy	Issues wheelchair. Washing and dressing practice. Home visit.	Day two after operation.
	Ward nurse	Provision of any necessary home equipment. Assists patients towards independent mobility and personal care.	Day five onwards. Daily.

Figure 3 Algorithm for selection of amputation level.

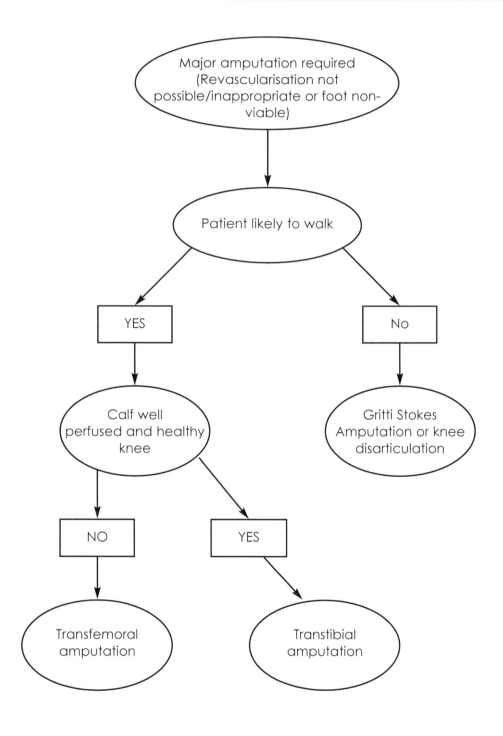

about 72 hours prior to amputation by epidural may reduce the intensity and frequency of post amputation phantom pains [21] **(II)**. Early involvement of the pain team in appropriate cases is most beneficial.

Early walking aids

There are three main types of early walking aids used in the UK. The best known is the pneumatic post amputation mobility aid (PPAMaid). The more recently introduced early walking aids are Amputee Mobility Aid (AMA) and Femurette. The AMA, designed for trans-tibial amputees, allows the patient to bend the knee and it also has a foot, rather than a rocker end, which allows a more natural gait. The Femurette is an excellent early walking aid for trans-femoral amputees.

These early walking aids allow stump desensitisation, improves standing and walking balance, assist in reduction of stump oedema and may promote wound healing [22] **(II)**. They are an excellent moral booster for the amputees and are also used as assessment tools to estimate amputees' potential or otherwise for walking.

Summary

♦ Whenever possible an ICP should be used for patients undergoing major amputation **(B)**.

♦ If an ICP is used it should start as early as possible, preferably in the out-patient department and certainly pre-operatively **(A)**.

♦ The ICP must be multi-disciplinary in its approach, with all members of the team committed to its use **(B)**.

♦ Preserve the knee joint whenever possible if the patient has the potential to walk or to use a prosthetic limb to assist transfers from chair/bed etc **(A)**.

♦ For the patient who is likely to remain wheelchair/bed bound, a Gritti-Stokes amputation is preferable to a trans-femoral or trans-tibial level **(B)**.

♦ Prompt and adequate control of stump and phantom pain is vital for successful early rehabilitation **(A)**.

♦ Early walking aids should be used routinely unless there are problems with wound healing **(B)**.

♦ Adaptation of the home so that it is wheelchair accessible is often the key to successful rehabilitation **(A)**.

Further Reading

1 Murdoch G, Ed. *Amputation surgery and lower limb prosthetics*. Blackwell Science, Oxford, 1988.

References (grade I evidence and grade A recommendations in bold)

1 Department of Health and Social Security. Review of artificial limb and appliance centre services. London: HMSO, 1996.

2 McWinnie DL, Gordon AC, Collin J, Gray DWR, Morrison JD. Rehabilitation outcome 5 years after 100 lower limb amputations. *Br J Surg* 1994; 81: 1596-1599.

3. Collin C, Collin J. Mobility after lower-limb amputation. *Br J Surg* 1995; 82: 1010-1011.

4 Department of Health and Social Security, Office of population and Surveys. Hospital inpatient enquiry. London: HMSO 1983-5.

5 De-Frang RD, Taylor LM, Porter JM. Basic data related to amputations. *Ann Vasc Surg* 1991; 5: 202-7.

6 Johnson B, Evans L, Datta D, Morris-Jones W, Beard JD. Surgery for limb threatening ischaemia. A reappraisal of costs and benefits. *Eur J Vasc Endovasc Surg*. 1995; 9: 181 - 188.

7 Callum K. Amputations. In: *Clinical problems in vascular surgery*. Galland RB, Clyne CAC, Eds. Edward Arnold, London, 1993; 79-88.

8 Johnson S, Dracass M, Vartan J, Summers S, Edington J. Setting standards using integrated care pathways. *Prof Nurse* 2000; 15: 640-3.

9 Currie L. Researching care pathway development in the United Kingdom: Stage 1. *NT Research* 1999; 4: 378-382.

10 Mikulaninec CE. An Amputee Critical Path. *J Vasc Nurs* 1992; 10: 6-9.

11 Ham R, Regan J, Roberts V. Evaluation of introducing the team approach to the care of the amputee: the Dulwich study. *Prosthetics and Orthotics* 1994; 6: 62-6.

12 Schaldach DE. Measuring quality and cost of care: evaluation of an amputation clinical pathway. *J Vasc Nurs* 1997; 15: 13-20.

13 Toogood GJ, Wilmott K, Jones L, Magee TR, Galland RB. Feasibility of pre-admission nurse clerking of patients with vascular disease. *J R Coll Surg Edinb* 1998; 43: 246-7.

14 Houghton AD, Taylor PR, Thurlow S, Rookes E, McColl I. Success rates for rehabilitation of vascular amputees: implications for preoperative assessment and amputation level. *Br J Surg* 1992; 79: 753-5.

15 Ruckley CV, Stonebridge PA, Prescott RJ. Skewflap versus long posterior flap in below-knee amputations: multicenter trial. *J Vasc Surg* 1991; 13: 423-7.

16 Houghton A, Allen A, Luff R, McColl I. Rehabilitation after lower limb amputation: a comparative study of above-knee and Gritti-Stokes amputations. *Br J Surg* 1989; 76: 622-4.

17 Campbell WB, Morris PJ. A prospective, randomised comparison of healing in Gritti-Stokes and through-knee amputations. *Ann R Coll Surg Engl* 1986; 69: 1-4.

18 Welch GH, Leiberman DP, Pollock JG, Angerson W. Failure of Doppler ankle pressure to predict healing of conservative forefoot amputations. *Br J Surg* 1985; 72: 888-91.

19 Savin S, Sharni S, Shields DA, Scurr JH, Coleridge-Smith PD. Selection of amputation level: a review. *Eur J Vasc Surg* 1991; 5: 611-20.

20 Isherwood PA, Robertson JC, Rossi A. Pressure measurements beneath below-knee stump bandages. Elastic bandaging, the Puddifoot dressing and a pneumatic bandaging technique compared. *Br J Surg* 1975; 62: 982-986.

21 Back S, Norenz MF, Tjellden NU. Phantom limb pain in amputees during the first twelve months following limb amputation after pre-operative lumbar epidural seventy-two hours pre-operation. *Pain.* 1988; 33: 297-301.

22 Ramsay EM. A clinical evaluation of the LIC Femurette as an early training device for the primary above knee amputee. *Physiotherapy.* 1988; 74: 12: 598 - 601.

Chapter 22

Elective abdominal aortic aneurysm repair

Donna Parkin Consultant Nurse
Jonothan J Earnshaw Consultant Vascular Surgeon
Brian Heather Consultant Vascular Surgeon

DEPARTMENT OF VASCULAR SURGERY,
GLOUCESTERSHIRE ROYAL HOSPITAL, GLOUCESTER, UK

Introduction

Elective repair of an abdominal aortic aneurysm (AAA) is undertaken in order to prevent death from future rupture. However, elective repair itself carries a 5 - 8% mortality risk [1-3] and must be weighed against the risk of rupture in the coming months or years. Traditional repair of an AAA involves an open operation, though there has been a move towards endovascular aneurysm repair. Endovascular repair is covered in a separate chapter. This chapter focuses on patients undergoing an elective open AAA repair. Figure 1 outlines an algorithm for the pre-operative management of such a patient.

The risk of death from a ruptured abdominal aortic aneurysm (AAA) is around 80% [4], making this the most serious vascular emergency that faces any vascular surgical team. For those who survive to reach hospital, immediate surgery is required to allow any chance of survival.

The chapter on transfer protocols discusses the initial management of a patient with a suspected ruptured AAA. The subsequent care pathway is similar to that for elective repair with the following exceptions:

- No time exists for a detailed pre-operative risk assessment. Therefore patients should proceed to surgery unless clearly unfit.

- More blood will be required and so the issue of autotransfusion becomes more important (see chapter on blood conservation).

- An ITU bed will always be required because of the need for cardiac, respiratory and renal support.

Indications for, and risks of elective AAA repair

Diagnosis

Most AAAs remain asymptomatic until they rupture. The most common symptoms of an acute presentation are abdominal and/or back pain [1]. Clinical examination confirming a pulsatile abdominal mass can detect the presence of an AAA but this alone will not identify everyone with an aneurysm. The advent of local screening programmes has generated a steady flow

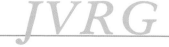

Figure 1 Preoperative AAA pathway.

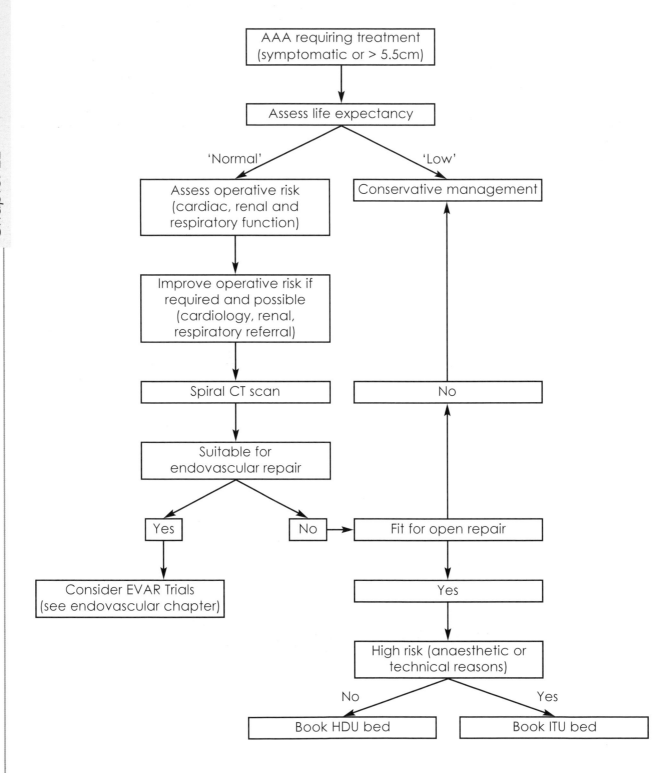

of aneurysms within a screened population in an attempt to reduce the number of preventable deaths from rupture [5,6]. More information with regard to screening programmes can be found in the relevant chapter on screening and surveillance.

AAAs are usually detected incidentally through abdominal ultrasound imaging or computed tomography (CT) when under investigation for another complaint [1]. In Gloucestershire, where we have a screening programme, an increasing proportion of elective repairs are undertaken on screen-detected AAAs (Figure 2).

Indications for surgical repair of an AAA

The decision to repair an AAA electively must be reached after careful consideration of the risks of surgery when balanced against the natural history of aneurysm disease, for which the evidence is less clear. The main factors that determine the indication for surgery are size of the aneurysm and the general fitness of the patient. The practice of different surgeons in their selection of patients for elective AAA repair cannot be compared directly as each will have a slightly different threshold of fitness at which they

Figure 2 Proportions of aneurysm surgery categories in Gloucestershire.

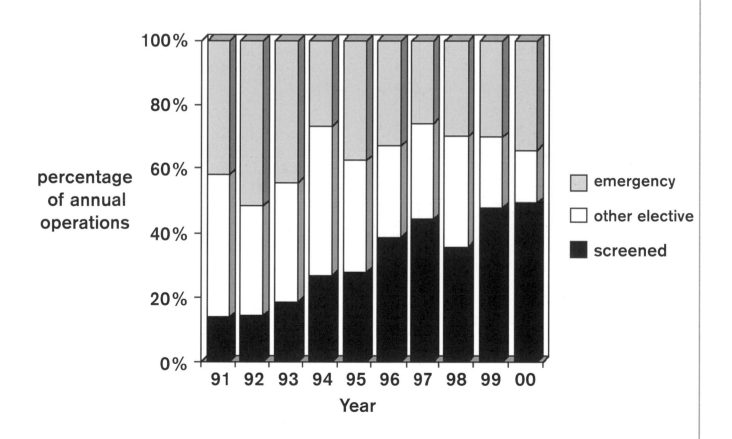

would consider operative repair. Brown *et al* in 1996 [7] advocated surgery on aneurysms of 4.5 - 5.0 cm diameter where an increase in size of 0.5 cm or more per year is witnessed. This contradicts an earlier uncontrolled study which recommended surveillance of aneurysms under 6 cm [8]. The latter is supported by the results of the UK Small Aneurysm Trial which concluded that aneurysms with a diameter of less than 5.5 cm, can safely be managed by continued ultrasonographic surveillance [3]. This trial showed no difference in mortality between the early surgery group for aneurysms 4.0 - < 5.5 cm in diameter and the surveillance group. Results from a similar study - the ADAM trial - (as yet unpublished) in North America reached a similar conclusion. No trials exist comparing surgery and surveillance of AAAs above 5.5 cm in diameter, but most vascular surgeons regard this size as an indication for operation **(B)**. Other indications include a growth rate of >1.0cm in one year, or the development of symptoms such as pain or distal embolisation [9].

Operative risk

The published mortality rate from elective AAA repair is 5 - 8%. However, this risk may be increased in the presence of other factors such as old age, ischaemic heart disease, chronic obstructive pulmonary disease and renal impairment [9,10].

Patients with an AAA have a high prevalence of symptomatic and asymptomatic cardiac disease. It is therefore not surprising that cardiac complications are the commonest causes of complication and death [2,3,11,12]. The risk of peri-operative myocardial infarction can be reduced by the administration of intra-operative heparin, without significantly increased blood loss [13] **(II)**. Other complications of AAA surgery include haemorrhage, respiratory failure, gut and limb ischaemia and multi-system organ failure [11].

The risk of post-operative renal dysfunction is higher in the presence of pre-existing renal impairment and where the aortic aneurysm arises at or above the level of the renal arteries, in which case a suprarenal clamp may be needed [12]. A pre-operative CT to determine the level at which the aneurysm arises is crucial when discussing the operative risk with a patient.

Pre-operative cardiac assessment

Although it is well documented that pre-existing cardiac disease is a significant risk factor, the methods by which it is assessed vary between surgeons and range from simple clinical assessment to more specific investigation such as ventricular ejection fraction and even coronary angiography.

The most common cardiac assessment requested by a vascular surgeon is the ventricular ejection fraction, followed by referral to a cardiologist if a patient is identified as having significant cardiac impairment [14]. However, the significant mortality associated with initial coronary artery bypass grafting along with the risk of aneurysm rupture whilst awaiting cardiac revascularisation, often proves too great to consider. In high risk patients it may be more appropriate not to offer surgery, especially as patients with large aneurysms deemed unfit for surgery have been shown to have a median survival of less than 2 years from causes other than aneurysm rupture [15]. Patients with asymptomatic cardiac disease may benefit from optimal medical treatment using peri-operative beta-blockade to reduce cardiac mortality and morbidity [16] **(I)**.

Renal assessment

Routine blood chemistry will highlight pre-existing renal impairment pre-operatively. If renal impairment is present prior to surgery, there is an increased risk of further deterioration especially if a suprarenal clamp is required [17]. This must be discussed with the patient prior to surgery. Conversely, for patients who are already established on dialysis, there is no additional contraindication to surgery. However, their pre and post-operative care will require joint management by the vascular and renal teams.

Respiratory assessment

Initial assessment of respiratory status is based on clinical history and a chest x-ray. In the presence of respiratory disease, pulmonary function tests and assessment by a chest physician is advisable. This may be followed by admission for pre-operative intensive physiotherapy to maximise lung function.

Risk scoring

The decision to offer surgical repair of an AAA is one that rests with the individual vascular surgeon in conjunction with cardiac, renal and respiratory specialists as well as the anaesthetist, based on the available evidence and balance of risk [18].

Support is growing for the use of simple cardiac risk scoring systems or statistical methods such as the POSSUM scoring system in order to predict outcome [19,20]. POSSUM, the Physiological and Operative Severity Scoring in the enUmeration of Mortality and morbidity, is a scoring system based on 14 standard pre-operative physiological variables and six operative variables relating to the extent and severity of the surgery performed. The Portsmouth modification of POSSUM, known as P-POSSUM uses the same variables but a different regression equation and analysis, and can also be used to predict outcome after elective AAA repair [21]. The Vascular Surgical Society of Great Britain and Ireland is recommending collection of POSSUM data items in order that a database is generated that could be used to compare the results of individual surgeons in different hospitals in a National Vascular Database [20] (B). The chapter on audit covers this in more detail.

An optimal pathway of care for elective AAA surgery

A pathway of care is based on published evidence or best current practice and combines all multi-disciplinary documentation into one core document which follows the patient during their hospital stay. This core document details the plan of care on a day to day basis, with any variations from this plan documented for future analysis. In the development stage of the pathway, the multi-disciplinary team must agree the outcomes to be measured and the criteria for future audit. This allows the team to review, update and improve their clinical practice in line with clinical governance strategies whilst promoting a multi-disciplinary approach to patient care which aids communication across the disciplines [22,23] (C).

Abdominal aortic aneurysm surgery is a high risk procedure which is associated with the well recognised complications. There is little documented evidence with regard to the influence of nursing management in the care of patients undergoing this major operative procedure. However, it is now accepted practice that patients undergoing AAA repair are nursed on a designated vascular ward where both nursing and medical staff are familiar with the expected pathway of care which should contain the following elements:

Preadmission clinic

Attendance at a preadmission clinic 1-2 weeks before surgery facilitates the preparation of the patient, both physically and psychologically. One of the main advantages of this clinic is to allow the detection of unexpected medical abnormalities in order that appropriate treatment may be instigated. This can range from uncontrolled hypertension to the detection of abnormal blood antibodies that may result in a delay in obtaining compatible blood in time for surgery.

The other main advantage is the allocation of sufficient time to counsel the patient and their family with regard to the intended operation, associated risks, post-operative care and expected length of stay, whilst identifying any potential social problems that may need addressing prior to discharge. It provides a second opportunity for the patient and family to ask questions and serves as an initial contact with another clinician who will have an input into their inpatient care.

Consent

All patients admitted for AAA repair will have had several discussions with the vascular surgeon who will be performing the surgery. The risks of surgery should be based on the clinical results of the individual surgeon which may vary between hospitals. Figure 3 demonstrates the 5 year cumulative mortality figures that are quoted locally by the vascular surgical teams in Gloucester (B).

Figure 3 5-year cumulative mortality for all elective AAA repairs 1991-2000.

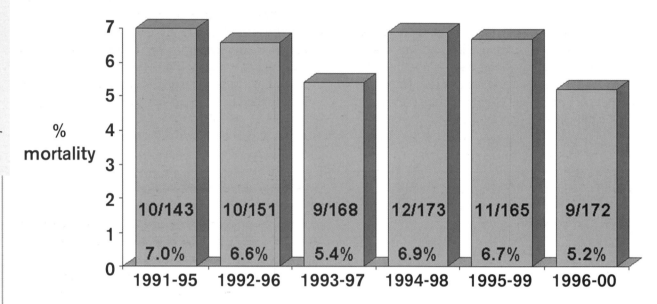

As aneurysms are often asymptomatic, it is important to emphasise that surgery is advised in an attempt to prevent risk of future rupture whilst highlighting the risks of death or morbidity from the surgery itself. Patients are often directed to the Gloucestershire Vascular Group website to allow those with access to the Internet the opportunity to obtain more detailed information. This also allows patients and their families to collect information at their own pace and to reinforce information already given by the surgeon or nurse specialist. The address for this site is: **http://members.aol.com/gvg97/**

An experienced member of the clinical team who has the knowledge and ability to counsel the patient and answer any further questions should obtain written consent prior to surgery. This should include the discussion and documentation of the risks associated with the surgical procedure.

Infection prophylaxis

Infection of a prosthetic aortic graft can have devastating consequences and carries a high morbidity and mortality [24]. The causative factors are direct contamination at operation, progression of an existing local wound infection and gut contamination [25].

With the increasing prevalence of MRSA (Methicillin Resistant *Staphylococcus Aureus*) in many hospitals, it is imperative that all possible precautions are taken in order to minimise the risk of contamination. Patients undergoing elective AAA repair should be admitted to an area where the risk of contamination is low. All patients should be prescribed (and receive) peri-operative antibiotic prophylaxis. Co-amoxiclav 1.2 g, or a cephalosporin e.g. cefuroxime 750 mg are the usual choices, but an agent effective against MRSA may be added in high risk units such as teicoplanin 200 mg **(C)**. The first dose should be given in theatre, with up to three subsequent doses to provide cover for the first 24 hours after surgery. Prolonged antibiotic therapy risks the development of pseudomembranous colitis and multiresistant organisms. The chapter on surgical site infections covers these issues in more detail.

Blood transfusion

Blood transfusion is often required in aortic surgery. Pre-operative haemodilution and the use of intra-operative red cell salvage can reduce the total blood requirement during surgery. Using a combination of techniques can avoid the requirement for homologous transfusion in approximately 50% of elective operations. In units where all ancillary methods are available, elective aortic aneurysm surgery can be carried out with a pre-operative crossmatch of only two units of blood. Further details about these ancillary methods can be found in the chapter on blood conservation.

Location

Most patients can be extubated immediately following surgery and therefore do not necessarily require an ITU bed. At the very least an HDU bed is required for intensive monitoring in the first 24-48 hours. Once stable the patient should then be transferred to a ward with an experienced team of nursing and medical staff who are familiar with caring for vascular patients. Many surgeons and anaesthetists will not commence an elective AAA repair unless a minimum of an HDU bed is available. Protected HDU beds for elective surgery reduce the risk of last-minute cancellation, which wastes valuable theatre time and distresses the patient. High risk patients who may require post-operative ventilation for anaesthetic or technical reasons (e.g. suprarenal AAA) will require an ITU bed post-operatively. The chapter on critical care referral and outreach practice discusses these matters in more detail.

Monitoring

Close observation of vital signs, urine output and oxygenation are required in order to detect any

abnormalities which, if left untreated, may lead to more serious complications. Immediate post-operative management will be undertaken in the ITU/HDU setting and usually involves intensive observation of vital signs every 30 - 60 minutes. Blood gases should be monitored 2-3 times a day and ventilatory requirements adjusted accordingly. Temporary deterioration of renal function may be managed by haemofiltration which can avoid the need for haemodialysis. However, continued deterioration of renal function may need the expertise of a renal physician. The vascular status of the feet should be assessed regularly, initially 2 hourly, along with the manual palpation of foot pulses or Doppler assessment, whilst observing for signs of distal embolisation.

Analgesia

Respiratory problems are one of the main risks after aneurysm repair and the use of epidural analgesia allows adequate chest expansion which, coupled with regular physiotherapy, can reduce the risk of chest infection. However, it is important to inspect the insertion site for signs of infection and to remove the epidural after 3 or 4 days, or as soon as the patient is able to cope with other forms of analgesia. Combination analgesics, which are stronger than paracetamol alone, are suitable alternatives that can be taken orally. Diclofenac which is a non-steroidal anti-inflammatory (NSAID) drug can also be used and has the advantage of a longer duration of action when administered 100 mg rectally every 18 hours. However, care must be taken when considering its use in patients with impaired renal function, asthma or previous history of gastro-intestinal bleed. Post-operative analgesia is discussed in the chapter on acute pain relief.

Hydration and nutrition

Following intra-operative handling of the bowel during AAA repair, it takes several days for effective peristalsis to be re-established. The routine insertion of a nasogastric (NG) tube will prevent the build up of gastric secretions. Allowing patients a small amount of oral fluid in the immediate post-operative period increases their comfort without leading to an increase in abdominal distension and is safe in the presence of an NG tube. Fluid balance needs particular care and the administration of intravenous fluids continued until the patient is able to tolerate oral fluids.

Once bowel sounds become active and NG tube drainage becomes minimal or the patient passes flatus, increasing amounts of oral fluid may be taken. At this stage high calorie supplements may be taken to improve nutrition and food commenced once the patient is tolerating free fluids. Once bowel motions recommence it is not uncommon for the patient to experience diarrhoea which usually settles within 24-48 hours. Should diarrhoea persist then careful monitoring of serum potassium levels is required and a stool sample should be sent for toxin assay and culture to exclude clostridium difficile overgrowth (pseudomembranous colitis). If rectal bleeding occurs, colonoscopy may be required to exclude ischaemic colitis.

Most patients undergoing aortic surgery do not need peri-operative nutrition. There may be advantages in introducing early enteral feeding via the NG tube to prevent small intestinal villous atrophy and enterotoxin absorption. Patients with prolonged complications after surgery will benefit from full enteral feeding. Total parenteral nutrition (TPN) is not usually required unless a prolonged ileus is encountered. The problem of lack of absorption of enteral feed via a NG tube is often due to gastric stasis, particularly if the patient is sedated and ventilated. This can be overcome by using a nasojejunal tube, inserted either at the time of surgery or endoscopically.

Immobilisation and thromboprophylaxis

Pressure area breakdown is a hazard of prolonged immobility. The use of epidural analgesia compounds this risk as discomfort in vulnerable areas is not felt by the patient. Pressure area care and the use of an appropriate pressure-relieving mattress will help to reduce the risk of pressure damage. Early mobilisation should be encouraged and monitored by the multi-disciplinary team.

Another hazard is the development of a deep vein thrombosis (DVT), and pulmonary embolism. This is a potentially life-threatening event and therefore its prevention is essential. The administration of subcutaneous unfractionated heparin (UFH) 5,000 units 2-3 times a day post-operatively, plus antiembolic stockings (unless contraindicated) is standard clinical practice after all major vascular surgery. In many units a once daily dose of low molecular weight heparin (LMWH), has replaced UFH.

Summary

◆ Elective surgery carries 5-8% mortality and must be weighed against factors such as age, aneurysm size, and other co-morbidities such as ischaemic heart disease, chronic obstructive pulmonary disease and renal impairment when determining a patient's fitness for surgery (I).

◆ The use of scoring systems may be the way forward when attempting to predict outcome and this has been supported by the Vascular Surgical Society of Great Britain and Ireland. Individual surgeons must discuss risks and expected outcomes based on their own results (B).

◆ The patient undergoing elective abdominal aortic aneurysm repair should be cared for by an experienced multi-disciplinary vascular team using the evidence available to support their current practice (A).

◆ Our vascular unit uses a care pathway for all patients undergoing an elective AAA repair to standardise nursing and medical treatment. This can be found on the website.

◆ Use of a pathway of care may have an impact on length of stay for patients undergoing elective AAA, but probably not in a well run vascular unit. Highlighting the expected care path can improve quality and consistency of care (C).

Further Reading

1   Calligaro KD, Dougherty ML, Hollier LH. *Diagnosis and Treatment of Aortic and Peripheral Arterial Aneurysms*. WB Saunders, Philadelphia, 1999.

References (grade I evidence and grade A recommendations in bold)

1   Fielding JWL, Black J, Ashton F, Slaney G, Campbell DJ. Diagnosis and management of 528 abdominal aortic aneurysms. *Br Med J* 1981; 283: 355-9.

2   Johnson KW. Multicenter prospective study of nonruptured abdominal aortic aneurysm. Part II. Variables predicting morbidity and mortality. *J Vasc Surg* 1989; 3: 437-47.

3   **The UK Small Aneurysm Trial Participants. Mortality results for a randomised controlled trial of early elective surgery or ultrasonographic surveillance for small abdominal aortic aneurysms. *Lancet* 1998; 352: 1694-1655.**

4   Johansson G, Swedenborg J. Ruptured abdominal aortic aneurysms: a study of incidence and mortality. *Br J Surg* 1986; 73: 101-3.

5   Heather BP, Poskitt KR, Earnshaw JJ, Whyman M, Shaw E. Population screening reduces the mortality rate from aortic aneurysms in men. *Br J Surg* 2000; 87: 750-53.

6   **Scott RAP, Wilson NM, Ashton HA, Kay DN. Influence of screening on the incidence of ruptured abdominal aortic aneurysm: 5-year results of a randomized controlled study. *Br J Surg* 1995; 82: 1066-1070.**

7   Brown PM, Pattenden R, Vernooy C, Zelt DT, Gutelius JR. Selective management of abdominal aortic aneurysms in a prospective measurement program. *J Vasc Surg* 1996; 23: 213-222.

8   Scott RAP, Wilson NM, Ashton HA, Kay DN. Is surgery necessary for abdominal aortic aneurysm less than 6 cm in diameter? *Lancet* 1993; 342: 1395-96.

9   Milne AA, Ruckley CV. Indications for elective surgery for abdominal aortic aneurysm. In: *The Evidence for Vascular Surgery*. Earnshaw JJ, Murie JA, Eds. tfm publishing, Shropshire, 1999.

10 Hollier LH, Taylor LM, Oschner J. Recommended indications for operative treatment of abdominal aortic aneurysms. Report of a subcommittee of the Joint Council for Vascular Surgery and the North American Chapter of the International Society for Cardiovascular Surgery. *J Vasc Surg* 1992; 15: 1046-56.

11 Galland RB. Mortality following elective infrarenal aortic reconstruction: a Joint Vascular Research Group study. *Br J Surg* 1998; 85: 633-36.

12 Johnson KW, Scobie TK. Multicenter prospective study of nonruptured abdominal aortic aneurysms. 1. Population and operative management. *J Vasc Surg* 1988; 7: 69-79.

13 **Thompson JF, Mullee MA, Bell PRF *et al*. Intraoperative heparinisation, blood loss and myocardial infarction during aortic aneurysm surgery: A Joint Vascular Research Group Study. *Eur J Endovasc Surg* 1996; 12: 86-90.**

14 Galland RB. Preoperative cardiac assessment in patients with peripheral vascular disease: is it worthwhile? *Eur J Endovasc Surg* 1999; 18: 466-68.

15 Jones A. Cahill D, Gardham R. Outcome in patients with a large abdominal aortic aneurysm considered unfit for surgery. *Br J Surg* 1998; 85: 1382-84.

16 **Poldermans D, Boersma E, Baxx JJ *et al*. The effect of bisoprolol on perioperative mortality and myocardial infarction in high risk patients undergoing vascular surgery. *N Engl J Med* 1999; 341: 1789-94.**

17 Allen BT, Anderson CB, Rubin BG, Flye MW, Baumann DS, Sicard GA. Preservation of renal function in juxtarenal and suprarenal abdominal aortic aneurysm repair. *J Vasc Surg* 1993; 17: 948-958.

18 Brady AR, Fowkes FG, Greenhalgh RM, Powell JT, Ruckley CV, Thompson SG. Risk factors for postoperative death following elective surgical repair of abdominal aortic aneurysm. *Br J Surg* 2000; 87: 742-49.

19 Irvine CD, Shaw E, Poskitt KR, Whyman MR, Earnshaw JJ, Heather BP. A comparison of the mortality rate after elective repair of aortic aneurysms detected either by screening or incidentally. *Eur J Vasc Endovasc Surg* 2000; 20: 374-78.

20 Prytherch DR, Ridler BMF, Beard JD, Earnshaw JJ. A Model for National Outcome Audit in Vascular Surgery. *Eur J Vasc Endovasc Surg* 2001; 21: 477-83.

21 Wijesinghe LD, Mahmood T, Scott DJA, Berridge DC, Kent PJ, Kester RC. Comparison of POSSUM and the Portsmouth predictor equation for predicting death following vascular surgery. *Br J Surg* 1998; 85: 209-12.

22 Barker SGE, Sachs R, Louden C, Linnard D, Abu-Own A, Buckland J, Murphy S. Integrated care pathways for vascular surgery. *Eur J Vasc Endovasc Surg* 1999; 18: 207-15.

23 Johnson S, Dracass M, Vartan J, Summers S, Edington J. Setting standards using integrated care pathways. *Prof Nurse* 2000; 15: 640-43.

24 Steed DL. Aneurysm cultures. In: *Vascular Graft Infections*. Bunt TJ, Ed. Futura, New York, 1994.

25 Ratliff DA. New initiatives in the prevention and treatment of graft infection. In: *The Evidence for Vascular Surgery*. Earnshaw JJ, Murie JA, Eds. tfm publishing, Shropshire, 1999.

Elective abdominal aortic aneurysm repair

Chapter 23

Thoracic aneurysm - *dissection and transection*

Peter R Taylor Consultant Vascular Surgeon

John F Reidy Consultant Radiologist

Marion Aukett Vascular Nurse Practitioner

DEPARTMENTS OF VASCULAR SURGERY & RADIOLOGY
GUY'S & ST. THOMAS' HOSPITAL, LONDON, UK

Introduction

Much less is known about pathology affecting the thoracic aorta compared with the infrarenal aorta, and traditional surgical repair has been associated with high morbidity and mortality. However, surgical methods are being refined, and since the advent of techniques such as cerebrospinal fluid drainage, partial cardiopulmonary bypass, sequential clamping, intercostal reimplantation and selective visceral and renal perfusion, surgical results have improved markedly. The recent development of endoluminal repair is also associated with low morbidity and mortality although the durability of the current devices remains unknown.

Epidemiology

Aneurysms of the descending thoracic aorta occur much less frequently than infrarenal abdominal aortic aneurysms. The incidence is six new aneurysms per 100,000 person-years in a population-based report from Rochester, Minnesota, between 1951-1980 [1]. This showed a 2-year survival rate of only 29% in patients who were not treated, with half of the deaths due to rupture. Similar findings were reported in 94 patients who did not undergo repair with a reported 5-year survival of 19% for patients with non-dissecting aneurysms and 7% for those with dissecting aneurysms, with the majority of deaths due to rupture [2]. One quarter of patients with a thoracic aneurysm also had an infrarenal abdominal aortic aneurysm. Thoracic aneurysmal disease has an equal sex ratio. In an autopsy study from Sweden the overall occurrence of thoracic aneurysms per 100,000 autopsies was 489 for men and 437 for women [3]. There is some evidence that the incidence of deaths from thoracic aneurysms is increasing in the UK. A series from England and Wales showed an increase of 17% in deaths from thoracic aneurysm between 1974 and 1984 [4]. A recent study from Rochester, Minnesota, showed an overall incidence of 10% for thoracic aneurysms per 100,000 person-years [5]. The incidence increased with age, and the average age at diagnosis was significantly higher in women (76 years) than in men (62 years), although the majority of ruptures occurred in women.

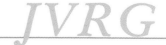

Aetiology

There is no agreement as to which is the commonest cause of thoracic aneurysms. Some suggest that it is medial degenerative disease, while others cite dissection or atherosclerosis. Medial degenerative disease includes a range of pathology including cystic medial necrosis, myxomatous or myxoid degeneration, senile aorta and Marfan's syndrome. Less common causes include aortitis, trauma and infection. Dissection of the aorta affects approximately 10 per 100,000 population per year [6]. Mortality from dissection is approximately 1% per hour for the first 48 hours with a higher mortality when the aorta proximal to the left subclavian is involved [7]. Proximal dissections may progress towards the heart causing myocardial ischaemia, aortic valve regurgitation and finally tamponade. Death may also be due to rupture into the pleural space, the mediastinum or the abdominal cavity. Stroke may follow proximal dissections that occlude the arteries to the head. Dissections distal to the left subclavian may cause death from rupture into the pleura and abdomen, and serious morbidity may accrue from branch vessel occlusion which may result in paraplegia, visceral and renal ischaemia and acute limb ischaemia. If laparotomy is required for bowel ischaemia after initial repair of a dissection, then the mortality increases to 80% [8]. One study on the long-term outcome for aortic dissection found that age greater than 70 years and post-operative patency of the false lumen of the thoracic aorta were significant factors in predicting late mortality [9].

Coarctation of the aorta may result in aneurysm formation. This can result from untreated coarctation that may not be severe enough to cause the classical clinical manifestations, but then presents in later years as aneurysmal disease. More commonly it is seen in the long-term follow-up of patients treated surgically for coarctation in early life and is due to pseudoaneurysm formation [10].

Traumatic rupture or transection of the thoracic aorta usually affects the proximal descending aorta and is invariably due to severe deceleration injuries. It is associated with a very poor prognosis unless operated on, with death often due to delayed rupture into the left pleural cavity [11].

Imaging

Many thoracic aneurysms are first noticed as incidental findings on chest x-ray. Computed tomography is then used to confirm the diagnosis and to accurately define the extent of the disease and its relation to important branches. Most specialised units would now use contrast-enhanced spiral or helical computed tomography. It is important to scan the whole length of the aorta including the iliac vessels. Three-dimensional image reconstructions, a technique known as multiplanar reformatting, are useful in delineating the extent of the aneurysm or dissection and are more comparable to conventional angiography [12-16]. Special types of reformatting such as maximum intensity projections and surface shaded display may help to define the extent of the aortic pathology. Further sophisticated three-dimensional reconstructive techniques are capable of displaying thrombus and calcified plaque separately based on the density of the different tissues. Multi-slice computed tomography is likely to replace conventional machines and has the advantage of very rapid acquisition of data sets with the ability to reconstruct thinner slices. Disadvantages of computed tomography include relatively high x-ray dose, and the nephrotoxic effects of the contrast medium. Magnetic resonance angiography involves no radiation and can provide cross-sectional images that can be easily reconstructed in any plane. Contrast enhanced scans use an intravenous injection of gadolinium to enhance the blood signal. Disadvantages include greater expense, limited availability compared with computed tomography, and the inability of patients with claustrophobia to tolerate the enclosed space within the machine.

In recent years computed tomographic angiography has largely replaced conventional angiography but centres carrying out endovascular procedures have continued to use aortography in their pre-procedural assessment. Aortography is useful to define the relationship of major branches to the aneurysm and their patency (Figure 1). The relationship of the true and false lumens to various branches and any connections between the two lumens can be defined if the catheter is placed sequentially in both lumens and injections made at different levels. A calibrated catheter with centimetre

Figure 1 Aortogram demonstrating an aneurysm of the descending thoracic aorta arising below the origin of the left subclavian artery (a) and after successful exclusion with a covered stent graft (b).

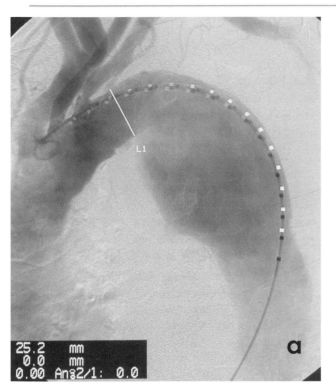

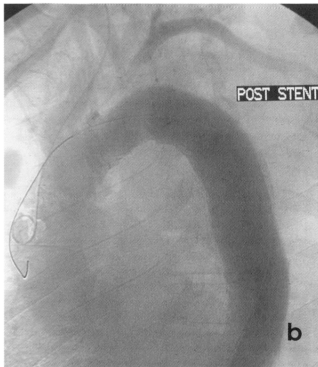

markings is used to measure length if an endoluminal graft is being contemplated. Angiography of the aortic arch carries a small risk of stroke [17] (**I**). Transoesophageal echocardiography can be very helpful in localising the proximal tear in aortic dissection, but may not be available in all hospitals. The appearance of linear artifacts within the aortic lumen can make the diagnosis of aortic dissection or traumatic disruption of the thoracic aorta difficult [18]. Transoesophageal echocardiography has been advocated to position thoracic stent grafts and, when used in combination with colour Doppler, it can detect perigraft flow that can be treated with further balloon dilatation [19]. However, in a comparative study evaluating transoesophageal echocardiography with magnetic resonance imaging in the follow-up of patients with dissection, echocardiography was found to be less accurate [20]. Intravascular ultrasound has also been used to assess aneurysms and dissections of the thoracic aorta [21,22]. One comparative study

suggested that it was less effective at detecting disease in the thoracic aorta than transoesophageal echocardiography [21]. However, a review of intravascular ultrasound showed that the technique is useful in complex anatomical problems, especially dissections when it can show the extent of the dissection, and the technique has been successfully used in percutaneous fenestration procedures of the dissection flap [22]. Intravascular ultrasound has been used in the assessment of infrarenal abdominal aortic aneurysms treated with stent grafts [23], and new developments include the addition of colour Doppler [24].

Timing of intervention

The risk:benefit ratio defines the timing of intervention. However, the risks of surgery to correct thoracic aortic pathology are high when compared to surgical intervention at other sites. Whereas open surgical correction may be the only option for some thoracoabdominal aneurysms, there are now an increasing number of reports of endovascular intervention. The natural history of some thoracic pathology is not well documented, which makes the decision on the timing of intervention difficult. In a study of 87 consecutive patients with thoracic aneurysms, the overall median expansion was 1.4mm/year, but this was greater with larger aortic diameters in an exponential manner [25]. Intraluminal thrombus, previous stroke, smoking and peripheral vascular disease were important factors associated with aneurysm growth. Some authorities have suggested that given the relatively high risks of open surgery, that the risk:benefit ratio only tilts in favour of surgery in aneurysms greater than 8 cm; aneurysms less than 5.5 cm can be safely observed and those between 5.5-7.5 cm should be closely observed [26]. In a review of 109 patients who did not undergo surgery, the risk of rupture of aneurysms above 7 cm was fourteen times greater than for aneurysms of 5 cm or less [27]. The authors therefore suggest that 6.5 cm should be the size at which intervention is justified **(B)**. One paper on the natural history of thoracic aneurysms has prospectively tried to calculate the risk of rupture of descending thoracic aneurysms and thoracoabdominal aneurysms using the patient's age, a history of chronic obstructive pulmonary disease, the presence of pain and the maximum thoracic and abdominal aortic diameters [28]. The threshold for intervention in asymptomatic thoracic aneurysms in the USA is lower than in the UK, with 30-day mortality figures of 8-10% being published [29-31]. Reports from the UK have much higher mortality rates ranging from 15-42% depending upon the extent of the aneurysm [32]. All single centre series tend to report excellent figures. However, a recent audit of cardiothoracic centres in the UK showed a mortality of 28% for procedures on the descending thoracic aorta [33] **(II)**. Saccular aneurysms have a higher risk of rupture and should probably be repaired at a smaller diameter than fusiform aneurysms. Symptomatic aneurysms should be repaired if the patient is fit enough as the average length of time to rupture has been estimated to be 2 years. An algorithm outlining the management of an asymptomatic and symptomatic aneurysm of the descending thoracic aorta are shown in Figures 2 and 3 respectively.

Intervention for dissection in Marfan's syndrome is dictated by the diameter of the aortic root. This has progressively decreased from 6 cm to 5 cm as the surgical results have improved with time [34-38]. Treatment of the descending thoracic aorta in Marfan's syndrome is often required following successful aortic root surgery [39-40]. This may be for further dissection, but may also be required for aneurysmal dilatation without dissection.

Traumatic injury to the descending thoracic aorta is associated with a mortality of 85% before the patient reaches hospital [41]. The in-hospital mortality thereafter is 1% per hour for the first 48 hours. Immediate repair is therefore justified if the patient's condition is not hopeless **(B)**.

Treatment

Surgery

Repair of aneurysms affecting only the descending thoracic aorta is differentiated from thoracoabdominal aneurysms (which also affect the abdominal aorta giving rise to the visceral vessels) in only a few series. The largest series of localised descending thoracic aortic aneurysms reported on 832 patients with a mortality of 8% using left heart bypass [42]. Paraplegia affected 5%, renal failure 7% and pulmonary complications occurred in 28%. Another large series of patients had higher rates of death and complications with a mortality of 14% and a paraplegia rate of 19% [43]. The main causes of death following surgery were due to cardiac and pulmonary complications [42-44] **(II)**. Mortality was increased significantly in cases of rupture or when the surgery was undertaken as an emergency. The presence of a dissection did not seem to influence the risk of surgery in this group of patients. Long-term results show a 5-year survival of 50-60% with a 10-year survival of 30-38% [42,43] **(II)**. The majority of late deaths are due to cardiac causes (31-39%), but rupture of other aneurysms is also an important cause (21-22%).

Thoracoabdominal aneurysms were classified by Crawford into four groups: type I affected the descending thoracic aorta distal to the left subclavian

Figure 2 Algorithm for the management of an asymptomatic aneurysm of the descending thoracic aorta.

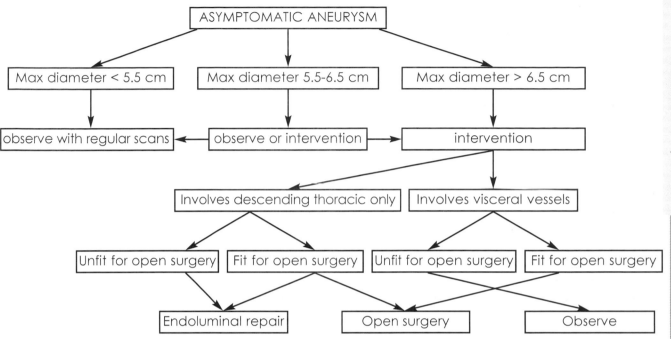

Chapter 23

Figure 3 Algorithm for the treatment of a symptomatic aneurysm of the descending thoracic aorta.

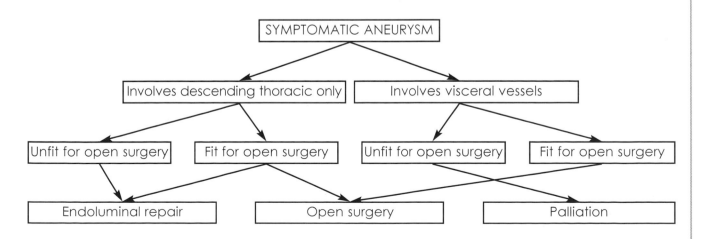

and involved the abdominal aorta bearing the visceral vessels, the infrarenal aorta being normal; type II affected the whole of the descending thoracic aorta and the infrarenal aorta to the origin of the common iliac arteries; type III had a normal segment of descending thoracic aorta and affected the distal descending thoracic aorta together with the abdominal aorta giving the visceral branches; and type IV started below the level of the diaphragm but affected the visceral arteries [45]. Thoracoabdominal aortic aneurysm repair is associated with much higher risks with mortality rates ranging from 8-28% [32,46] **(II)**. The most feared complication is paraplegia which occurs in approximately 10% of patients with reported series ranging from 4-21% [30,47] **(II)**. Other major complications include cardiac complications, coagulopathy, renal failure and respiratory problems [30,32] **(II)**. Many centres have abandoned the technique of "cross-clamp and go" popularised by Crawford [48], and have introduced adjuvant techniques to try to increase the safety of the procedure. These include cerebrospinal fluid drainage and distal aortic perfusion with moderate hypothermia [49-51] **(II)**. In a randomised trial of cerebrospinal fluid drainage in Crawford type I and II repairs, the incidence of paraplegia was 12% in the control group and 3% in the treatment group [52] **(II)**. A recent overview has also confirmed the efficacy of cerebrospinal fluid drainage in the prevention of paraplegia during thoracoabdominal aneurysm repair [53] **(II)**. Intercostal artery reattachment has also been shown to be important in the prevention of paraplegia, particularly those in the lower thoracic region [54]. Some authorities have recommended the use of motor evoked potentials to identify important intercostals which should be reimplanted [55]. Selective visceral perfusion and cooling reduces the risk of post-operative organ failure, and may also be important in preventing coagulopathy [56]. The role of perfusion in the prevention of renal dysfunction is controversial, with some finding a beneficial role and others finding that it causes deterioration in renal function [57,58]. Post-operative pulmonary complications and stay in the intensive care unit can be reduced by not completely transecting the diaphragm [59]. The use of partial cardiopulmonary bypass allows sequential aortic clamping so that the operation can be performed in stages in an unhurried manner. The long-term results show a survival of 53-60% at 5 years with the main causes of death being related to the cardiac and pulmonary systems [29, 60].

The immediate management of patients with dissection is dependent upon the site of the primary tear, and the extent of the dissection. Those that affect the ascending aorta and the arch (Stanford A) should be repaired surgically to prevent rupture and tamponade which cause immediate death in about 40% of patients [61] **(B)**. Those which have the primary tear distal to the left subclavian (Stanford B) are treated medically in the first instance as the immediate death rate is about 10% which is lower than the mortality associated with immediate surgery **(B)**. The most important part of initial treatment for Type B dissections is effective hypotensive therapy. Beta blockers and nitrates are usually the first-line of treatment. Surgery is indicated if there is any evidence of rupture. The majority of patients have some fluid in the left chest which is usually a transudate secondary to the dissection, and this needs to be differentiated from rupture. Once rupture is excluded, the next step is to look for evidence of ischaemia. This may be amenable to percutaneous techniques such as the placement of stents, stent grafts and balloon fenestration [62-65] **(B)**. One further reason to intervene in patients with dissection is the presence of continuing pain following good control of blood pressure with hypotensive agents. In an international registry of acute aortic dissection, the mortality of patients with type A having surgery was 26%; those who were treated conservatively because of age or serious comorbidity had a mortality of 58% [66]. The mortality of type B in the 80% of patients treated medically was 11%, and in the 20% who had surgery the mortality was 31%. An algorithm outlining the management of an acute dissection of the thoracic aorta is outlined in Figure 4.

Following the acute event, approximately one third of patients will progressively dilate the false lumen which may eventually lead to rupture. In a study on the long-term survival of patients with Stanford B dissections treated medically, 20% of patients died of rupture [67]. The mortality from rupture of chronic dissection is 90%. Another study of 50 patients followed long-term found that 10 patients died of rupture and 10 patients had surgery to prevent rupture [68]. Factors found to be significantly associated with rupture were age, chronic obstructive pulmonary disease and elevated mean blood pressure. Patients with rupture of dissections were found to have slightly smaller diameter aneurysms compared with degenerative aneurysms [67].

Figure 4 Algorithm for the management of an acute dissection of the thoracic aorta.

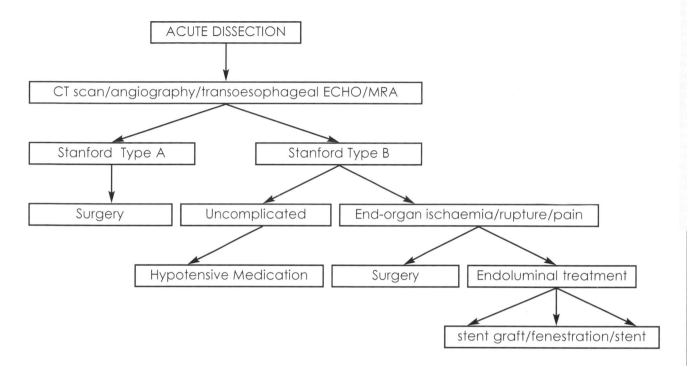

Surgical repair of traumatic aortic transection can usually be achieved by use of a graft interposition, using simple cross-clamping of the aorta, or with atriofemoral bypass, or passive shunts. Occasionally, if the tear involves the arch then total cardiopulmonary bypass with hypothermic circulatory arrest is required. In a meta-analysis of 1492 patients with blunt aortic trauma who had surgery, simple aortic cross-clamping was associated with a mortality rate of 16% and paraplegia in 19%; passive shunts had a mortality of 12% and paraplegia of 11%; and partial left heart bypass a mortality of 15% and a paraplegia rate of 2% [69] **(II)**. A recent report using left atrial to femoral artery bypass cites much better results with no cases of paraplegia or death in 30 patients [70].

Endovascular intervention

Dake and his colleagues at Stanford have the largest experience of thoracic stent grafts. Originally they used "home-made" stent grafts made from woven polyester grafts sutured to stainless steel, self-expanding Z-shaped stents with polypropylene sutures [71]. They reported on 103 patients with aneurysms of the descending thoracic aorta. Complete thrombosis of the aneurysm sac was achieved in 83% of patients, with an early mortality was 9%. Paraplegia occurred in 3% and stroke in 7%. At an average follow-up of 3.7 years only 53% of patients were free from treatment failure. Our own early experience has been reported using commercially produced stent grafts [72]. A total of 18 degenerative aneurysms were treated with no deaths or paraplegia (Figure 1). Encouraging results were also reported from Japan in a series of 50 patients [73]. Phase II studies are currently underway in the United States to compare the results of commercially produced devices with open surgery. Stent grafts bearing multiple branches have been advocated and used in a few cases to treat thoracoabdominal aneurysms which involve the origins of the visceral and renal vessels, but these are in their infancy [74].

The main aim of endovascular treatment of acute type B dissections is to cover the primary entry tear [64]. A small series of 19 patients all with tears in the descending thoracic aorta were treated by first generation stent grafts. Complete thrombosis of the false lumen of the thoracic aorta was achieved in 79% of patients, and revascularization of ischaemic branches occurred in 76%. There were no deaths, and no patient suffered from aortic rupture during the short (average 13 month) follow-up period. Another small series of patients with chronic dissection compared 12 patients treated with stent grafts to 12 matched controls treated with surgery [65]. There were no deaths and no serious morbidity in the stent graft group compared with four deaths and five serious adverse events in the surgical group. Percutaneous balloon fenestration and stenting can be very useful in patients presenting with acute aortic dissection causing end organ ischaemia [63]. Successful revascularization was achieved in 93% of patients. However, the 30-day mortality rate was 25% which was secondary to irreversible ischaemia of intra-abdominal organs. This should be contrasted with the much higher mortality in patients after thoracic aneurysm surgery who then require laparotomy for intra-abdominal ischaemia [8]. Stent grafts for type A dissections have been produced; however, they are not yet a realistic treatment option [75].

Endoluminal repair of aortic transections has been performed with encouraging results [72,76]. These two series reported no deaths or paraplegia albeit in a small number of patients. Aneurysms related to previous coarctation repair can also be treated with stent grafts with minimal morbidity and mortality [72], however, the durability of stent grafts remains unproven in the long-term [77].

Optimal care

Consent

All patients with thoracic aortic pathology should be made aware of the risks involved in treatment. These include death, myocardial infarction, paraplegia, stroke, renal failure, visceral ischaemia, distal embolisation, pulmonary failure and infections. If procedures include exposure of the aortic bifurcation then impotence should be discussed. Endoluminal treatment also has a mortality rate and can be complicated by paraplegia, stroke, renal failure, distal embolisation and damage to the arteries used for access. The risks involved in treatment must be compared with the natural history of the disease so that the risk:benefit equation can be fully understood by the patient.

Anaesthesia/analgesia

Patients having open surgery require general anaesthesia. Post-operatively they can be converted to patient controlled analgesia using intravenous morphine. Endoluminal procedures can be performed under regional or local anaesthesia, and post-operatively patients usually require only oral analgesia.

Situation

All patients having open surgery should have an intensive care unit bed, so that adequate monitoring can be performed. Patients should be warned that the operation may have to be postponed if no intensive care unit bed is available on the day of their surgery. They can be moved to a high dependency unit when they are no longer ventilated. The stay in hospital is usually between 1 and 3 weeks, depending on the complexity of the case. Patients having endoluminal treatment are usually kept in recovery for 2 hours then moved to the ward for discharge at 48 hours.

Monitoring

Open surgical patients require close monitoring of vital signs, with regular assessment of cardiac output, respiratory function, urine output, blood gases, acid base balance, blood chemistry and haematology. All abnormalities should be corrected and any adverse trends treated quickly. The drain for cerebrospinal fluid should be left in for at least 72 hours. Removal before this time can be associated with paraplegia. The height of the container collecting the fluid should be 10-12 cm above the level of the spinal cord when the patient is lying flat. If the patient develops any evidence of paraplegia after the drain has been withdrawn, it should be replaced immediately.

Patients having endoluminal procedures should have their wounds checked and their distal pulses palpated. If there is any doubt about the distal circulation then Doppler pressures should be measured. Patients developing paraplegia should have a cerebrospinal drain inserted urgently.

Hydration

Patients having open surgery often have an ileus and therefore require intravenous hydration until this resolves. Patients having endoluminal procedures under regional or local anaesthesia can drink in recovery and eat on their return to the ward.

Mobilisation

Patients with open surgery usually require ventilation for the first 1 to 3 days depending upon their respiratory function. They may sit out in a chair when this is practical, usually when they are extubated. They should be encouraged to walk as soon as most of their lines and catheters have been removed. Patients having endoluminal repair can be allowed out of bed as soon as the regional anaesthetic has worn off.

Summary

- There is a lack of good randomised trials in the treatment of thoracic aortic pathology. The majority of the evidence is based upon observational data from large single centre series **(II)**.

- Diseases of the descending thoracic aorta, although rare, are usually life-threatening if not treated. Careful assessment should be made of the risk:benefit ratio associated with intervention **(A)**.

- The results of open surgery have improved in recent years with the introduction of adjunctive techniques including partial cardiopulmonary bypass, sequential clamping, intercostal reimplantation, cerebrospinal fluid drainage, visceral and renal perfusion and cooling **(II)**.

- Endoluminal repair is associated with much lower morbidity and mortality when compared with surgery. However, there are serious concerns regarding the long-term durability of stent grafts. Endoluminal repair using such technology must be followed for life to identify problems which require correction **(III)**.

Further reading

1 Beard JD, Gaines PA, Eds. *Vascular and Endovascular Surgery*. Second Edition. WB Saunders, London, 2001.
2 Branchereau A, Jacobs M, Eds. *Surgical and Endovascular Treatment of Aortic Aneurysms*. Futura Publishing Company, Armonk NY, 2000.
3 Dyet JF, Ettles DF, Nicholson AA, Wilson SE, Eds. *Textbook of Endovascular Procedures*. Churchill Livingstone, London, 2000.

References (grade I evidence and grade A recommendations in bold)

1 Bickerstaff LK, Pairolero PC, Hollier LH *et al.* Thoracic aortic aneurysms: a population-based study. *Surgery* 1982; 92: 1103-1108.
2 Crawford ES, DeNatale RW. Thoracoabdominal aortic aneurysm: observation regarding the natural course of the disease. *J Vasc Surg* 1986; 3: 578-582.
3 Svensjo S, Bengtsson H, Bergqvist D. Thoracic and thoracoabdominal aortic aneurysm and dissection: an investigation based on autopsy. *Br J Surg* 1996; 83: 68-71.
4 Fowkes FG, MacIntyre CC, Ruckley CV. Increasing incidence of aortic aneurysms in England and Wales. *Br Med J* 1989; 298: 33-35.
5 Clouse WD, Hallett JW Jr, Schaff HV *et al.* Improved prognosis of thoracic aortic aneurysms. *JAMA* 1998; 280: 1926-1929.
6 Svensson LG, Crawford ES. Aortic dissection and aortic aneurysm surgery: clinical observations, experimental investigations and statistical analyses. Part II. *Curr Probl Surg* 1992: 29: 915-1057.

7   Miller DC, Mitchell RS, Oyer PE *et al.* Independent determinants of operative mortality for patients with aortic dissections. *Circulation* 1984; 70: 1153-64.

8   Fann JI, Sarris GE, Mitchell RS *et al.* Treatment of patients with aortic dissection presenting with peripheral vascular complications. *Ann Surg* 1990; 212: 705-13.

9   Bernard Y, Zimmerman H, Chocron S *et al.* False lumen patency as a predictor of late outcome in aortic dissection. *Am J Cardiol* 2001; 87: 1378-1382.

10 Parks WJ, Ngo TD, Plauth WH Jr *et al.* Incidence of aneurysm formation after Dacron patch aortoplasty for coarctation of the aorta: long-term results and assessment utilizing magnetic resonance angiography with three-dimensional surface rendering. *J Am Coll Cardiol* 1995; 26: 266-271.

11 Pickard LR, Mattox KL, Espada R *et al.* Transection of the descending thoracic aorta secondary to blunt trauma. *Journal of Trauma-Injury Infection and Critical Care* 1977; 17: 749-753.

12 Rubin GD, Walker PJ, Dake MD *et al.* Three-dimensional spiral computed tomographic angiography: an alternative imaging modality for the abdominal aorta and its branches. *J Vasc Surg* 1993; 18: 656-665.

13 Balm R, Eikelboom BC, van Leeuwen MS *et al.* Spiral CT-angiography of the aorta. *Eur J Vasc Surg* 1994; 8: 544-551.

14 Van Hoe L, Baert AL, Gryspeerdt S *et al.* Supra- and juxtarenal aneurysms of the abdominal aorta: preoperative assessment with thin-section spiral CT. *Radiology* 1996; 198: 443-448.

15 Broeders I, Blankensteijn J, Olree M *et al.* Preoperative sizing of grafts for transfemoral endovascular aneurysm management: a prospective comparative study of spiral CT angiography, arteriography and conventional CT imaging. *J Endovasc Surg* 1997; 4: 252-261.

16 Urban BA, Bluemke DA, Johnson KM, Fishman EK. Imaging of thoracic aortic disease. *Cardiology Clinics* 1999; 17: 659-682.

17 Executive Committee for the Asymptomatic Carotid Atherosclerosis Study. Endarterectomy for asymptomatic carotid artery stenosis. *JAMA* 1995; 273: 1421-1461.

18 Vignon P, Spencer KT, Rambaud G *et al.* Differential transesophageal echocardiographic diagnosis between linear artifacts and intraluminal flap of aortic dissection or disruption. *Chest* 2001; 119: 1778-1790.

19 Rapezzi C, Rocchi G, Fattori R, *et al.* Usefulness of transesophageal echocardiographic monitoring to improve the outcome of stent-graft treatment of thoracic aortic aneurysms. *Am J Cardiol* 2001; 87: 315-319.

20 Cesare ED, Giodano AV, Cerone G *et al.* Comparative evaluation of TEE, conventional MRI and contrast-enhanced 3D breath-hold MRA in the post-operative follow-up of dissecting aneurysms. *International Journal of Cardiac Imaging* 2000; 16: 135-147.

21 Buck T, Gorge G, Hunold P, Erbel R. Three-dimensional imaging in aortic disease by lighthouse transesophageal echocardiology using intravascular ultrasound catheters. Comparison to three-dimensional transesophageal echocardiology and three-dimensional intra-aortic ultrasound imaging. *Journal of the American Society of echocardiography* 1998; 11: 243-258.

22 Manninen HI, Rasanen H. Intravascular ultrasound in interventional radiology. *European Radiology* 2000; 10: 1754-1762

23 van Sambeek MRHM, Gussenhoven EJ, van Overhagen H *et al.* Intravascular ultrasound in endovascular stent-grafts for peripheral aneurysm: a clinical study. *J Endovasc Surg* 1998; 5: 106-112.

24 Irshad K, Reid DB, Miller PH *et al.* Early clinical experience with color three-dimensional intravascular ultrasound in peripheral interventions. *J Endovasc Therapy* 2001; 8: 329-338.

25 Bonser RS, Pagano D, Lewis ME *et al.* Clinical and patho-anatomical factors affecting expansion of thoracic aortic aneurysms. *Heart* 2000; 84: 277-283.

26 Pitt MPI, Bonser RS. The natural history of thoracic aortic aneurysm: an overview. *J Card Surg* 1997; 12: 270-278.

27 Coady MA, Rizzo JA, Hammond GL *et al.* Surgical intervention criteria for thoracic aortic aneurysms: a study of growth rates and complications. *Ann Thorac Surg* 1999; 67: 1922-1926.

28 Junoven T, Ergin MA, Galla JD *et al.* Prospective study of the natural history of thoracic aortic aneurysms. *Ann Thorac Surg* 1997; 63: 1533-1545.

29 Svensson LG, Crawford ES, Hess KR *et al.* Experience with 1509 patients undergoing thoracoabdominal aortic operations. *J Vasc Surg* 1993; 17: 357-368.

30 Hollier LH, Money SR, Haslund TC *et al.* Risk of spinal cord dysfunction in patients undergoing thoracoabdominal aortic replacement. *Am J Surg* 1992; 164: 210-213.

31 Safi HJ, Campbell MP, Miller CC 3rd *et al.* Cerebral spinal fluid drainage and distal aortic perfusion decrease the incidence of neurological deficit: the results of 343 descending and thoracoabdominal aneurysm repairs. *Eur J Vasc Endovasc Surg* 1997; 14: 118-124.

32 Gilling-Smith GL, Worswick L, Knight PF *et al.* Surgical repair of thoracoabdominal aortic aneurysms: 10 years' experience. *Br J Surg* 1995; 82: 624-629.

33 Keogh BE, Kinsman R. National adult cardiac surgical database report 1998 of the Society of Cardiothoracic Surgeons of Great Britain and Ireland, Concord Services London 1999.

34 Gott VL, Pyeritz RE, Cameron DE *et al.* Composite graft repair of Marfan aneurysm of the ascending aorta: results in 100 patients. *Ann Thorac Surg* 1991; 52: 38-45.

35 Coady MA, Rizzo JA, Hammond GL *et al*. What is the appropriate size criterion for resection of thoracic aortic aneurysms? *J Thorac Cardiovasc Surg* 1997; 113: 476-479.

36 Kouchokos NT, Dougenis D. Surgery of the thoracic aorta. N Engl J Med 1997; 336: 1876-1888.

37 Gott VL, Greene PS, Alejo DE *et al*. Replacement of the aortic root in patients with the Marfan syndrome. *N Engl J Med* 1999; 340: 1307-1313.

38 Ergin MA, Spielvogel D, Apaydin A *et al*. Surgical treatment of the dilated descending aorta: when and how? *Ann Thorac Surg* 1999; 67: 1834-1839.

39 Finkbohner R, Johnson D, Crawford ES *et al*. Marfan syndrome: long-term survival and complications after aortic aneurysm repair. *Circulation* 1995; 91: 728-733.

40 Kawamoto S, Bluemke DA, Traill TA *et al*. Thoracoabdominal aorta in Marfan syndrome: MR imaging findings of progression of vasculopathy after surgical repair. *Radiology* 1997; 203: 727-732

41 Parmley L, Mattingly T, Marian W *et al*. Non-penetrating traumatic injury of the aorta. *Circulation* 1958; 17: 1086.

42 Svensson LG, Crawford ES, Hess KR *et al*. Variables predictive of outcome in 832 patients undergoing repairs of the descending thoracic aorta. *Chest* 1993; 104:1248-1253.

43 Lawrie GM, Earle N, DeBakey ME. Evolution of surgical techniques for aneurysm of the descending thoracic aorta: twenty-nine years experience with 659 patients. *J Card Surg* 1994; 9: 648-661.

44 Coselli JS, Konstadinos AP, La Francesca S *et al*. Results of contemporary surgical treatment of descending thoracic aortic aneurysms: experience in 198 patients. *Ann Vasc Surg* 1996; 10: 131-137.

45 Crawford ES. Thoracoabdominal and abdominal aortic aneurysm involving renal, superior mesenteric and celiac arteries. *Ann Surg* 1974; 179; 763-772.

46 Coselli JS, LeMaire SA. Left heart bypass reduces paraplegia rates after thoracoabdominal aortic aneurysm repair. *Ann Thorac Surg* 1999; 67: 1931-1934.

47 Cox GS, O'Hara PJ, Hertzer NR *et al*. Thoracoabdominal aneurysm repair: a representative experience. *J Vasc Surg* 1992; 15: 780-788.

48 Crawford ES, Crawford JL, Safi HJ *et al*. Thoracoabdominal aortic aneurysms: preoperative and intraoperative factors determining immediate and long-term results of operations in 605 patients. *J Vasc Surg* 1986; 3: 389-404.

49 Safi HJ, Bartoli S, Hess KR *et al*. Neurological deficit in patients at high risk with thoracoabdominal aortic aneurysms: the role of cerebral spinal fluid drainage and distal aortic perfusion. *J Vasc Surg* 1994; 20: 434-443.

50 Safi HJ, Hess KR, Randel M *et al*. Cerebrospinal fluid drainage and distal aortic perfusion: reducing neurologic complications in repair of thoracoabdominal aortic aneurysm types I and II. *J Vasc Surg* 1996; 23: 223-229.

51 von Segesser LK, Marty B, Mueller X *et al*. Active cooling during open repair of thoracoabdominal aortic aneurysms improves outcome. *Eur J Cardiothorac Surg* 2001; 19: 411-415.

52 Coselli JS, LeMaire SA, Schmittling ZC *et al*. Cerebrospinal fluid drainage in thoracoabdominal aortic surgery. *Seminars in Vascular Surgery* 2000; 13: 308-14.

53 Ling E, Arellano R. Systematic overview of the evidence supporting the use of cerebrospinal fluid drainage in thoracoabdominal aneurysm surgery for prevention of paraplegia. *Anesthesiology* 2000; 93: 1115-1122.

54 Safi HJ, Miller CC 3rd, Carr C *et al*. Importance of intercostal artery reattachment during thoracoabdominal aortic aneurysm repair. *J Vasc Surg* 1998; 27: 58-68.

55 Jacobs MJ, Meylaerts SA, De Haan P *et al*. Strategies to prevent neurologic deficit based on motor-evoked potentials in type I and II thoracoabdominal aortic aneurysm repair. *J Vasc Surg* 1999; 29: 48-59.

56 Safi HJ, Miller CC 3rd, Yawn DH *et al*. Impact of distal aortic and visceral perfusion on liver function during thoracoabdominal and descending thoracic aortic repair. *J Vasc Surg* 1998; 27: 145-153.

57 Jacobs MJ, Eijsman L, Meylearts SA *et al*. Reduced renal failure following thoracoabdominal aortic aneurysm repair by selective perfusion. *Eur J Cardio Thor Surg* 1998; 14: 201-205.

58 Safi HJ, Harklin SA, Miller CC *et al*. Predictive factors for acute renal failure in thoracic and thoracoabdominal aortic aneurysm surgery. *J Vasc Surg* 1996; 24: 338-45.

59 Engle J, Safi HJ, Miller CC 3rd *et al*. The impact of diaphragm management on prolonged ventilator support after thoracoabdominal aneurysm repair. *J Vasc Surg* 1999; 29: 150-156.

60 Schepens MA, Vermeulen FE, Morshuis WJ *et al*. Impact of left heart bypass on results of thoracoabdominal aortic aneurysm repair. *Ann Thorac Surg* 1999; 67: 1963-1967.

61 Daily PO, Trublood HW, Stinson EB *et al*. Management of acute aortic dissections. *Ann Thorac Surg* 1970; 10: 237-247.

62 Slonim SM, Nyman U, Semba CP *et al*. Aortic dissection: percutaneous management of ischemic complications with endovascular stents and balloon fenestration. *J Vasc Surg* 1996; 23: 241-251.

63 Slonim SM, Miller DC, Mitchell RS *et al*. Percutaneous balloon fenestration and stenting for life-threatening complications in patients with acute aortic dissection. *J Thorac Cardiovasc Surg* 1999; 117: 1118-1127.

64 Dake MD, Kato N, Mitchell RS *et al*. Endovascular stent-graft placement for the treatment of acute aortic dissection. *N Engl J Med* 1999; 340: 1546-1552.

65 Nienaber CA, Fattori R, Lund G *et al*. Nonsurgical reconstruction of thoracic aortic dissection by stent-graft placement. *N Engl J Med* 1999; 340: 1539-1545.

66 Hagan PG, Nienaber CA, Isselbacher EM *et al*. The international registry of acute aortic dissection (IRAD): new insights into an old disease. *JAMA* 2000; 283: 897-903.

67 Griepp RB, Ergin MA, Galla JD *et al*. Natural history of descending thoracic and thoracoabdominal aneurysms. *Ann Thorac Surg* 1999; 67: 1927-1930.

68 Juvonen T, Ergin MA, Galla JD *et al*. Risk factors for rupture of chronic type B dissections. *J Thorac Cardiovasc Surg* 1999; 117: 776-786.

69 Von Oppell UO, Dunne TT, De Groot MK *et al*. Traumatic aortic rupture: twenty-year meta-analysis of mortality and risk of paraplegia. *Ann Thorac Surg* 1994; 58: 585-593.

70 Szwerc MF, Benckart DH, Lin JC *et al*. Recent clinical experience with left heart bypass using a centrifugal pump for repair of traumatic aortic transection. *Ann Surg* 1999; 230: 484-490.

71 Dake MD, Miller DC, Mitchell RS *et al*. The "first generation" of endovascular stent-grafts for patients with aneurysms of the descending thoracic aorta. *J Thorac Cardiovasc Surg* 1998; 116: 689-703.

72 Taylor PR, Gaines PA, McGuinness CL, Cleveland TJ, Beard JD, Cooper G, Reidy JF. Thoracic aortic stent grafts - early experience from two centres using commercially available devices. *Eur J Vasc Endovasc Surg* 2001; 22: 70-76.

73 Kawaguchi S, Ishimaru S, Shimazaki T *et al*. Clinical results of endovascular stent graft repair for 50 cases of thoracic aortic aneurysms. *Jap J Thoracic Cardiovasc Surg* 1998; 46: 971-975.

74 Chuter TA, Gordon RL, Reilly LM *et al*. Multi-branched stent-graft for type III thoracoabdominal aneurysm. *J Vasc Interven Radiol* 2001; 12: 391-392.

75 Inoue K, Hosokawa H, Iwase T *et al*. Aortic arch reconstruction by transluminally placed endovascular branched stent graft. *Circulation* 1999; 100 (suppl 19): II 316-321.

76 Rousseau H, Soula P, Perreault P *et al*. Delayed treatment of traumatic rupture of the thoracic aorta with endoluminal covered stent. *Circulation* 1999; 99: 498-504.

77 Colin J, Murie JA. Endovascular treatment of abdominal aortic aneurysm: a failed experiment. *Br J Surg* 2001; 88: 1281-1282.

Chapter 24

Renal artery intervention

John E Scoble Consultant Nephrologist
Peter R Taylor Consultant Vascular Surgeon
John F Reidy Consultant Radiologist
Marion Aukett Vascular Nurse Practitioner

DEPARTMENTS OF NEPHROLOGY, SURGERY & RADIOLOGY
GUY'S & ST. THOMAS' HOSPITAL, LONDON, UK

Introduction

Renal artery narrowing was shown by Goldblatt in experimental animals to cause hypertension which was reversible when the renal artery narrowing was treated. This led to an enormous interest in intervention in renal artery stenosis. At present there are few randomised trials to guide the management of such patients.

Renal artery narrowing can occur with many disease processes. In Europe the two major pathologies are atherosclerotic and fibromuscular disease. Atherosclerosis is common in older patients who may have evidence of widespread disease. Fibromuscular disease is less common and occurs in younger, predominantly female patients. Other causes of renal artery narrowing are too uncommon to be discussed in this chapter. Renal artery stenosis can present in a number of ways and clinical issues are important in deciding the course of management. These are discussed separately in this chapter and a protocol is given for intervention in both hypertension and renal dysfunction.

Flash pulmonary oedema

This condition was only recognised relatively recently [1], and is a clinical diagnosis made in patients with relatively good cardiac function who present with acute unprovoked pulmonary oedema. The association with renal artery stenosis was shown by Pickering et al [1] who demonstrated that intervention could cure the condition. Patients were admitted on average three times before the diagnosis was made and they often required a period of ventilation. This condition is now widely regarded as an absolute indication for intervention **(B)** although there are no case-controlled studies to support this **(II)**. However, clinical observation in a large number of cases suggests that cure can be achieved in most patients. Flash pulmonary oedema is more likely to be found in bilateral renal artery stenosis or stenosis in a single functioning kidney [2]. It seems to be only seen in atherosclerotic disease of the renal artery, although it can present in renal transplant recipients due to iliac atherosclerotic disease.

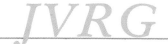

Hypertension

Early work in this area suggested that revascularization might be a method of curing hypertension but this has been found to be overly optimistic. Hypertension is a common problem and the incidence increases with age. It is common practice to fully investigate patients with hypertension below the age of 30 years but not to do so over the age of 60 years. However any patient presenting with accelerated or malignant hypertension should also undergo thorough investigation **(III)**.

The age of presentation gives some indication as to the cause. Patients with hypertension under the age of 30 years or presenting with malignant hypertension should have screening for phaeochromocytoma, Conn's syndrome and renal arterial disease **(C)**. Currently magnetic resonance angiography is the best screening test for the renal arteries. Nuclear medicine investigation has previously been used but problems include exposure to radiation and the indirect nature of the assessment of renal artery stenosis. Nuclear medicine tests should not be the first line investigation if both tests are available.

If renal artery stenosis is found in a young patient with hypertension the most likely cause is fibromuscular dysplasia. Angioplasty has been shown to be highly effective in this condition with a high probability of producing a cure [3]. This should therefore be offered to these patients **(A)**. Figure 1 outlines an algorithm for the management of patients with suspected renovascular hypertension.

The situation is more complex in older patients who have hypertension and are found on investigation to have renal artery stenosis. There are three randomised controlled studies that have failed to show an advantage of angioplasty over best medical treatment [4-6] **(I)**. Each trial has its own limitations but hypertension alone is probably not an indication for intervention **(A)**. However there are special situations where intervention may, in the future, be shown to be justified. Angiotensin Converting Enzyme Inhibitors (ACEI) have been shown to be beneficial in a number of conditions such as insulin dependent diabetes with nephropathy and heart failure. They have also been shown to cause an important decline in renal function in patients with renal artery stenosis. It is possible that in future renal intervention might be indicated in patients with hypertension and renal artery narrowing in order that an ACEI can be prescribed for their treatment **(C)**.

Renal dysfunction

This is an area of considerable debate. In younger patients renal artery narrowing is a rare cause of renal dysfunction unless it induces malignant hypertension. In older patients with atherosclerotic disease, hypertension and renal artery narrowing due to atheroma can frequently occur in combination with renal dysfunction. Non-randomised studies in patients with progressive renal dysfunction have suggested that renal revascularisation may improve outcome. These have usually been in patients with either bilateral disease or unilateral disease with a single kidney. In this instance it can be surmised that renal artery narrowing may have a pivotal role in the progression of renal dysfunction. However, other investigators have suggested that in these patients there is a process termed atherosclerotic nephropathy in which renal artery narrowing is only one of the many pathophysiological processes in play.

Atherosclerotic renovascular disease as a cause of renal dysfunction should be suspected in a patient who also has peripheral vascular disease. Studies have shown that this is the most consistent association [7]. The initial screening should include clinical examination for signs of peripheral vascular disease. Clinical experience has suggested that femoral bruits are important in indicating potential renovascular disease. Other features that suggest atherosclerotic renovascular disease are asymmetry of renal size or a deterioration of renal function when the patient is prescribed an ACEI.

Screening can be performed using the most frequently used test in each individual unit. Intra-arterial angiography remains the investigation of choice in many units although it is likely that magnetic resonance angiography will replace this within the next few years.

At present there are no randomised controlled trials to establish the efficacy of intervention in these patients **(III)**. Figure 2 outlines a pragmatic

Figure 1 Algorithm for the management of renovascular hypertension.

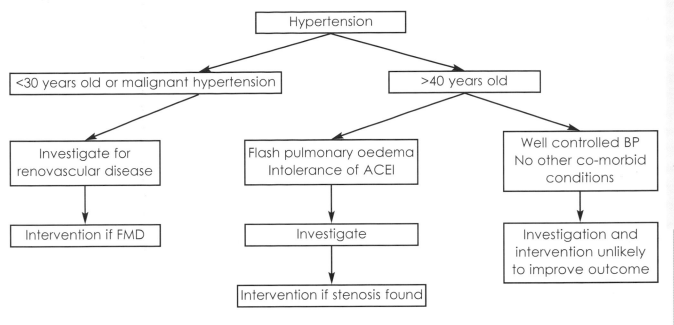

Figure 2 Algorithm for the management of renal dysfunction.

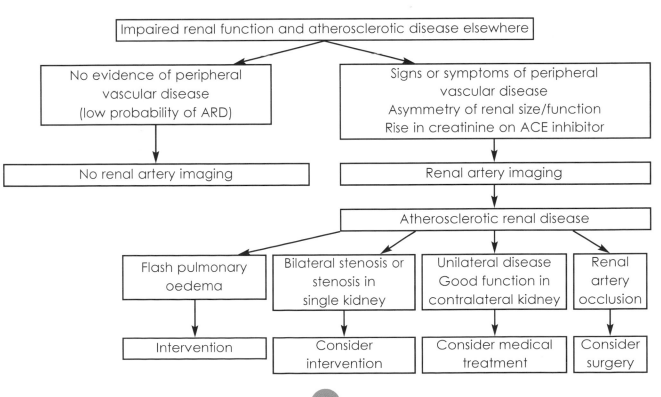

Figure 3 Arteriogram demonstrating a right renal ostial stenosis and a left renal artery occlusion in a young patient with renovascular hypertension and impaired renal function (a). The stenosis on the right was treated successfully with a stent (b).

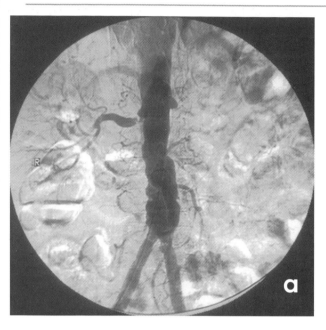
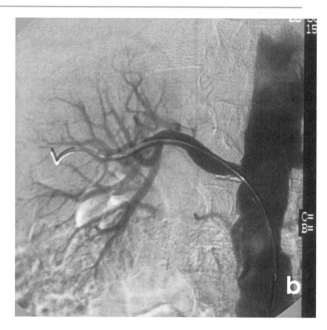

management pathway for such patients but this is not supported by grade I evidence. Currently there are trials underway to address this issue and suitable patients should be entered into such trials where possible **(C)**. The lack of clarity as to intervention in these patients also applies to atherosclerotic renovascular disease found on investigation of patients with peripheral vascular disease which can be expected to be found in 50% of cases.

Hypertension and renal dysfunction in a renal transplant recipient

Renal transplant artery stenosis can occur at any time after grafting although it is more common in the first year. With the use of donor aortic patches in cadaveric transplantation, stenosis at the site of anastomosis is rare. The underlying mechanism for the narrowing is unclear.

Hypertension and graft dysfunction are both frequently found in renal transplant patients. Hypertension is seen in the vast majority of renal transplant recipients. However, new worsening of hypertension or a rise in plasma creatinine with an ACEI are indications for screening. In most cases Doppler angiology can be performed and the diagnosis excluded. If suspected then at present intra-arterial angiography is the investigation of choice with angioplasty with or without stent placement as the preferred treatment. Renal dysfunction occurring in transplant recipients should be investigated with colour Doppler ultrasound to detect any stenoses occurring in either the native vessels or the transplant arteries. It is important to realise that renal dysfunction can occur over 10 years after grafting and that treatment of stenoses may reverse the renal dysfunction **(II)**. If renal artery stenosis is proven on imaging then intervention to improve renal function or hypertension should be considered **(B)**.

Intervention

The choice of intervention lies between balloon angioplasty (with or without stent) and surgery. Balloon angioplasty is very effective for fibromuscular dysplasia [3]. Angioplasty without stent placement is probably also effective for non-ostial stenoses of the renal artery or its major branches. However, there is a significant risk of restenosis. The risk of restenosis is much higher in ostial stenoses occurring in 15-40% of patients. One randomised study comparing angioplasty with angioplasty plus stent placement for ostial lesions has found that restenosis is significantly less with stenting [8] (I). However, there are no data to show that the long-term outcome of intervention is better in angioplasty with or without stent placement (Figure 3).

One prospective randomised trial has shown no difference between surgery and angioplasty where both are possible [9] (I). Given the morbidity and cost it would appear that in most cases angioplasty is the method of choice. However, there are some situations in which surgery may be required for failed angioplasty [10]. These include technical failures and urgent complications such as acute thrombosis or rupture of the renal artery (C).

If surgical repair is required, then the status of the aorta and the fitness of the patient should be taken into account. If the aorta is normal in a fit patient, then aortorenal bypass can be performed with autogenous vein or a prosthetic graft. If the aorta is diseased but the patient is fit enough to withstand aortic clamping, then aortorenal endarterectomy can be performed. If the patient is unfit, then a non-anatomic bypass can be used, using the hepatic, renal or iliac arteries. In patients with coexisting renal artery stenoses and aortic aneurysms, then repair of the aortic aneurysm can be combined with renal artery reconstruction using either a bypass graft or endarterectomy [11]. Simultaneous repair of asymptomatic renal artery stenosis in patients who require infrarenal aortoiliac reconstruction either for stenosing or aneurysmal disease is not justified and should not be performed [12].

In certain circumstances, the kidney may be kept alive by collaterals after the renal arteries have occluded, the so-called hibernating kidney. These patients may be dialysis dependent, but have functioning kidneys on nuclear medicine scans. Surgery to revascularise the kidney may allow the patient to remain free from dialysis [13]. In patients with irreparable ischaemic injury where nuclear medicine scans show that the kidney is contributing less than 10% of the total renal function, and when the length of the kidney is less than 5 cm with evidence of cortical infarction, then nephrectomy is appropriate if removal of the kidney will result in a benefit to the patient. This is usually when there is difficulty in controlling hypertension.

Optimal Care

Consent

All patients should be made aware that there are risks involved in endovascular renal intervention. The most serious being loss of the kidney with subsequent reliance on dialysis. Other risks include problems at the access site including bleeding, false aneurysm formation, dissection and thrombosis.

Monitoring

Pulse, blood pressure and urine output should be kept under close review in the first few hours following intervention. However, loin pain is often the first indication that renal infarction is occurring. This is usually severe and requires opiate analgesia. If there is any doubt about the blood supply to the kidney then an urgent Doppler ultrasound scan should be performed. If the warm ischaemia time is less than 60 minutes, then urgent angiography should be performed as thrombolysis or urgent surgery could salvage renal function. Daily weight is important in patients who are at risk of renal failure.

Pressure area care

Patients who have renal intervention for atherosclerotic renal artery stenosis often have occlusive arterial disease affecting the arteries to the lower limb. These patients are particularly at risk of developing ulcers and gangrene usually of the heel. Care must be paid to these pressure areas to prevent such complications.

Summary

- Flash pulmonary oedema is an indication for revascularization **(II)**.

- Patients with hypertension who are less than 30 years old should be fully investigated for renal artery stenosis **(III)**.

- Hypertension due to fibromuscular dysplasia is an indication for revascularization **(II)**.

- There is no indication for intervention to cure hypertension due to atherosclerotic renovascular disease **(II)**.

- Patients who have renal dysfunction can be considered for revascularization if they have bilateral renal artery stenoses or if they have a stenosis in a single kidney **(II)**.

- Patients who have a stenosis in a transplant should be considered for revascularization if they have hypertension or renal dysfunction **(II)**.

- Balloon angioplasty with stent should be considered in ostial disease **(I)**.

- Surgery should be considered if angioplasty is not possible or when it fails **(III)**.

Further reading

1 Novick AC, Scoble J, Hamilton G, Eds. *Renal Vascular Disease*. WB Saunders, London, 1996.

2 Earnshaw JJ, Murie JA, Eds. *The Evidence for Vascular Surgery*. tfm Publishing Ltd, Shropshire, 1999.

3 Beard JD, Gaines PA, Eds. *Vascular and Endovascular Surgery*. Second Edition, WB Saunders, London, 2001.

References (grade I evidence and grade A recommendations in bold)

1 Pickering TG, Herman L, Devereux RB, *et al*. Recurrent pulmonary oedema in hypertension due to bilateral renal artery stenosis: treatment by angioplasty or surgical intervention. *Lancet* 1988; 2: 551-552.

2 Bloch MJ, Trost DW, Pickering TG, Sos TA, August P. Prevention of recurrent pulmonary edema in patients with bilateral renovascular disease through renal artery stent placement. *American Journal of Hypertension* 1999; 12: 1-7.

3 Ramsay LE, Waller PC. Blood pressure response to percutaneous transluminal angioplasty for renovascular hypertension: an overview of published series. *Br Med J* 1990; 300(569-572).

4 Webster J, Marshall F, Abdalla M, *et al*. Randomised comparison of percutaneous angioplasty vs continued medical therapy for hypertensive patients with renal artery stenosis. *Journal of Human Hypertension* 1998; 12: 329-335.

5 Plouin PF, Chatellier G, Darne B, Raynaud A. Blood pressure outcome of angioplasty in atherosclerotic renal artery stenosis. *Hypertension* 1998; 31: 823-829.

6 van Jaarsveld BC, Krijnen P, Pieterman H, *et al*. The effect of balloon angioplasty on hypertension in atherosclerotic renal-artery stenosis. *New Engl J Med* 2000; 342: 1007-1014.

7 Choudhri AH, Cleland JGF, Rowlands PC, Tran TL, McCarthy M, Al-Kutoubi MA. Unsuspected renal artery stenosis in peripheral vascular disease. *Br Med J* 1990; 301: 1197-1198.

8 van de Ven PJG, Kaatee R, Beutler JJ *et al*. Arterial stenting and balloon angioplasty in ostial atherosclerotic renovascular disease: a randomised trial. *Lancet* 1999; 353: 282-286.

9 Weibull H, Bergqvist D, Bergentz SE, Jonsson K, Hulthen L, Manhem P. Percutaneous transluminal renal angioplasty versus surgical reconstruction of atherosclerotic renal artery stenosis: a prospective randomised study. *J Vasc Surg* 1993; 18: 841-852.

10 Wong JM, Hansen KJ, Oskin TC *et al*. Surgery after failed percutaneous renal artery angioplasty. *J Vasc Surg* 1999; 30: 468-482.

11 Davis M, Dawson K, Hamilton G. Renal and intestinal vascular disease. In: *Vascular and Endovascular Surgery*. Beard JD, Gaines PA, Eds, 2nd Edition. WB Saunders, London, 2001

12 Williamson WK, Abou-Zamzam AM Jr, Noeta GL *et al*. Prophylactic repair of renal artery stenosis is not justified in patients who require infrarenal aortic reconstruction. *J Vasc Surg* 1998; 28: 14-20.

13 Cohen DL, Townsend RR, Kobrin SD *et al*. Dramatic recovery of renal function after 6 months of dialysis dependence following surgical correction of total renal artery occlusion in a solitary functioning kidney. *Am J Kidney Diseases* 2001; 37: E7.

Chapter 25

Carotid endarterectomy

Gareth D Griffiths Consultant Vascular Surgeon [1]
Carolyn Johnstone Vascular Nurse Specialist [1]
Marilyn Horner Vascular Nurse Specialist [2]
Cliff Shearman Professor of Vascular Surgery [2]

[1] DEPARTMENT OF VASCULAR SURGERY, NINEWELLS HOSPITAL, DUNDEE, UK
[2] DEPARTMENT OF VASCULAR SURGERY, SOUTHAMPTON GENERAL HOSPITAL, SOUTHAMPTON, UK

Introduction

Stroke is a major cause of morbidity and mortality with an annual incidence in the UK of 1 in 500 [1] **(I)** superseded only by coronary heart disease and malignancy [2] **(I)**. Carotid endarterectomy has the potential to reduce the risk of stroke in a relatively small, but well-defined group of patients. However, the margins of benefit and cost effectiveness of the operation are small and only with careful patient selection, excellent surgical results and best use of resources can these benefits be realised [3]. This chapter examines the steps involved in carotid endarterectomy and how these may be optimised to ensure correct selection of patients for surgery, minimise the risks of the procedure and to ensure all the important aspects of care are delivered.

Carotid endarterectomy is a good model for an Integrated Care Pathway (ICP) as it is a common procedure and the majority of patients have a short, predictable hospital stay [4,5]. An ICP which starts in the out-patient department and continues through the whole of the in-patient stay can address all the issues relating to possible complications and can ensure that all steps are taken to minimise the risks [6]. It can also ensure that unnecessary procedures or investigations are avoided (Figure 1).

Pre-operative preparation

The aim of pre-operative preparation is to deliver a fully optimised patient to the operating theatre with the minimal delay. This process starts with the first out-patient visit and should ensure the best possible medical conditions for anaesthesia and surgery and that the patient is fully mentally and medically prepared for the forthcoming procedure.

Out-patient preparation

The indication for surgery should be established and the need for any further imaging determined (see chapter on the investigation of TIAs and stroke). Involvement of a neurologist in all cases is not always practicable but must be considered where there is any doubt about the aetiology of the neurological event **(A)**.

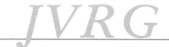

Figure 1 Algorithm illustrating some of the important steps in the management of a patient undergoing a carotid endarterectomy.

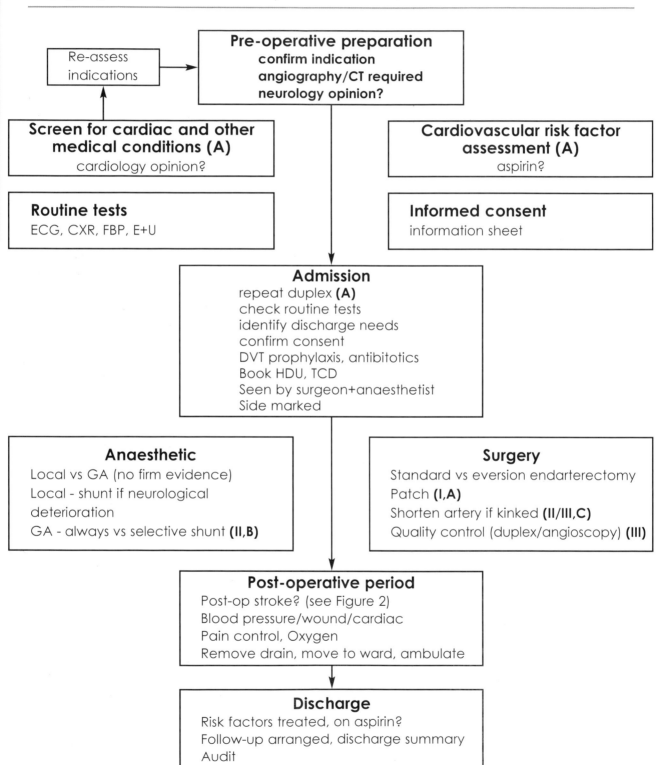

It is important to identify and when possible correct any medical conditions that could have an adverse effect **(A)**. The evidence for the benefit of this is overwhelming but it is poorly applied to clinical practice **(I, A)**. Ischaemic heart disease is common in patients presenting with cerebrovascular disease and the commonest cause of death after carotid endarterectomy is myocardial infarction or dysrhythmia [7] **(II)**. Not all patients need cardiological review, but those with symptoms are at higher risk of peri-operative cardiac events, especially if they have poor ventricular function [8]. All patients require a resting ECG **(A)**. Some centres will also perform an exercise ECG, resting or stress echocardiogram or a dipyridamole-thallium scan. A cardiologist should review patients with cardiac failure, symptomatic arrthymias, poor ventricular function, unstable angina or those who have had a myocardial infarction within the last 30 days **(B)**. In some patients their medical treatment can be optimised, but it may be necessary to consider cardiac revascularisation or review the decision to undertake carotid endarterectomy **(B)**. Although currently unproven, carotid stenting may become the best option for such patients.

It is important to identify and document any pre-existing neurological deficit the patient may have prior to surgery. The timing of surgery after non-disabling stroke remains controversial. Recent evidence suggests surgery within 30 days does not confer excess risk as previously thought and reduces the risk of a further embolic stroke while the patient is waiting for surgery [9]. However, patients must have neurological function worth preserving before being offered surgery [10,11] **(I) (A)**.

Other medical conditions such as chronic chest disease, diabetes, hypertension and hypercholesterolaemia should be identified and treated **(A)**. Smoking is a major risk factor for further cardiovascular events and encouragement and support to stop should be given **(A)**. Care should be taken to ensure that the patient is taking an antiplatelet agent such as aspirin at this stage. Combination therapy with clopidogrel should be stopped pre-operatively as there have been several reports of excessive intra-operative bleeding in patients on such combination therapy **(III)**. The ICP can record all of these factors and show action has been taken and when omissions have occurred **(A)**.

Most routine pre-operative investigations such as chest x-ray and blood tests can be carried out during the out-patient visit or a pre-admission visit. This allows time for the results to be reviewed and will reduce unnecessary delays and cancellations.

Informed consent

Carotid endarterectomy is a prophylactic procedure and not intended to improve the patient's current state of health. The sole aim of the operation is to reduce the risk of disabling or fatal stroke compared to the risk of such a stroke with medical treatment alone. It is important that this concept is explained to the patient and also that the patient understands the relative stroke risks of medical and surgical treatment. This must be discussed at a point when the patient and their family and carers have time to consider their decision to proceed and not left immediately prior to surgery. The ECST and NASCET trials demonstrated a 6-10 fold reduction in the long term risk of stroke for carotid endarterectomy and best medical treatment compared to best medical treatment alone [10,11] **(I)**. This fact may be presented in many different ways but it is important to explain it to the patient in terms appropriate to their level of understanding. Patients should be aware that although the long-term stroke risk is lower with surgery, the short-term (30 day) post-operative risk is higher - 5.8% to 7.5% for death and all stroke or 2.1% to 3.7% for death and disabling stroke [10,11] **(I)** - compared to medical treatment alone.

The nature of the surgery should be explained and this can then be used to explain the local complications that can result. Local nerve trauma (hypoglossal, mandibular branch of the facial, recurrent laryngeal, cutaneous branches of the cervical plexus) occurred in 7.6% of cases in the NASCET trial [11] **(I)**. This should be mentioned with the explanation that sensory loss over the angle of the mandible could be permanent. Although haematoma resulting in laryngeal oedema, stridor and respiratory arrest is rare, the serious nature of this risk requires that it should be mentioned. Systemic complications such as myocardial infarction should also be discussed.

The patient should receive an information leaflet outlining all of the above (see website) and should be encouraged to discuss surgery with his/her family. It is advisable to include the current track record for the unit. The ICP should document the whole process of consent and show that a person with the appropriate knowledge of the procedure obtained it **(A)**.

In-patient preparation

In-patient preparation should confirm medical fitness and consent, answer any remaining questions the patient may have, identify specific nursing requirements and prepare for discharge.

Medical preparation

The patient undergoes a routine history and examination and the results of the routine investigations are checked. If not already undertaken, blood should be sent for grouping, but formal cross matching is generally unnecessary. If there is any significant change from the out-patient assessment the ICP should serve to bring this to the attention of the surgical team. Prophylaxis against deep venous thrombosis is prescribed. Infection in carotid endarterectomy is uncommon but the results can be devastating so antibiotic prophylaxis is recommended especially if a prosthetic patch is used **(B)**. An anaesthetic assessment is carried out including a full explanation to the patient of the anaesthetic proposed (local or general). Any peri-operative investigation such as transcranial Doppler ultrasound should be booked and if high dependency or intensive care facilities are required these should be arranged.

It is important to confirm the patency of the internal carotid artery in patients with a pre-occlusive (>95%) stenosis with a repeat duplex scan immediately prior to surgery. Up to 3% of patients can progress from a tight stenosis to a pre-operative asymptomatic internal carotid occlusion in which case surgery would be inappropriate [12] **(II) (A)**. Scanning can be confined to the side to be operated on to reduce time.

The pre-operative information is vital to build up a picture of the case-mix and is a useful audit tool. The data should be collected in a way that allows incorporation into the unit audit system **(A)**.

Nursing preparation

The ICP should include a section on the patient's family, background details and home circumstances. This allows the nurse to develop an understanding of the patient and what their requirements are likely to be. An assessment is made of the patient's ability to care for themselves. This will include nutritional status, pressure area risk assessment and manual handling requirements. While these are not useful in isolation, when taken in conjunction with a full nursing assessment they help determine the level of care the patient is likely to require [13] and provide a more interactive assessment of risk.

Getting to know the patient in this way allows the nurse to make a judgement of the patient's level of understanding regarding the risks and benefits of carotid endarterectomy. The nurse is well placed to identify any areas the patient is unsure of and to help the patient understand them or draw them to the attention of senior surgical staff as appropriate [14]. This is an important part of the process of informed consent **(A)**.

Peri-operative factors

Anaesthetic technique

After appropriate pre-operative preparation and suitable sedative pre-medication the patient should arrive in theatre relaxed and normotensive. The aims of anaesthesia are to maintain these conditions, give the surgeon good operating conditions and to maintain normal cerebral perfusion. Most commonly this has been achieved with general anaesthesia. Blood pressure, PaO_2 and $PaCO_2$ are maintained as closely as possible to the pre-operative values for that patient. One drawback of general anaesthesia is the inability to directly assess cerebral function during carotid cross clamping. This has led to a variety of methods of indirect cerebral monitoring.

Local anaesthetic (superficial and deep cervical plexus block augmented by local infiltration as necessary) has the advantage of allowing conscious cerebral monitoring by talking to the patient, asking them to count up to ten and by asking them to perform tasks with the appropriate hand (such as squeezing a squeaky toy). Inadequate cerebral perfusion can thus be positively identified and a shunt inserted. This reduces the use of shunts and shunt related complications to those patients in whom an absolute need is identified. Cerebral blood flow autoregulation is also preserved under local anaesthesia and there is generally a compensatory rise in blood pressure on carotid clamping. The disadvantages of local anaesthesia are perceived to be an inability of the patient to lie still in an uncomfortable position, patient anxiety leading to high catecholamine levels and a higher blood pressure [15] **(I)**. Many patients tolerate local anaesthetic very well and operating conditions are as good as under general anaesthesia. There is a suggestion based on meta-analysis evidence that cardiac mortality, stroke and death are reduced with local anaesthetic [16] **(I)**, but the trials available for the analysis had flaws and the randomised trial referred to above [15] **(I)** showed no difference in mortality or stroke rate. At present there is no evidence to choose one technique in favour of the other and the choice rests with the experience of the surgical team and the preferences of the patient **(C)**.

Surgical techniques

Careful surgical technique and experience are essential. It is suggested that each surgeon carrying out carotid endarterectomy should perform a minimum number per year [17,18,19] **(III) (C)**. The minimum number seems difficult to define, but at least ten procedures per year are required for a meaningful audit of outcome.

General points

A skin crease incision or one running along the anterior border of sternocleidomastoid may be used. The former results in a more cosmetic scar and is less likely to injure the mandibular branch of the facial nerve but may limit exposure, particularly if the bifurcation is high.

The dissection is performed with minimal manipulation of the arteries to reduce the risk of embolisation. Transcranial Doppler has been helpful in identifying embolisation during this phase allowing a modification in dissection technique.

Systemic heparinisation is almost universally practised although the dose varies. Commonly 5000 units are given prior to carotid cross clamping although in some small patients it is better to calculate the dose relative to the body weight (70 units per kg body weight). The balance of evidence suggests that this should not be reversed with protamine for fear of increasing stroke risk [20] **(II) (B)**.

Careful attention is paid to the endarterectomy site, ensuring it is clear of all loose material and that the proximal and distal end points are securely attached, with tacking sutures if necessary **(A)**.

On completion of the closure, the artery is thoroughly irrigated with heparinised saline and the internal carotid is allowed to back bleed as the suture line is finally closed to flush out any remaining debris **(A)**.

Shunting

Shunts enable continued internal carotid perfusion and so may reduce the frequency of stroke secondary to hypoperfusion. There is no proof for this, however, and this potential advantage has to be off set against the risks of intimal trauma, air or particulate embolism, shunt thrombosis and the fact that the shunt can get in the way. Many surgeons therefore prefer to use a shunt only when it is perceived to be necessary.

"Awake" testing during carotid clamping under local anaesthetic makes it clear when a patient requires a shunt and only a minority do. There is difficulty in identifying these patients under general anaesthesia and a variety of cerebral function and blood flow monitors have been devised in an attempt to identify those patients who require a shunt. Although some surgeons employ selective shunting based on changes in the monitored parameters there is no evidence to show the level of cerebral function or blood flow below which a shunt is required to prevent a stroke. Cerebral function and blood flow parameters correlated with awake testing cannot be extrapolated to general anaesthesia where the capacity for cerebral autoregulation is reduced or lost [21]. For this reason, other surgeons advocate routine shunting when operating under general anaesthetic **(II)**. A Cochrane review showed that there is currently insufficient evidence to say whether a shunt should be used routinely or selectively under general anaesthetic, although there was a trend towards a lower stroke and death rate when a shunt was used [22] **(I) (C)**.

Carotid endarterectomy under local anaesthesia allows direct monitoring of cerebral function. Deterioration of cerebral function (which can be subtle) is almost always reversed by shunt insertion and so can be used as the "ideal" indicator of whether a shunt is required. The advocates of local anaesthesia point out that it is the only reliable method of allowing selective shunting. However, rapid shunt insertion in agitated or confused patients can be difficult.

Cerebral monitoring

Short of "awake" testing, it is not clear which is the most appropriate method of cerebral monitoring or at what level action (shunt insertion) should be taken **(III)**.

Cerebral function
Under general anaesthesia the alternatives are the electroencephalogram (EEG) or the detection of sensory evoked potentials. The EEG is very sensitive not only to hypoxia but also to many other factors. This can result in excessive shunt use either for unimportant degrees of hypoxia or even for conditions unrelated to low blood flow. The EEG also requires either a skilled technician or sophisticated software for analysis.

The detection of cortical sensory evoked potentials after a peripheral stimulus indicates that the whole pathway to the cortex is functioning normally. A reduction in the amplitude of the cortical potential or delayed conduction can indicate cerebral hypoxia [23] **(II)**.

Cerebral perfusion
The simplest measure is the degree of back bleeding from the internal carotid artery. This may be pulsatile, non-pulsatile or absent and can be quantified by measuring the stump pressure. These measures bear little relation to intracerebral blood flow and can vary depending on conditions in the Circle of Willis and on the precise state of intracerebral blood flow regulation.

Measurement of the velocity of blood in the middle cerebral artery by transcranial Doppler is widely used. It is valuable in detecting emboli, so allowing early internal carotid cross clamping when necessary, and in monitoring shunt flow when one is used. It can also be used to determine the need for a shunt - a 50-80% velocity reduction (the exact level varies between units) from pre-clamping levels may suggest hypoperfusion **(II)**.

Near infrared spectrophotometry (NIRS) allows indirect measurement of the oxygen saturation of blood in the cortex. The majority of the blood volume in the brain is venous and so oxygen saturation levels measured by NIRS are around 75%. This measure correlates well with middle cerebral artery velocity [24] **(II)** but again it is not known what level of fall in saturation should trigger shunt insertion. A 10% fall from pre-clamping levels is suggested, with the absolute value not being useful.

Standard or eversion endarterectomy?

Standard endarterectomy through a longitudinal arteriotomy has the advantage of allowing direct visualisation of the end points and of ensuring the removal of all loosely adherent plaque. If the end point of the endarterectomy did not "feather" well or is not secure, "tacking" sutures can be placed to ensure it does not dissect distally when blood flow is restored. Eversion endarterectomy involves division of the internal carotid artery at its origin and removal of the plaque by peeling back the adventitia and outer media as one layer from the plaque. The end point of the endarterectomy is therefore "feathered" but is not directly visualised. The internal carotid is then anastomosed back to the defect in the common carotid. If the plaque extends significantly into the common carotid this defect may need to be extended and a standard common carotid endarterectomy performed. Eversion endarterectomy requires a more extensive circumferential dissection compared to standard endarterectomy but is generally quicker to perform.

No difference has been shown between standard and eversion endarterectomy with respect to 30-day stroke, 30-day mortality, early thrombosis, technical defects at operation or the need for surgical revision [25] (I).

In some patients the internal carotid is long and tortuous. After carrying out the dissection and endarterectomy this may result in unacceptable kinking of the artery. Under these circumstances the internal carotid may need to be shortened. In the eversion technique this is easily performed prior to reanastomosis. In the standard technique a continuous plication-tacking suture may be used at the distal end point to achieve a modest degree of shortening [26] (II) (C). If more shortening is required the internal carotid may be divided at the level of the end point, the excess artery excised from the endarterectomised section and re-anastomosis performed using the suture line to tack the distal end point. Other methods of reconstruction are also available according to the prevailing circumstances [27] (III), but interposition grafting is probably best reserved for revisional surgery (C).

Patching

Primary closure of the arteriotomy after standard endarterectomy may narrow the lumen and lead to early thrombosis or late restenosis. The aim of patch closure is to reduce these risks. Early thrombosis is rare (2-3%) but a major cause of stroke [28] (II). Late restenosis (>70%) or occlusion is more common (9%) but rarely causes problems [29] (II) possibly because the pathology of restenosis is intimal hyperplasia. Using a patch lengthens clamp or shunt time, and exposes the patient to the low risks of patch rupture (if vein is used) or infection (if a prosthesis is used). Some surgeons have therefore advocated selective patching for small arteries [30] (II) (for example, internal carotid diameter less than 5mm).

A Cochrane review of randomised trials [31] (I) and an additional prospective randomised trial [32] (I) both found statistical support for the routine use of patches. There were reduced rates of early thrombosis, early and late stroke and late restenosis in patients treated with a patch. In spite of some caveats with this conclusion, it is becoming generally accepted that patch closure should be employed (A). No difference has been found in results from different types of patch [33] (I).

Quality control

The aim of quality control is to minimise the frequency of correctable defects leading to stroke. The most important of these are residual thrombus in the lumen and a distal intimal flap. These are obviously best assessed prior to restoration of blood flow and this can be done using either an angioscope or flexible hysteroscope [34] (II). After flow has been restored, assessment can be made by angiography or duplex [35] (II). The drawback is that the complication may have already occurred once flow has been restored.

There is no consensus on whether quality control should be performed, particularly as the pick up rate of defects is higher than the expected stroke rate without quality control. Equally, there is no agreement on what type of quality control to use (III).

Post-operative care

This involves the early detection and treatment of complications, nursing assistance as required, patient education and arterial risk factor treatment. The major complications to be addressed are stroke, myocardial infarction, labile blood pressure and wound haematoma.

Post-operative complications

Stroke

Strokes can be classified into those that occur prior to flow restoration and those that occur after flow restoration. Stroke prior to flow restoration is apparent either during the procedure (under local anaesthetic) or on recovery from general anaesthesia. It is more common than subsequent stroke after flow restoration [36] **(II)** when the patient develops a neurological deficit after a full initial recovery.

Stroke prior to flow restoration is caused by embolisation (during dissection or from a shunt) or hypoperfusion either alone or in combination. It occurs most often in high-risk patients (pre-existing neurological deficit or contralateral carotid occlusion) who are very vulnerable to cerebral hypoxia. Due to the aetiology, surgery has nothing to offer for stroke prior to flow restoration.

Stroke after flow restoration most commonly results from thrombosis of the endarterectomy site. Intracerebral haemorrhage is a less common cause (1-2% of all carotid endarterectomies) [37] **(II)**. There is evidence that early carotid thrombosis may be heralded by small asymptomatic emboli into the middle cerebral artery [38]. These can be detected by transcranial Doppler in the early recovery period and can be stopped by the infusion of the anti-platelet agent, dextran [39] **(I)(A)**. Should they continue, surgical re-exploration can correct the source of the problem **(A)**. If transcranial Doppler is not available dextran may be used routinely, but is associated with increased bleeding complications **(C)**. Under these circumstances immediate surgical re-exploration is indicated at the first sign of a new post-operative neurological deficit **(A)**. This has the potential to limit or reverse the neurological deficit. The more severe the neurological deficit the more likely that the internal carotid and middle cerebral arteries have completely thrombosed which is not correctable surgically [40] **(II)**.

There is some difficulty when a patient wakes up with a stroke after general anaesthesia (Figure 2). While this is most likely to be due to stroke prior to flow restoration, it is possible that the stroke resulted from thrombosis forming on the endarterectomy site during wound closure and so is, in fact, a stroke after flow restoration. The distinction can be made by duplex ultrasonography or by specific flow patterns on transcranial Doppler. A duplex scan may take some time to organise and although it may avoid an unnecessary re-exploration, any delay may reduce or

remove the potential for recovery in a patient with thrombosis of the endarterectomy site. If there is any delay in obtaining the test, immediate re-exploration is indicated in a patient waking up from general anaesthesia with a new neurological deficit **(A)**. Under local anaesthesia, this difficulty is avoided as it is clear whether the stroke occurred before or after flow restoration.

Labile blood pressure

Post-operative hypertension is common. It is important to treat common causes such as pain or bladder distension. Hypertension should otherwise be controlled with short acting drugs such as intravenous Esmolol (short-acting beta-blocker) or sublingual nifedipine to reduce the risk of myocardial infarction, or cerebral haemorrhage due to reperfusion syndrome [37]. The aim should be to maintain the post-operative blood pressure at a level below the pre-operative level **(B)**. Hypotension can also occur and may be more likely after carotid sinus blockade when it can be associated with bradycardia. Bradycardia may also occur in isolation. Treatment with atropine is indicated for a heart rate less than 40 or for a symptomatic bradycardia. Other causes of hypotension (hypovolaemia, dysrhythmias or myocardial infarction for example) should be sought and investigations suggested in the ICP. Treatment is directed at the cause, but if none is found the patient should simply be monitored unless the hypotension becomes symptomatic in which case vasopressor agents may be used cautiously. Patients with labile post-operative blood pressure require invasive blood pressure monitoring in a high dependency unit **(B)**.

Myocardial infarction

Peri-operative myocardial infarction has clinical sequelae in 1% of patients. Oxygen should be prescribed post-operatively and should be continuous for 24 hours. Thereafter it should be given for two further nights, as the commonest time for myocardial infarction is the third post-operative night. ECG monitoring and biochemical testing should be suggested in the ICP and used when appropriate. Management of myocardial infarction or dysrhythmia

Figure 2 Algorithm for the management of a patient with a new post-operative neurological deficit.

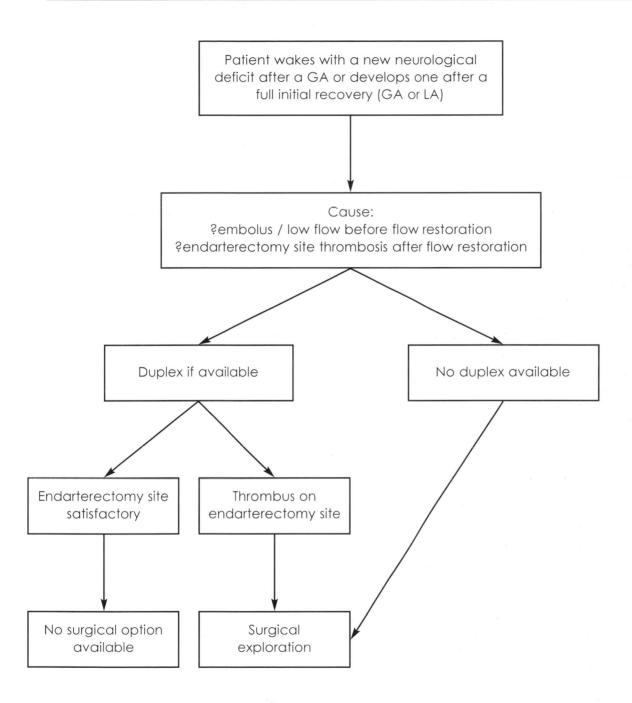

follows standard lines (with the obvious exception of thrombolysis) and appropriate indications for cardiology referral should be included in the ICP.

Post-operative haematoma

Significant bleeding may cause a haematoma which, through venous congestion, reduces venous drainage and results in oedema. If laryngeal oedema occurs the patient will develop stridor. This can develop quickly and may progress to respiratory arrest. Monitoring and treatment for this complication should be part of the ICP. An experienced anaesthetist should be called and the patient reassured. The patient should be sat up to minimise venous congestion and should already be breathing humidified oxygen. An adrenaline nebuliser may be given to reduce oedema formation in the larynx. If the stridor does not improve then the skin closure and any deeper wound sutures should be removed on the ward. Partial evacuation of the haematoma may then be possible. If there is still no improvement, the patient should be anaesthetised and intubated, which can be very difficult. If the airway cannot be secured in this way then cricothyroidotomy is the treatment of choice. Formal evacuation of the haematoma is always required but in most instances it is possible to transfer the patient to theatre in a controlled manner for anaesthesia and intubation. Post-operative care is generally on the Intensive Care Unit with ventilation until the laryngeal oedema settles (C).

Recovery and discharge

The ICP should identify the key steps in routine recovery. These include introduction of oral fluids and food, removal of drain and when the patient can ambulate. Adequate pain control should be confirmed and action taken if poor. The surgical and nursing team should agree the timing of these events when setting up the ICP and continually review them. The reason for patients not achieving these "milestones" should be recorded as variances and when possible corrected. The ICP can also ensure that an appropriate reduction in the level of care occurs; for example discontinuation of intravenous fluids and move from a High Dependency Unit to the ward.

The key medical and nursing factors that need to be achieved before a patient is discharged from hospital should be agreed. When the ICP confirms that these have been satisfactorily met the patient can leave the hospital. This reduces unnecessary delay such as waiting for senior medical review and gives the patient and the team clear focused targets. The ICP should confirm that agreed follow-up plans have been put into place including reduction of cardiovascular risk factors. Finally the ICP should be fed back into the unit audit process to identify variances in the way that the patient was treated which may suggest areas where care could be improved.

Summary

♦ There are over 140 key steps that must be undertaken by the team looking after a patient undergoing a carotid endarterectomy.

♦ Failure to successfully complete any of these steps may result in a poor outcome for the patient and negate the whole point of the operation, which is to prevent stroke.

♦ An ICP provides a method to ensure that no vital steps are missed, avoids uneccessary delays, and indicates areas where care can be improved (B).

♦ The risk of stroke and cranial nerve injury must be discussed with the patient, preferably aided by an information sheet, and documented in the ICP (A).

♦ Vascular surgeons performing carotid endarterectomy must perform the operation regularly and be aware of their own results (B).

♦ Local anaesthesia avoids the need for cerebral monitoring, and reduces the need for a shunt due to preservation of cerebral autoregulation (B).

♦ Eversion endarterectomy is useful when the internal carotid artery is tortuous (C).

◆ A patch should usually be used to close a standard endarterectomy to reduce the risk of post-operative thrombosis and late restenosis **(A)**.

◆ An immediate duplex scan should be performed on any patient who develops a post-operative stroke, and re-exploration undertaken if this reveals thrombus on the endarterectomy site **(B)**.

◆ Post-operative hypertension must be controlled to reduce the risk of myocardial infarction or cerebral haemorrhage **(B)**.

Further reading

1 Callow AD. *Surgery of the carotid and vertebral arteries for the prevention of stroke*. Williams and Wilkins, 1996.

2 Naylor AR, Mackey WC. *Carotid artery surgery: a problem-based approach*. WB Saunders, 2000.

References (grade I evidence and grade A recommendations in bold)

1 **Bamford J, Sandercock P, Dennid M, Burn J, Warlow CP. A prospective study of acute cerebrovascular disease in the community. The Oxfordshire Community Stroke Project 1981-1986. (1) Methodology, demography and incident cases of first ever stroke. *J Neurol Neurosurg Psychiatry* 1988; 51: 1373.**

2 **Warlow CP. Stroke, transient ischaemic attack and intracranial thrombosis. In: *Brain's diseases of the nervous system*. Donaghy M, Ed. Oxford University Press, Oxford 2001; 777-789.**

3 Naylor AR, Rothwell P. Should cost-effectiveness influence patient selection for carotid surgery? In: *Carotid Artery Surgery*. Naylor AR, Mackey WC, Eds. Harcourt Publishers Limited, London, 2000; 66-72.

4 Christensen CR. Carotid endarterectomy clinical pathway: a nursing perspective. *Journal of Vascular Nursing* 1997; 15:1-7.

5 Middleton S, Roberts A. *Integrated Care Pathways - A Practical Approach to Implementation*. Butterworth Heinemann, Oxford, 2000.

6 Wilson J. *Integrated Care Management - The Path to Success*. Butterworth Heinemann, Oxford, 1997.

7 Riles TS, Kopelman I, Imparato AM. Myocardial infarction following carotid endarterectomy: A review of 683 operations. *Surgery* 1979; 85: 249-252.

8 Eagle KA, Brundage BH, Chaitman BR *et al*. Guidelines for perioperative cardiovascular evaluation for non-cardiac surgery: report of the American College of Cardiology/American Heart Association task force on practice guidelines (committee on perioperative cardiovascular evaluation for non-cardiac surgery.) *J Am College Cardiol* 1996; 27: 910-948.

9 Gasecki AP, Ferguson GG, Elisaziw M *et al*. Early endarterectomy for severe carotid artery stenosis after non-disabling stroke: results from the North American Symptomatic Carotid Endarterctomy Trial. *J Vasc Surg* 1994; 20: 288-295.

10 **European Carotid Surgery Trialists Collaborative Group. MRC European Carotid Surgery Trial: interim results for symptomatic patients with severe (70-99%) or with mild (0-29%) carotid stenosis. *Lancet* 1991; 337: 1235-1241.**

11 **North American Symptomatic Carotid Endarterectomy Trial Collaborators. Beneficial effect of carotid endarterectomy in symptomatic patients with high grade stenosis. *N Engl J Med* 1991; 325: 445-453.**

12 Griffiths GD, Tootill R, Dodd PDF, Wilde LM, Walker MG. Value of carotid duplex scanning the day before carotid endarterectomy. *J Vasc Inv* 1998; 4: 11-13.

13 Morison MJ. *The Prevention and Treatment of Pressure Ulcers*. Mosby, Edinburgh, 2001.

14 Arthur J. Carotid disease. In: *Vascular Disease - Nursing and Management*. Murray S, Ed. Whurr Publishers, London, 2001; 369-385.

15 **Forsell C, Takolander R, Bergqvist D, Johansson A. Local versus general anaesthesia in carotid surgery: a prospective randomised study. *Eur J Vasc Surg* 1989; 3: 503-509.**

16 **Tangkanakul C, Counsell C, Warlow CP. Local versus general anaesthesia in carotid endarterectomy: a systematic review of the evidence. *Eur J Vasc Surg* 1997; 13: 491-499.**

17 Michaels J, Palfreyman S, Wood R. Evidence-based guidelines for the configuration of vascular services. *Journal of Clinical Excellence* 2001; 3: 145-153.

18 Cebul RD, Snow RJ, Pine R, Hertzer NR, Norris DG. Indications, outcomes and provider volumes for carotid endarterectomy. *JAMA* 1998; 279: 1282-1287.

19 Hannan EL, Popp AJ, Tranmer B, Fuestel P, Waldman J, Shah D. Relationship between provider volume and mortality for carotid endarterectomies in New York State. *Stroke* 1998; 29: 2292-2297.

20 Fearn SJ, Parry AD, Picton AJ, Mortimer AJ, McCollum CN. Should heparin be reversed after carotid endarterectomy? A randomised prospective trial. *Eur J Vasc Surg* 1997; 13: 394-397.

Chapter 25

21   McCleary AJ, Dearden NM, Dickson DH, Watson A, Gough MJ. The differing effects of regional and general anaesthesia on cerebral metabolism during carotid endarterectomy. *Eur J Vasc Surg* 1996; 12: 173-181.

22   Counsell C, Salinas R, Warlow CP, Naylor AR. The role of carotid artery shunting during carotid endarterectomy: a systematic review of the randomised trials of routine and selective shunting and the different methods of intra-operative monitoring. Stroke Module of the Cochrane database of Systematic Reviews. Warlow CP, van Gijn J, Sandercock P. BMJ Publishing Group, London, 1996.

23   Naylor AR, Bell PRF, Ruckley CV. Monitoring and cerebral protection during carotid endarterectomy. *Br J Surg* 1992; 79: 735-741.

24   Mason PF, Dyson EH, Sellars V, Beard JD. The assessment of cerebral oxygenation during carotid endarterectomy utilizing near infra-red spectroscopy. *Eur J Vasc Surg* 1994; 8: 590-594.

25   Cao P, Giordano G, de Rango P, *et al*. Collaborators of the EVEREST study group. A randomized study on eversion versus standard carotid endarterectomy: Study design and preliminary results: The EVEREST Trial. *J Vasc Surg* 1998; 27: 595-605.

26   Makhdoomi KR, McBride M, Brittenden J, Bradbury AW, Ruckley CV. A prospective study of internal carotid artery plication during carotid endarterectomy: early clinical and duplex outcome. *Eur J Vasc Endovasc Surg* 1999; 18:391-4.

27   Fearn SJ, McCollum CN. Shortening and reimplantation for tortuous internal carotid arteries. *J Vasc Surg* 1998; 27: 936-9.

28   Takolander R, Bergentz SE, Bergqvist D, Persson NH. Management of early neurologic deficits after carotid endarterectomy. *Eur J Vasc Surg* 1987; 1: 67-71.

29   Naylor AR, John T, Howlett J, Gillespie I, Allan P, Ruckley CV. Surveillance imaging of the operated artery does not alter clinical outcome following carotid endarterectomy. *Br J Surg* 1996; 83: 522-526.

30   Golledge J, Cuming R, Davies AH, Greenhalgh RM. Outcome of selective patching following carotid endarterectomy. *Eur J Vasc Surg* 1996; 11 :459-463.

31   Counsell C, Salinas R, Warlow CP, Naylor AR. The role of routine patch angioplasty in carotid endarterectomy: a systematic review of the randomised controlled trials. Stroke Module of the Cochrane database of Systematic Reviews. Warlow CP, van Gijn J, Sandercock P. BMJ Publishing Group, London, 1995.

32   Aburahma AF, Khan JH, Robinson PA, *et al*. Prospective randomized trial of carotid endarterectomy with primary closure and patch angioplasty with saphenous vein, jugular vein and polytetrafluoroethylene: Perioperative (30 day) results. *J Vasc Surg* 1996; 24: 998-1007.

33   Counsell C, Salinas R, Warlow CP, Naylor AR. A comparison of different types of patch in carotid endarterectomy: a systematic review of the randomised trials. Stroke Module of the Cochrane database of Systematic Reviews. Warlow CP, van Gijn J, Sandercock P. BMJ Publishing Group, London, 1996.

34   Gaunt ME, Smith JL, Martin PJ, Ratliff DA, Bell PRF, Naylor AR. A comparison of quality control methods applied to carotid endarterectomy. *Eur J Vasc Surg* 1996; 11: 4-11.

35   Walker RA, Fox AD, Magee TR, Horrocks M. Intraoperative duplex scanning as a means of quality control during carotid endarterectomy. *Eur J Vasc Surg* 1996; 11: 364-367.

36   Krul JMJ, van Gijn J, Ackerstaff RGA, Eikelboom BC, Theodorides T, Vermeulen FE. Site and pathogenesis of infarcts associated with carotid endarterectomy. *Stroke* 1989; 20: 324-328.

37   Naylor AR, Ruckley CV. The post-carotid endarterectomy hyperperfusion syndrome. *Eur J Vasc Surg* 1995; 9: 365-367.

38   Gaunt ME, Ratliff DA, Martin PJ, Smith J, Bell PRF, Naylor AR. On table diagnosis of incipient carotid artery thrombosis during carotid endarterectomy by transcranial Doppler scanning. *J Vasc Surg* 1994; 20: 104-107

39   Lennard N, Smith J, Dumville J, *et al*. Prevention of postoperative thrombotic stroke after carotid endarterectomy: the role of transcranial Doppler ultrasound. *J Vasc Surg* 1997; 26: 579-584.

40   Naylor AR, Sandercock P, Sellar RJ, Warlow CP. Patterns of vascular pathology in acute first-ever cerebral infarction. *Scot Med J* 1993; 38: 41-44.

Chapter 26

Thoracic sympathectomy

John F Thompson Consultant Surgeon

Vanessa Ducker Staff Nurse

Andrew R Warin Consultant Dermatologist

EXETER VASCULAR SERVICE, ROYAL DEVON AND EXETER HOSPITAL, EXETER, UK

Introduction

Interruption of the ganglionated dorsal sympathetic chain results in sympathetic denervation of the upper limb and head, with subsequent vasodilation and anhydrosis. Sympathetic outflow from the lateral grey column of the spinal cord enters the chain via the ventral roots of the T6-T2 spinal nerves as myelinated white rami, which may synapse at the same level, or else travel upwards. Outflow to the head, neck and hand *must* pass through the T2 ganglion, so destruction of this crossroads will treat these regions. Interruption of the sympathetic chain between the first and second ganglia using scissors, with no diathermy, is particularly safe and can avoid Horners syndrome [1]. The exception to the pathway is the nerve of Kuntz, which may join the T2 segmental nerve some distance laterally. Outflow to the axilla passes through the T3 and T4 ganglia.

This chapter looks at the indications and care pathway for thoracic sympathectomy.

Indications

Palmar and axillary hyperhidrosis: sympathectomy, performed with modern video assisted thoracic surgery (VATS) techniques achieves success rates approaching 100% for the hand and 75% for the axilla. The lower axilla may still sweat, but this can be treated by alternative methods (see later). Interestingly, pedal sweating may also improve after the procedure [2] **(I)**.

Vasospasm: primary vasospasm, as seen in Raynaud's disease, does not lead to tissue loss. There are no data regarding the long-term efficacy of VATS sympathectomy for Raynaud's Disease, as the open operation fell into disrepute for this indication, but it is not recommended. In Raynaud's syndrome, usually due to a mixed connective tissue disease, caution is advised. There may be situations, however, when VATS sympathectomy can increase blood flow to tissues of marginal viability. Selective digital artery sympathectomy and prostanoid infusions are an alternative. In vasospasm associated with thoracic outlet syndrome, a T2 ganglionectomy is useful as an adjunct to first rib resection **(III)**.

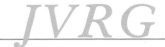

Facial flushing: socially disabling facial flushing is emerging as an interesting indication [3]. The cranial outflow is interrupted by trunkotomy using scissors at the lower border of the T1 ganglion. Diathermy is avoided to reduce the risk of Horner's syndrome. In a large series from Boras, Sweden, Visual Analogue Scores for flushing fell from 8.7 +/- 0.1 to 2.2 +/- 0.2, $P < 0.0001$. Increased sweating of the trunk occurred in 75% of cases. Overall, 85% of the patients were satisfied with the result and 15% were to some degree dissatisfied, mainly due to an insufficient effect, but only four patients (2%) regretted the procedure **(II)**.

Angina pectoris: sympathetic denervation of the heart has had good results in a small group of patients who had intractible pain despite maximal medical treatment and non-reconstructable coronary artery atherosclerosis [4] **(III)**.

Peripheral arterial disease (PAD): the indications here are doubtful, but may include the patient who has agreed to stop smoking and who requires digital amputation in the face of distal disease although this is rarely seen in the upper limb **(III)**.

Complex Regional Pain Syndrome (CRPS): the results of sympathectomy in this difficult condition are unpredictable [5]. In patients with CRPS-II (i.e. following trauma), further surgery can make the condition worse. Occasional successes in individuals may justify the procedure as long as they have responded to stellate ganglion or intravenous guanethidine blocks (whose role is actually unproven) and who have been treated by a multi-disciplinary pain team for at least 12-18 months to allow for spontaneous improvement **(III)**. Even then the patient should be counselled carefully and the details recorded in the notes for medico-legal reasons **(A)**.

Selecting the appropriate patient

Those presenting with disabling hyperhidrosis must convince the surgeon of the severity of their predicament. Examples from everyday life should convince the sceptic; for example, we have treated a computer engineer who dripped sweat into his "chips" and a guitarist whose strings rusted. A warm dry handshake is important to those in contact with others.

Psychological problems such as anxiety and phobic crises should be appreciated. There is no doubt that they may cause hyperhidrosis and that they can be treated appropriately, but some individuals with severe hyperhidrosis develop anxiety as a result of their condition. Their lives may be genuinely helped with surgery [6].

All patients should be reassured and given adequate time for sweating to reduce as part of the normal hormonal maturation seen during the teenage years. Similarly, patients from some ethnic backgrounds may have higher basal levels of sweating, whereas those from others may have a reduced threshold for acceptable sweating; papers from the Far East describe thousands of patients.

Medical conditions known to be associated with sweating such as diabetes, thyrotoxicosis, drugs and alcohol abuse should be excluded. Severe COAD or asthma that might preclude the operation should be excluded. Physical examination should be directed towards the exclusion of secondary diagnoses, documentation of upper limb pulses and examination of the chest plus respiratory function tests, if there are any concerns about chest disease. Anticoagulation and antiplatelet treatment are best withdrawn to minimise the risk of bleeding.

Selecting the appropriate procedure

Non-surgical options should be explored before recommending VATS. Simple advice about hygiene and the avoidance of perfumed soaps or cosmetics, which can cause irritation, should be given if appropriate. The advantages and disadvantages of the treatments that are available are shown in Table 1.

Complications of sympathectomy

Sympathectomy results in a degree of compensatory sweating in almost all patients. It usually occurs between the shoulder blades and beneath the breasts and is related to the extent of the

Table 1 Treatments available for hyperhydrosis.

Intervention	Advantages	Disadvantages
Aluminium containing roll-on or sprays	Easy, cheap, safe, effective for mild cases especially axilla	Skin sensitivity, less effective for severe cases. Lasts 12-24hrs
Anti-cholinergic creams (glycopyrrolate etc)	Easy, moderately cheap, less invasive	Side effects (dry mouth, blurred vision). Messy, lasts 12hrs approx.
Iontopheresis	Less invasive, safe (blocks sweat glands), useful for feet and hands	Painful for young women! Specialised equipment Expensive, lasts "a few weeks". Patients can purchase - "Drionic"
Botulinum toxin	Safe, effective, avoids surgery, no compensatory sweating Good for axillae	Expensive (£250), injections x 12-20, limited to axillae, not funded. Lasts 6-9 months
Excision of axillary skin or eccrine glands	Permanent, effective	Painful, poor cosmesis, wound complications (Draconian!)
VATS sympathectomy	Permanent, effective, safe, cheaper in long-term, high satisfaction, best for hands	General anaesthetic, compensatory hyperhidrosis, small risk of complications costs £850

Table 2 Extent of sympathectomy relating to required outcome.

Operative intent	Sympathectomy procedure
Dry confident handshake	Unilateral T2 + nerve of Kuntz
Bilateral dry hands	As above but bilateral
Bilateral dry hands and axillae	As above but T2 - 4
Abolish facial flushing	T1/2 trunkotomy

sympathectomy. It may be troublesome in 15-20% of cases; patients need to be warned. In one study, 90% of patients were affected and 11% of the patients regretted their operation [7]. The sweating usually diminishes in time, does not involve unpleasant odour and can be treated with sprays. In some cases the hands may become too dry afterwards so that gripping smooth objects is difficult. A unilateral sympathectomy preserves the sweating on the other side which can act as a reservoir of moisture for the dry hand to use if required. The procedure performed should be the minimum that will achieve the patient's wishes to reduce the risk of compensatory hyperhidrosis (Table 2).

Horner's syndrome (meiosis, anhydrosis, ptosis, enopthalmos) is rare (< 1%) and usually due to excessive diathermy. It can be avoided if diathermy is not used to divide the chain. Pain following the operation is moderate and should be controlled with local anaesthetic infiltration, combined with opioid/non-steroidal oral analgesia. Patients undergoing bilateral procedures should be warned about a deep seated mediastinal ache, which is sometimes mis-interpreted as a heart attack and is common after the procedure.

Patients undergoing unilateral sympathectomy may be treated as day cases; however it is advisable to admit bilateral sympathectomies overnight. The patient should be fully informed about compensatory sweating, Horner's syndrome, failure to relieve sweating, incomplete or asymmetrical results, chest pain, pneumothorax, haemothorax and the possible need for a chest drain [8]. These complications should be included in an information leaflet about the procedure (see website). The discussion about complications and receipt of the information leaflet must be documented in the medical record **(A)**.

Technical considerations

Although it is possible to perform the operation using a laryngeal mask or high flow jet ventilation, most anaesthetists welcome the opportunity to practice selectively ventilating both lungs and most surgeons appreciate the superior views obtained, rather than fighting back the lung. Port sizes, position and number depend on the equipment used. Five millimetre ports are preferred (2 mm have been reported [9]). One port is used when a resectoscope is employed (diathermy is obligatory throughout), two if scissors are to be used to section the upper chain (preferred) and three if a retractor is needed to reach T4. Multiple ports are required if adhesions are encountered. Ports should be placed behind the pectoralis major, especially in women, where Langers' line incisions should be made to avoid unsightly scars. We do not recommend anterior placed ports for cosmetic reasons.

The patient is placed supine on the table in a "hammock" position (to improve venous return) with the hands supported on a vein board in the "surrender" position (Figure 1). Both sides are prepped and the leads for the VATS equipment fed out over the head, so that they can be transferred to the other side. This is quick, convenient and avoids the need to redrape.

We obtain the pneumothorax using a Verres needle and insufflate 0.5l CO_2. No further gas is required and the ports are inserted using a blunt technique. The right side is treated first as the anatomy is more complex in view of the azygos and hemiazygos veins. This side takes slightly longer to perform when a T4 sympathectomy is required and the patient may become hypoxic due to intrapulmonary shunting during the second half of the procedure. The anatomy is established and the pleura opened to expose the chain. The upper extent of the dissection is defined by sharp scissor transection of the highest extent of the chain above T2. The chain can then be divided by diathermy, scissors or harmonic scalpel (which may be less painful). Diathermy should continue along the second rib to interrupt the nerve of Kuntz. Diathermy should be limited to the area over the neck of the rib to avoid damage to the intercostal nerves and arteries between the ribs, causing pain or bleeding. Some surgeons resect the chain to prevent late recurrence, but this is unproven.

If bleeding occurs direct pressure is usually effective. A section of ganglion can be used to promote haemostasis as neural tissue is strongly thrombogenic, or else a pledget of Surgicel is used. In theory, the surgeon and nursing team should be able and prepared to perform anterolateral thoracotomy [10].

Figure 1 Operative position. The arms are elevated but *not* beyond 90 degrees to avoid traction to the brachial plexus. The forearm is supported in 30 to 40 degrees of internal rotation (a). The VATS leads come in from above so that they may be switched to the other side half way through the procedure (b).

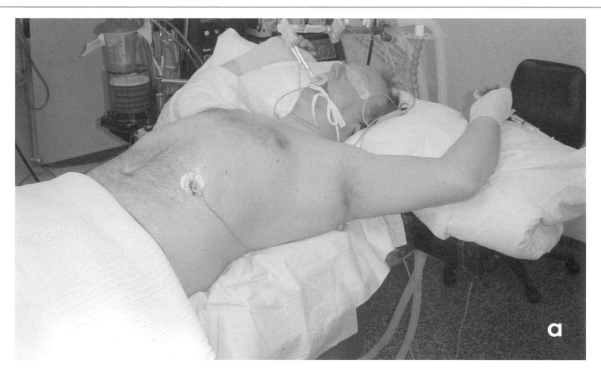

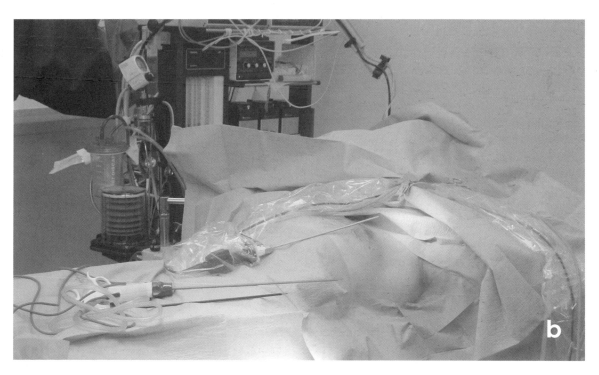

Local anaesthetic is instilled into the pleural cavity and we use 10ml bupivacaine 0.5% with adrenaline through the upper port. Another 10ml is used for the wounds, which are closed with suture strips. Expansion of the lung is confirmed endoscopically and the ports removed under a forced Valsalva manoeuvre, using the flap valve created when inserting the ports (above the rib).

Post-operative care

A chest x-ray is obtained in recovery. A significant pneumothorax can be aspirated through the second intercostal space in the mid-clavicular line. Assessment of the patient's pain is made and this can be controlled with patient controlled analgesia (PCA), rectal diclofenac and then oral paracetamol/codeine. Pain control is fully discussed in the chapter on acute pain.

Table 3 Care pathway for thoracic sympathectomy.

	Medical	Nursing	Anaesthesia
Pre- admission	Clerk, explain consent, bloods, mark side. Document discussed complications.	Assess needs, orientate to ward, PCA education.	Pre-op visit, explain, examine, consent to agreed analgesia and explain PCA.
Operation	As described	NA	As described
Recovery	Check CXR and observations. Reassure and phone spouse/family.	Analgesia, observations as discussed.	Check CXR and observations. Prescribe appropriate analgesia.
Ward	Treat problems as they arise. Examine and reassure about chest. Document complications, extent of anhydrosis.	Chest physio and incentive spirometer, ensure analgesia is effective. Assess as above. Educate re-smoking and refer to cessation programme if required.	Post-operative visit and feedback to departmental audit if appropriate.
Discharge planning	Prescribe TTAs & check GP summary/ follow-up appointment.	Check wounds, TTAs. District/practice nurse referral. Provide information leaflet & contact phone number.	NA

On return to the ward the patient is monitored closely for signs of respiratory compromise, tachycardia or hypotension. The main concerns being:

Haemothorax; tachypnoea, tachycardia, hypotension, cold sweating, thirst, anxiety, decreased/absent air entry and stony dullness to percussion. Chest x-ray to confirm. If more than 2-300 ml insert chest drain and transfuse if Hb < 7.0g/dl in fit patients. The drained blood may be autotransfused. If more than 500 ml/h return to theatre.

Pneumothorax; tachypnoea, tachycardia, hypoxia, anxiety, decreased air entry and hyper-resonance. If <10-20% with little respiratory embarrassment, leave alone. If worse, either aspirate or insert apical chest drain through the camera port.

Tension pneumothorax; as above, plus severe hypoxia and tracheal deviation away from the affected side. Requires emergency insertion of a large intravenous cannula in 2nd or 3rd space followed by chest drain as above.

Nursing observations should include:

- Respiration rate and Oxygen saturation.

- Checking for symmetrical chest expansion.

- BP/Pulse every 15 min for 1hr, every 30 min for 2hrs, hourly for 4hrs and then 4hrly.

- Wound site inspections.

- Limb status (motor, sensory and bloodflow).

- Observing for signs of Horner's syndrome; ptosis, enopthalmos.

Patients may commence oral fluids and diet as soon as they have recovered from the anaesthetic. Physiotherapy is useful and the incentive spirometer particularly so.

Discharge arrangements include provision of take home analgesia (TTAs), written leaflet advice including a 24hour contact telephone number, a computer generated summary for the GP and out-patient review at 4-6 weeks. Post-operative complications are recorded in the notes and validated at local audit review meetings.

Table 3 outlines a complete care pathway for the procedure.

Summary

- Sympathectomy is a safe, reliable operation for hyperhidrosis with durable results **(A)**.

- Patient selection is the key to success. Complications, especially compensatory hyperhidrosis, should be discussed and documented **(A)**.

- Compensatory hyperhidrosis may be severe and disabling **(A)**.

- Plan the minimal procedure to achieve the patient's wishes to reduce the incidence of the above **(B)**.

- Provide the patient with written information in clinic **(A)**.

- Sympathectomy is not a minor procedure. It can be technically demanding and have major implications for the patient and their surgeon **(A)**.

Further reading

1   Thompson JF, Kinsella DC. Vascular disorders of the upper limb. In: *Vascular and Endovascular Surgery*, 2nd Edition. Beard J, Gaines P, Eds. WB Saunders, London, 2001.

References (grade I evidence and grade A recommendations in bold)

1   Fox AD, Hands L, Collin J. The results of thoracoscopic sympathetic trunk transection for palmar hyperhidrosis and sympathetic ganglionectomy for axillary hyperhidrosis. *Eur J Vasc Endovasc Surg* 1999 Apr;17 (4): 343-6.

2   **Andrews BT, Rennie JA. Predicting changes in the distribution of sweating following thoracoscopic sympathectomy. *Br J Surg* 1997 Dec; 84 (12): 1702-4.**

3   Drott C, Claes G, Olsson-Rex L, Dalman P, Fahlen T, Gothberg G. Successful treatment of facial blushing by endoscopic transthoracic sympathectomy. *Br J Dermatol* 1998 Apr;138 (4): 639-43.

Chapter 26

4   Khogali SS, Miller M, Rajesh PB, Murray RG, Beattie JM. Video-assisted thoracoscopic sympathectomy for severe intractable angina. *Eur J Cardiothorac Surg* 1999 Sep;16 Suppl 1:S95-8.

5   Schott GD. Interruption of the sympathetic outflow in causalgia and reflex sympathetic dystrophy. *Br Med J* 1998; 316: 792-3.

6   Telaranta T. Treatment of social phobia by endoscopic thoracic sympathectomy. *Eur J Surg* Suppl 1998; (580): 27-32.

7   Cameron AE. Complications of endoscopic sympathectomy. *Eur J Surg* Suppl 1998; (580): 33-5.

8   Fredman B, Zohar E, Shachor D, Bendahan J, Jedeikin R. Video-assisted transthoracic sympathectomy in the treatment of primary hyperhidrosis: friend or foe? *Surg Laparosc Endosc Percutan Tech* 2000 Aug;10 (4): 226-9.

9   Gossot D, Kabiri H, Caliandro R, Debrosse D, Girard P, Grunenwald D. Early complications of thoracic endoscopic sympathectomy: a prospective study of 940 procedures. *Ann Thorac Surg* 2001 Apr; 71 (4): 1116-9.

10 Sung SW, Kim YT, Kim JH. Ultra-thin needle thoracoscopic surgery for hyperhidrosis with excellent cosmetic effects. *Eur J Cardiothorac Surg* 2000 Jun;17 (6): 691-6.

Chapter 27

Vascular access for haemodialysis

Jane Andrew Community Dialysis Sister [1]

Chris Gibbons Consultant Vascular and General Surgeon [2]

[1] RENAL UNIT, MORRISTON HOSPITAL, SWANSEA, UK.
[2] DEPARTMENT OF VASCULAR SURGERY, MORRISTON HOSPITAL, SWANSEA, UK.

Introduction

Patients with end-stage renal failure require renal replacement therapy by haemodialysis, peritoneal dialysis or renal transplantation. An integrated approach involving all three modalities maximises life expectancy but most will require at least a period of haemodialysis (Figure 1).

Some patients present electively with deteriorating renal function, allowing the need for dialysis to be predicted. Others present acutely and require emergency haemodialysis using a double-lumen central venous catheter until permanent dialysis access has been established. The subsequent choice between haemodialysis and continuous ambulatory peritoneal dialysis (CAPD) may depend on patient preference, life-style and ability to cope. CAPD is often preferred in diabetics and allows greater mobility and independence but requires more patient participation, proving impossible in some elderly patients.

The principles of haemodialysis access

To allow effective haemodialysis, blood must pass through the dialysis machine at a rate of at least 200ml/min with sufficiently separate arterial inflow and venous return to avoid recirculation [1].

A double lumen central venous catheter (CVC) permits adequate flow when positioned within a central vein (usually the superior vena cava) and the separation of the openings of each lumen prevents recirculation.

An AV fistula increases the flow within a superficial vein allowing blood to be withdrawn through one needle near the fistula and returned to the circulation via a more proximal needle. When only a short length of vein is available a single needle may be used for alternating withdrawal and return of blood but dialysis times are prolonged. Fistula flow may initially be insufficient but increases after a few weeks as both the arterial inflow and the venous outflow dilate [2]. The vein also becomes thicker and more elastic allowing safer and easier needle placement.

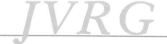

Figure 1 Pathway of care for end stage renal failure.

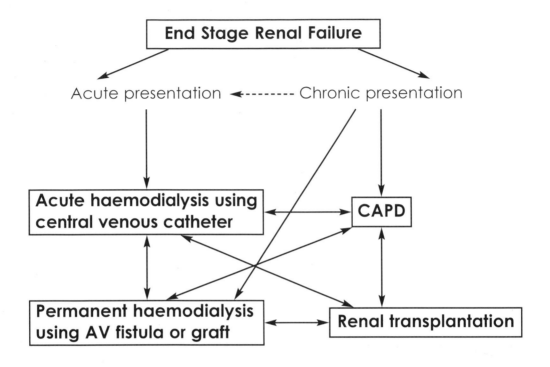

When no suitable superficial vein is available a prosthetic (e.g. PTFE or Dacron) AV bridge graft may be placed subcutaneously between a suitable artery and a deep vein. Needles are inserted directly into the graft for dialysis.

With effective access, patients undergo regular haemodialysis, for about four hours three times per week, usually as an out-patient, although some may be trained to dialyse themselves at home.

Organisation of vascular access

Whereas access by central venous catheter is usually accomplished by the nephrology physician, AV fistulae and grafts require specific surgical expertise. In the early days of dialysis self-taught renal physicians often constructed arteriovenous fistulae. Subsequently, transplant surgeons and urologists took over access surgery but vascular surgeons have become increasingly involved since the establishment of peripheral dialysis units. However, in many hospitals local expertise is lacking and patients must travel to other centres. Together with the general under-provision of access services, this leads to long periods of central venous catheter use with the added patient discomfort and accompanying risks outlined below. An increased number of surgeons performing access surgery and protected operating lists are required.

In some units an access coordinator has proved beneficial to identify problems, prioritise patients and organise operating lists [3]. Others advocate a specific clinic for assessment, organisation of pre-operative investigations and post-operative follow-up [4]. Radiologists with a specific interest are becoming increasingly involved for the placement and repositioning of catheters, and for the detection and treatment of failing access.

Chapter 27

Temporary or emergency haemodialysis access

The Scribner Shunt

The first haemodialysis access device was the Scribner shunt in 1960 [5]. However, repeated thrombosis and infection, poor patency [6], and patient discomfort led to its replacement by CVCs for emergency and AV fistulae for permanent access [7].

Temporary central venous lines

The central venous catheter is the linchpin of short term or emergency haemodialysis access. Insertion is usually performed under local anaesthesia with a post-procedural chest x-ray to check the position [8].

◆ **The internal jugular vein** in the neck is the best site for a CVC, [8,9] **(A)**.

◆ **Subclavian lines** have an increased risk of pneumothorax or haemothorax on insertion and may cause subclavian vein thrombosis or stenosis, leading to the loss of upper limb access sites [8,9].

◆ **Femoral lines** have a greater incidence of infection, may cause recirculation of blood and carry a small risk of retroperitoneal haematoma or inferior vena cava thrombosis [8,10]. They are uncomfortable for longer-term use and are usually reinserted for each dialysis.

Patients may be allowed home with a temporary CVC whilst awaiting permanent access. However, the waiting time on "lines" should be minimised because of the ever-present risk of septicaemia and central venous thrombosis [11,12] **(A)**. The USA National Kidney Foundation Dialysis Outcomes Quality Initiative (NKF-DOQI) guidelines recommend that less than 10% of patients should be dialysed on lines beyond three months [11,12] **(B)**. CVCs are associated with a relative mortality of 1.7 in non-diabetics and 1.54 in diabetics compared with autologous AV fistulae [13] **(I)**. In the UK more than 50% of patients start dialysis with a CVC in contrast to a European average of 33% [14,15], reflecting the under-provision of access surgery in the NHS.

Permanent central venous catheters

When other options for permanent access have been exhausted, a permanent double-lumen catheter (e.g. PermCath or Vascath) may be used. These have a dacron cuff within a subcutaneous tunnel to allow sutureless fixation and to act as a barrier to infection. However, they have a relatively short life span, most requiring removal or replacement within 18 months [16], although secondary patency varies greatly between centres [19]. The risks of infection and central venous thrombosis are much greater than for AV fistulae [17, 18, 19] **(I)**.

Complications of central venous catheters

Complications of insertion

These are infrequent but include pneumothorax, haemorrhage from inadvertent arterial puncture, chylothorax from thoracic duct puncture, brachial plexus trauma and air embolism [8].

Air embolus

Air embolus causes hypotension and tachypnoea. It can be avoided by cannulating the internal jugular or subclavian veins in the Trendelenberg position with careful occlusion of the catheter hub when manipulating the line. Treatment is by placing the patient in Durant's position (head down and left lateral) and 100% or hyperbaric oxygen [8].

Infection

Infection is the cause of death in 16-36% of dialysis patients and is access related in 50-70% [17,18] **(I)**. Bacteraemia is most frequent with central lines with an incidence of 1-6.5 episodes per 1000 catheter days and is most commonly due to *Staphylococcus aureus* [17] **(I)**. This may lead to metastatic infections such as bacterial endocarditis, mycotic aneurysms, osteomyelitis or septic arthritis. It can be minimised by careful aseptic technique when inserting, changing or using lines and the early establishment of permanent access. If there are early signs of infection systemic antibiotics should be given [11,12] **(II)** but if infection becomes established the catheter should also be removed temporarily [11,12,17,18] **(A)**. Antibiotic prophylaxis is not recommended [20-22] **(I)**.

Nursing strategies to prevent catheter related infection are diverse but UK guidelines have been published by the Department of Health [23]. The frequency of catheter access must be minimized, and ideally confined to dialysis as each manipulation could introduce infection **(A)**.The catheter site is examined for inflammation and exudate before each dialysis. Exit sites and bungs are cleaned with chlorhexidine, which is superior to povidone iodine [24,25] **(I)** and a dry dressing applied using careful aseptic technique [26] **(A)**.

Thrombosis

Local thrombolysis (e.g. using Urokinase instilled and left for 30 minutes) may clear an occluded line [27] but if this is unsuccessful the catheter may be replaced over a guide wire. Occasionally a fibrin cuff, which forms around the intravascular part of the line, may be removed by thrombolysis or "stripping" under angiographic control using a percutaneously introduced snare [19].

Protocols for the prevention of catheter thrombosis are stipulated by individual CVC manufacturers but are generally similar: before dialysis, the catheter should be fast flushed with a minimum of 10ml normal saline. After dialysis, a heparin lock, equal to the volume of each lumen, is inserted. Maintaining positive pressure whilst applying catheter clamps prevents reflux of blood into the line and avoids catheter thrombosis without systemic heparinisation. Microbal adherence may also be reduced [28] **(I)**.

Central venous thrombosis and subclavian stenosis

These are serious complications precluding further access in the upper limbs. Percutaneous angioplasty may restore patency but recurrence is common. Stent insertion is recommended for recurrent or resistant stenoses [11,12,29]. As a last resort, venous bypass (e.g. internal jugular turndown or right atrium - subclavian bypass) may restore patency but is a major undertaking [30-32].

Catheter displacement

A displaced or malpositioned CVC usually requires repositioning. Temporary lines should be secured by a suture and an appropriate dressing. Re-suturing of loose catheters extends their life and prevents the occasional patient arriving for dialysis with the dressing and catheter in their hand.

Patient education

During the pre-dialysis stage patients are introduced to the options for renal replacement, dialysis and vascular access. They must understand the need for a CVC, its care and the necessity for secure anchorage **(B)**. Patients who are discharged home require specific information regarding the safe handling of their line.

They are advised to contact the renal unit if there are signs of sepsis, bleeding or tenderness around the catheter exit site. They must take care when washing and showering, replacing any wet dressings and avoid tight clothing, which could dislodge the catheter.

Permanent vascular access

Vascular access planning

Permanent access is best provided by an arteriovenous fistula (AVF), although in the absence of adequate superficial veins a prosthetic AV bridge graft may be used [11,12] **(A)**. Maximum use should be made of available sites, starting as distally as possible. The non-dominant arm is used preferentially to allow tasks such as writing during dialysis and self-needling if home dialysis is anticipated **(A)**.

When access sites on the non-dominant arm are unavailable, the dominant arm and, as a last resort, the leg can be used.

The arterial inflow must be good, but considerable adaptation may occur so that even small vessels such as the distal radial artery may be used. In diabetics or patients with long-standing renal failure, the radial artery may be calcified, preventing adaptation and necessitating a brachiocephalic fistula. Any haemodynamically significant (>70%) upstream arterial stenosis will impair inflow and may cause thrombosis or failure of maturation.

The vein must be superficial, of good quality and without stenosis. In obese patients forearm veins may be difficult to locate necessitating a more proximal fistula or graft.

Pre-operative investigation

Generally, patients presenting for primary access with a good radial pulse and good forearm veins need no further investigation and can proceed to AV fistula formation with an excellent chance of success (C). Prior to a radiocephalic AVF, it is standard advice to perform an Allen test [11,12] (observation of digital perfusion with the radial artery occluded - blanching indicating an inadequate ulnar artery) but there is little evidence that it is necessary in practice.

A pre-operative upper limb arterial duplex scan is wise for secondary or tertiary procedures or if the radial pulse appears weak (B). Duplex of superficial veins is more difficult but can be facilitated by a venous tourniquet. Duplex scanning of the basilic/brachial venous complex is advisable prior to a basilic vein transposition fistula.

A duplex scan or venogram of the axillary and subclavian veins has been advocated in all patients with subclavian lines [11] and is mandatory in patients with signs of venous engorgement, oedema or venous collateral formation in the arm [11, 12] (B).

Pre-operative preparation

The cephalic vein must be avoided for drips and venepunctures and the dorsum of the hand should be used preferentially for intravenous infusions [11,12] (B).

The options for dialysis and the procedures involved should be carefully explained, backed up by written information and a video presentation. The operating surgeon should obtain informed consent.

Aspirin (75-300mg daily) ± dipyridamole (100mg t.d.s.) is given pre-operatively for at least 24 hours and continued post-operatively to reduce the risk of thrombosis [33-35] (I).

Peri-operative management

The procedure should be performed using magnifying loupes in a fully equipped and staffed operating theatre with adequate lighting. Local anaesthesia does not usually require an anaesthetist but an anaesthetic nurse should remain with the patient throughout. Full monitoring including ECG, pulse oximetry, blood pressure and pulse rate is essential, and 40% Oxygen is usually given by mask.

Local anaesthetic with a long acting agent such as bupivocaine (0.25 or 0.5%) is sufficient for most upper limb procedures except brachio-axillary grafts and basilic vein transposition fistulae. Some surgeons prefer axillary block, believing that the resulting vasodilatation improves fistula flow (III), but a qualified anaesthetist is usually required.

Intravenous sedation (e.g. diazepam 5-10mg) is helpful, especially with anxious patients. Prophylactic antibiotics (e.g. cefuroxime 750mg i.v.) are given at the start of surgery.

Post-operatively, the arm is warmed in a gamgee sleeve to promote vasodilatation. A glyceryl trinitrate patch is sometimes placed over the vein near the fistula in an attempt to improve patency (III) as this is known to reduce thrombosis after intravenous catheter insertion [36].

Possible fistula sites (Figure 2)

The radiocephalic (Breschia-Cimino) AVF

The classical wrist fistula was first described in 1966 and remains the gold standard [11,12,37] (B).

Figure 2 Access sites in the upper limb. (Commonly used sites in bold)

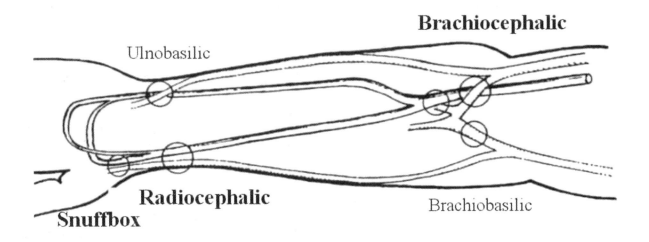

Chapter 27

Originally a side-to-side configuration was described but end-to-side (vein to artery) fistulae may be preferable to reduce distal venous hypertension. 30% of the flow into the fistula is retrograde from the distal radial artery, leading some to advocate an end-to-end configuration with distal arterial and venous ligation to minimise digital ischaemia [38]. A primary radiocephalic fistula is possible in over 60% of patients and becomes usable in 80% within 6 weeks with good long-term patency (65-70% at 1 year) [39, 40]. If it fails further radiocephalic fistulae may be possible in the forearm provided the arterial inflow is satisfactory.

The snuffbox AVF

A more distal radiocephalic fistula in the "anatomical snuffbox" [41,42] is possible in 50% of patients requiring primary access and is the preferred procedure in Swansea [41]. Patency is similar to the standard radiocephalic fistula [39,41], which, in the event of failure, can still be constructed in 45% [41].

The brachiocephalic AVF

If forearm veins are inadequate, the cephalic vein or one of its tributaries in the antecubital fossa can be anastomosed to the brachial artery to produce an excellent high-flow fistula. Needles are placed in the upper arm cephalic vein for dialysis [7,43].

Other autologous fistulae

Brachiocephalic or brachiobasilic forearm vein loops may be constructed when the forearm veins are adequate but the arteries poor: the distal cephalic or basilic vein is looped back in a subcutaneous tunnel and anastomosed to the brachial artery, leaving options open for a standard brachiocephalic AVF in the event of failure.

An ulnobasilic AVF is often possible as the basilic vein is less accessible and rarely used for intravenous infusions [7]. It is not precluded by a previously failed radiocephalic or brachiocephalic AVF, even if the radial artery is occluded, as the interosseous artery provides a good collateral supply to the hand **(III)**. However, needle placement can be more difficult.

A brachiobasilic AVF in the antecubital fossa only permits single needle dialysis as the median basilic vein runs deeply after 2-3 cm. However, rerouting the basilic vein in a subcutaneous tunnel in the upper arm renders it available for needling [44-47]. Such basilic vein transposition fistulae may have better patency than upper arm prosthetic grafts [48] **(II)**.

Prosthetic AV bridge grafts

Prosthetic grafts are invaluable for tertiary access in patients without suitable superficial veins. The usual configurations are brachial AV forearm loops, straight radio-basilic grafts or brachio-axillary grafts [7]. If access is impossible in the arms a femoro-femoral AV loop may be constructed in the thigh [7,49]. Usually 6mm PTFE is used but tapered or stepped grafts with the smaller end at the arterial anastomosis have been advocated to limit flow and reduce steal (see below) **(III)**. A central externally supported section prevents kinking in looped grafts.

Long saphenous vein can also be used but prosthetic grafts such as PTFE are easier to needle and can be used within 2-3 weeks [50]. However, they require long periods of compression following removal of dialysis needles. In comparison with autologous fistulae, PTFE grafts have poorer patency [6, 16, 51-53], require more frequent revisions [16], and have higher rates of infection (9% c.f. 1% per annum) [13, 16-18, 52] and greater mortality, especially in diabetics [13] **(I)**.

Despite their drawbacks, prosthetic grafts have been popular in the USA, even for primary access, and in 1993, 73% of all access in the USA was prosthetic [54, 55]. NKF-DOQI recommended that more than 50% of primary access procedures should be autologous fistulae **(B)**. In Europe, prosthetic graft usage is much lower (<30%) [56]. In Swansea, prosthetic grafts were used in only 2.3% of all 976 access procedures and in only 0.3% of 597 primary procedures in 12 years [57].

Complications of AV fistulae

Thrombosis

This is the most common cause of access failure. It usually results from an inadequate inflow due to upstream arterial stenosis or thrombosis/stenosis in the venous outflow following previous intravenous infusions or scarring after traumatic dialysis needle placement. Intimal hyperplasia may occur and is particularly common beyond the venous anastomosis in prosthetic grafts [58]. Thrombosis can also result from dehydration or hypercoagulability during intercurrent illness.

Fistula failure is more common with small vessels (<1.6mm diameter) and low fistula flows [2] **(II)**. It is also more frequent in women [40,41,59] **(II)** and prosthetic grafts [52,53] **(I)**. Diabetes has been implicated by some [40] but not others [41,60] **(III)**. Dialysis patients are generally anaemic and have reduced platelet "stickiness" which may explain why AV grafts and fistulae in patients without renal failure have a greater tendency to thrombose [61]. Fears that erythropoeitin therapy to increase blood haemoglobin might also reduce fistula patency have not been realised in practice [40,62,63] **(II)**. Antiplatelet agents such as aspirin and dipyridamole prolong fistula patency and are used routinely [33-35] **(I)**. Anticoagulation with warfarin reduces AVF thrombosis in patients with hypercoagulable states [64] but more widespread use is unwise in view of the risk of haemorrhagic complications in dialysis patients [65] **(II)**.

Treatment of fistula thrombosis is either by thrombolysis using streptokinase or rTPA and percutaneous angioplasty (PTA) under angiographic control or by surgical revision. The choice between surgery and interventional radiology depends partly on local expertise but the patency of AV bridge grafts may be better after surgical revision [53, 66] **(II)**.

Steal

Beyond a high flow fistula the arterial pressure is reduced, impairing or even reversing distal arterial flow. If the distal collateral supply is inadequate, ischaemia results, causing rest pain, paraesthesiae and numbness or even digital gangrene. Steal (so-called because blood is "stolen" from the extremity) may also result from a significant upstream arterial stenosis. It occurs in 1-8% of haemodialysis access procedures and is more common with proximal fistulae or bridge grafts [67-71].

The diagnosis is confirmed by the absence of a radial pulse and by measuring the pressure at the wrist using continuous-wave doppler [72] or in the fingers by photoplethysmography. By analogy with lower limb ischaemia, a wrist pressure of <50mmHg or a finger pressure of <40mmHg may indicate critical ischaemia [73].

Fistula ligation is curative but results in loss of access. Reduction of fistula flow by banding or interposition of a narrowed segment of graft is unreliable [74]. Distal ligation of the artery beyond the AVF together with revascularisation by a saphenous vein graft from the proximal brachial artery to the brachial artery beyond the fistula (the DRIL procedure) is the procedure of choice [67,68] **(II) (B)**.

Ischaemic monomelic neuropathy

Disabling neuropathic pain occasionally occurs after AV fistula placement. It can be confirmed by electrophysiology but treatment is difficult [75].

Infection

Bacteraemia is frequent in patients undergoing haemodialysis and may respond to systemic antibiotics. Local infection is more common in prosthetic bridge grafts than autologous fistulae [13, 17, 18]. In post-operative graft infection the whole prosthesis is usually involved and should be excised. Later, localised infection at needle sites may be treated by partial graft excision and bypass through a "clean" area but total excision may eventually become necessary [18,76]. Infection in autologous fistulae usually responds to antibiotics but grossly purulent needle sites may result in uncontrollable haemorrhage requiring fistula ligation.

Haemorrhage

Bleeding can occur after repeated needling at the same site especially in prosthetic grafts, which often require prolonged compression after removing needles. Haematoma formation (the "blown" fistula), results in scarring, stenosis and fistula failure, and

should be avoided. Self-sealing grafts may reduce leakage but have poorer patency [77] **(II)**.

Aneurysm

The venous dilatation proximal to an AVF sometimes becomes excessive. This is rarely a problem but pain, thrombosis or impending rupture may necessitate fistula ligation with creation of a more proximal AVF.

Venous hypertension

Distal venous flow in a side-to-side AVF occasionally causes swelling of the radial aspect of the hand or even ulceration of the thumb. Ligation of the distal venous outflow is usually curative. It is rare after end-to-side (vein to artery) fistulae **(II)**. Subclavian vein thrombosis or stenosis may cause gross arm swelling and can be treated by angioplasty with or without a stent [31] but if this fails fistula ligation may be required.

High output cardiac failure

This may occur with proximal fistulae or bridge grafts where flow often exceeds 1 litre per minute. Digital occlusion of the fistula may cause a reduction in pulse rate (Branham's sign) [38]. Treatment is either by fistula ligation or by interposing a narrow segment of prosthetic graft [78] **(C)**.

Needle placement

A new AV fistula should be allowed to mature for 1 to 3 months prior to use [11,12] **(B)** and, initially, cannulation should only be undertaken by experienced staff. Minimizing trauma to new fistulae prolongs their life and obviates the need for CVC access.

The skin should be prepared with chlorhexidine or povidone iodine. Some patients require local anaesthetic (e.g. lignocaine 2%), and a tourniquet may be used to distend the vessel prior to needle insertion. The needle gauge is carefully selected to

Figure 3 Strategies for needling AV fistulae. Crosses represent needle sites.

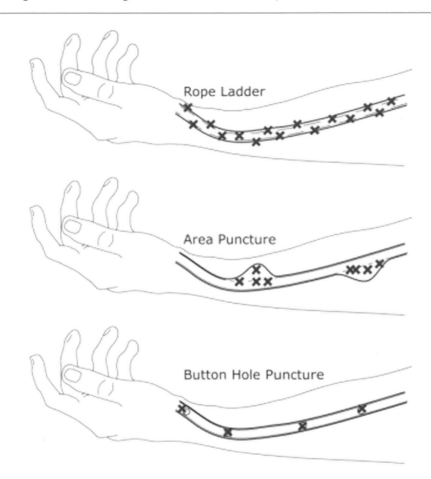

ensure optimum flows. Initially smaller needles (16-17g) may be used but larger gauges (14-15g) may be required for high blood flows [79]. Needles are introduced aseptically at 45° to the skin, inserting the whole shaft into the vessel and securing the butterfly wing with tape [80]. A syringe placed at the end of the needle serves to check the position and provides an assessment of flow.

Cannulation is by one of three methods [81] (Figure 3):

♦ **Rope ladder:** Systematic evenly spaced cannulation along the length of the vein draining the fistula causes mild and well-distributed dilatation throughout an autologous fistula and is recommended for prosthetic graft cannulation.

♦ **Area puncture:** Repeated cannulation over short segments of the vein causes localised dilatation and, sometimes, interspersed stenoses. It is useful for encouraging dilatation in a new fistula but inadvisable for long-term use.

♦ **Buttonhole:** Repeated puncture through the same needle site causes little dilatation and reduces pain of cannulation but is not recommended for prosthetic grafts.

If cannulation is unsuccessful after two or three attempts, assistance should be sought so that further trauma is prevented. If the site becomes swollen, the area should be temporarily avoided.

Figure 4 Algorithm showing usual sequence of haemodialysis access. Most common procedures are shown in a bold large font.

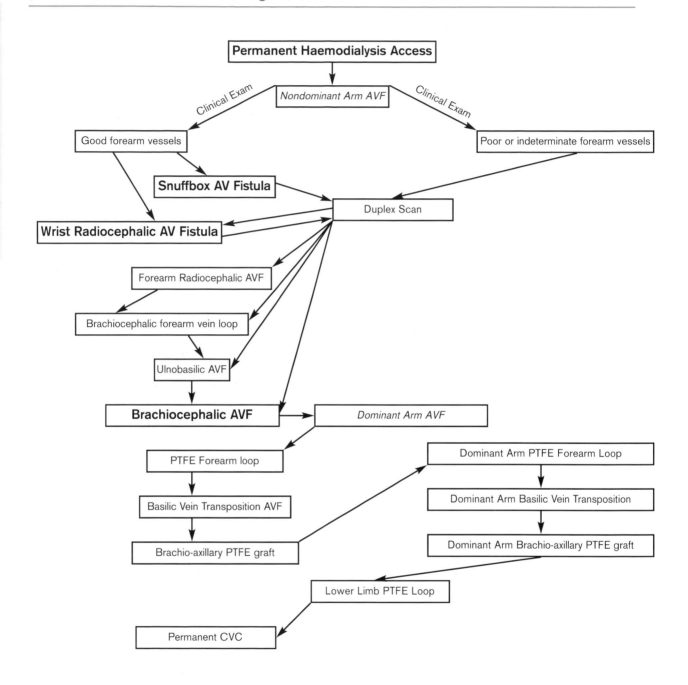

Vascular access surveillance

In some patients, a reduction in the palpable thrill or in dialysis flow rates, or an increase in venous pressure on dialysis may herald fistula failure. In others, thrombosis occurs suddenly for no apparent reason. Many such fistulae have asymptomatic stenoses, which, with timely detection, could have been treated prophylactically by angioplasty or surgery. Surveillance by duplex scanning, static and dynamic pressure measurements within the fistula and measurement of access blood flow have all been advocated to detect such stenoses [82]. However, there is no good evidence that autologous fistula patency is prolonged whereas, for prosthetic grafts, patency is known to be improved and hospitalisation reduced by some form of surveillance [82] **(III)**.

Care of the vascular access patient

As the need for dialysis approaches, the patient is counselled by nursing and medical staff, with the aid of booklets, leaflets, videos and help from patient organisations, to reduce anxiety and improve compliance [83, 84]. Careful explanations of procedures, reassurance regarding the discomfort of needle placement, and sensitivity to the concerns of patients about scarring and altered body image are important. Supplementary information acquired through the Internet can provide extra patient-centred information (www.kidneywise.com). Provision of information that encourages patient interactivity can improve patient outcomes [85]. Patients are advised to wear watches and bracelets on the opposite wrist and to avoid drips and venepunctures on the fistula arm. They should also be shown how to apply digital pressure in the event of needle-site haemorrhage.

Vascular access in children

Children present particularly difficult access problems. Transplantation is ideal and achieves optimal growth and development. CAPD is the next best choice but haemodialysis is often required. Distal autologous fistulae are more difficult to perform and necessitate microsurgical skills but several European units have shown that they are preferable [86-88] **(B)**.

However many units rely on permanent central venous lines or prosthetic grafts risking the loss of available access sites.

Summary and conclusions

◆ An integrated approach to the treatment of end-stage renal failure involving haemodialysis, CAPD and renal transplantation is required to maximise life expectancy (Figure 1) **(A)**.

◆ Early AV fistula construction minimises the use of central venous catheters reducing infection, hospitalisation and mortality **(A)**.

◆ Careful planning of fistula sites and avoidance of AV grafts maximises life on dialysis and minimises access problems. The preferred sequence of haemodialysis access procedures is summarised in Figure 4 **(A)**.

◆ The AV fistula is the patient's lifeline and must be preciously preserved.

◆ Safe and atraumatic cannulation of the veins draining an AV fistula is dependent not only on the quality of the fistula but also the skill and experience of the dialysis nurse.

◆ Patients must be well educated in fistula care and may need to inform carers whose experience may lie elsewhere **(A)**.

◆ Dialysis is a long-term commitment and patients require psychological support in the face of repeated setbacks.

Further Reading

1   Conlon PJ, Schwab SJ, Nicholson ML, Eds. *Haemodialysis Vascular Access: Practice and Problems*. Oxford University Press, Oxford, 2000.

2   NKF-K/DOQI Clinical Practice Guidelines for Vascular Access: Update 2000. *Am J Kidney Dis.* 2001; 37(1) Suppl 1: S137-81.

3   Emery J. Nursing Care of Patients with dialysis access. In: *Dialysis Access: Current Practice*. Akoh TA, Hakaim NS, Eds. Imperial College Press, London, 2001; 371-395.

Chapter 27

Chapter 27

References (grade I evidence and grade A recommendations in bold)

1. Nicholson ML, Murphy GJ. Surgical considerations in vascular access. *In: Haemodialysis Vascular Access: Practice and Problems.* Conlon PJ, Schwab SJ, Nicholson ML, Eds. Oxford University Press, Oxford, 2000; 101-123.

2. Wong V, Ward R, Taylor J, Selvakumar S, How TV, Bakran A. Factors associated with early failure of arteriovenous fistulae for haemodialysis access. *Eur J Vasc Endovasc Surg* 1996; 12: 207-213.

3. Kalman PG, Pope M, Bhola C, Richardson R, Sniderman KW. A practical approach to vascular access for haemodialysis and predictors of success. *J Vasc Surg* 1999; 30; 727-733.

4. Manas DM. The access clinic. In: *Dialysis Access: Current Practice.* Akoh TA, Hakaim NS, Eds. Imperial College Press, London, 2001; 67-87.

5. Quinton WE, Dillard D, Scribner BH. Cannulation of blood vessels for prolonged haemodialysis. *Trans Am Soc Artif Intern Organs* 1960; 6: 104-113.

6. Burger H, Kluchert SA, Koostra G, Kitslaar PJEHM, Ubbink DTH. Survival of arteriovenous fistulas and shunts for haemodialysis. *Eur J Surg* 1995, 161, 327-334.

7. Bell PRF, Wood RFM. *Surgical Aspects of Haemodialysis.* Churchill Livingstone, Edinburgh, 1983.

8. **Farrell J, Abraham KA, Walshe JJ. Acute vascular access. In:** *Haemodialysis Vascular Access: Practice and Problems.* **Conlon PJ, Schwab SJ, Nicholson ML, Eds. Oxford University Press, Oxford, 2000; 3-22.**

9. **Cimochowski GE, Worley E Rutherford WE,** *et al.* **Superiority of the internal jugular vein over subclavian access for temporary haemodialysis.** *Nephron* **1990; 54: 154-156.**

10. Zaleski GX, Funaki B, Lorenz JM, *et al.* Experience with tunnelled femoral dialysis catheters. *Am J Roentgenol* 1999; 172: 493-496.

11. **NKF-DOQI clinical practice guidelines for vascular access. National Kidney Foundation-Dialysis Outcomes Quality Initiative.** *Am J Kidney Dis* **1997; 30 (4) Suppl 3: S150-S191.**

12. **NKF-K/DOQI Clinical Practice Guidelines for Vascular Access: Update 2000.** *Am J Kidney Dis.* **2001; 37(1) Suppl 1: S137-81.**

13. **Dhingra RK, Young EW, Hulbert-Shearon TE, Leavey SF, Port FK. Type of vascular access and mortality in U.S. hemodialysis patients.** *Kidney Intl* **2001; 60: 1443-1451.**

14. Goodkin DA, Mapes DL, Held PJ. The dialysis outcomes and practice patterns study (DOPPS): how can we improve the care of hemodialysis patients? *Semin Dial* 2001; 14:157-159.

15. The Kidney Alliance. *End Stage Renal Failure - A Framework for Planning and Service Delivery.* Munro and Forster, London, 2001.

16. Hodges TC, Fillinger MF, Zwolak RM, Walsh DB, Bech F, Cronenwett JL. Longitudinal comparison of dialysis access methods: factors for failure. *J Vasc Surg* 1997; 26: 1009-1019.

17. **Nasser GM, Ayus JC, Infectious complications of haemodialysis access.** *Kidney International* **2001; 60: 1-13.**

18. **Kirkland KB, Sexton DJ. Dialysis-access infection. In:** *Haemodialysis Vascular Access: Practice and Problems.* **Conlon PJ, Schwab SJ, Nicholson ML, Eds. Oxford University Press, Oxford, 2000; 84-100.**

19. Blankenstijn PJ. Cuffed tunnelled catheters for long-term vascular access. In: *Haemodialysis Vascular Access: Practice and Problems.* Conlon PJ, Schwab SJ, Nicholson ML, Eds. Oxford University Press, Oxford, 2000; 67-84.

20. **Bock SN, Lee RE, Fisher B,** *et al.* **A prospective randomised trial evaluating prophylactic antibiotics to prevent triple-lumen catheter - related sepsis in patients treated with immunotherapy.** *J Clin Oncol* **1990; 8: 161-169.**

21. **Al-Sibai MB. The value of prophylactic antibiotics during insertion of long-term indwelling silastic right atrial catheters in cancer patients.** *Cancer* **1987; 60: 1891-1895.**

22. **Ranson MR, Oppenheim BA, Jackson A, Kamthan AG, Scarffe JH. Double-blind placebo controlled study of vancomycin prophylaxis for central venous catheter insertion in cancer patients.** *J Hosp Infect* **1990; 15: 95-102.**

23. **Department of Health. Guidelines for preventing infections associated with the insertion and maintenance of central venous catheters.** *J Hosp Infect* **2001; 47 (Suppl): S47-S67.**

24. **Maki DG, Ringer M, Alvardo CJ. Prospective randomised trial of povidone-iodine, alcohol, and chlorhexidine for prevention of infection associated with central venous and arterial catheters.** *Lancet* **1991; 338: 339-343.**

25. **Mimoz O, Pieroni L, Lawrence C, Edouard A, Costa Y, Samii K, Brun-Buisson C. A prospective, randomised trial of two antiseptic solutions for prevention of central venous or arterial catheter colonization and infection in intensive care unit patients.** *Crit Care Med* **1996; 24: 1818-1823.**

26. **Conly JM, Grieves K, Peter B. A prospective, randomised study comparing transparent and dry gauze dressings for central venous catheters.** *J Infect Dis* **1989; 159: 310-319.**

27. Northsea C. Using urokinase to restore patency in double lumen catheters. *ANNA J* 1994; 21: 261-264.

28. **Randolph AG, Cook DJ, Gonzales CA, Andrew M. Benefit of heparin in peripheral venous and pulmonary artery catheters: a meta-analysis of randomised controlled trials.** *Chest* **1998; 113: 165-171.**

29 Shoenfeld R, Hermans H, Novick A, Brener B, Cordero P, Eisenbud D, Mody S, Goldenkranz R, Parsonnet V. Stenting of proximal venous obstructions to maintain haemodialysis access. *J Vasc Surg* 1994; 19: 532- 538.

30 Bhatia DS, Money SR, Oschner JLCrockett DE, Chatman D, Dharamsey SA, Mulingtapang RF, Shaw D, Ramee SR. Comparison of surgical bypass and percutaneous balloon dilatation with primary stent placement in the treatment of central venous obstruction in the dialysis patient: One-year follow-up. *Ann Vasc Surg* 1996; 10: 452-455.

31 Criado E, Marston WA, Jaques PF, Mauro MA, Keagy BA. Proximal venous outflow obstruction in patients with upper extremity arteriovenous dialysis access. *Ann Vasc Surg* 1994; 8: 530-535.

32 Tordoir JHM, Leunissen KML. Jugular vein transposition for the treatment of subclavian vein obstruction in haemodialysis patients. *Eur J Vasc Surg* 1993; 7: 335-338.

33 **Hakkim R, Himmelfarb J. Haemodialysis failure: A call to action. *Kidney International* 1998; 54:1029-1040.**

34 **Andrassy K, Malluche H, Bornfeld H,Comberg Mritz E, Jessdinsky H, Mohring K. Prevention of PO clotting of AV. Cimino fistulae with acetylsalicyl acid: Results of a prospective double blind study. *Klin Wochenschr* 1974; 52: 348-349.**

35 **Sreedhara R, Himmelfarb J, Lazarus JM, Hakim RM. Antiplatelet therapy in graft thrombosis: results of a prospective randomised double blind study. *Kidney Intl* 1994; 45: 1477-1483.**

36 Wright A, Hecker JF, Lewis GB. Use of transdermal glyceryl trinitrate to reduce failure of intravenous infusion due to phlebitis and extravasation. *Lancet* 1985; 2: 1148-1150.

37 Breschia MJ, Cimino JE, Appel K, Hurwich BJ. Chronic hemodialysis using venepuncture and a surgically created arteriovenous fistula. *N Eng J Med* 1966; 275: 1089-1092.

38 Gelabert HA, Freischlag JA. Haemodialysis access. In: *Vascular Surgery*. Rutherford RB, Ed. 5th Ed. Saunders, Philadelphia, 2000; 1466-1477.

39 Marx AB, Landmann J, Harder FH. Surgery for vascular access. In: *Curr Probl Surg* 1990; Jan: 3-48.

40 Golledge J, Smith CJ, Emery J, Farrington K, Thompson HH. Outcome of primary radiocephalic fistula for haemodialysis. *Br J Surg* 1999; 86: 211-216.

41 Wolowczyk L, Williams AJ, Gibbons CP. The snuffbox arteriovenous fistula for vascular access. *Eur J Vasc Endovasc Surg* 2000; 19: 70-76.

42 Rassat JP, Moscovtchenko JF, Perrin J, Traeger J. La fistule artero-veineuse dans la tabatiere anatomique. *Journal d' Urologie et de Nephrologie*. 1969; 75: Suppl.12: 482.

43 Livingston CK, Potts JR. Upper arm arteriovenous fistulas as a reliable access alternative for patients requiring chronic hemodialysis. *Am Surg* 1999; 65: 1038-1042.

44 Dagher F, Gerber R, Ramos E *et al*. The use of basilic vein and brachial artery as an AV fistula for long-term haemodialysis. *J Surg Res* 1976; 20: 373-376.

45 LoGerfo FW, Menzoian KO, Kumaki DJ *et al*. Transposed basilic vein brachial arteriovenous fistula. *Arch Surg* 1978; 113: 1008-1010.

46 Rivers SP, Scher LA, Sheehan E, Lynn R, Veith FJ. Basilic vein transposition: an underused autogenous alternative to prosthetic dialysis angioaccess. *J Vasc Surg* 1993; 18: 391-396.

47 Hakaim AG, Oldenberg WA. Basilic vein transposition for chronic haemodialysis. *Adv Vasc Surg* 2000, 8: 125-130.

48 Matsuura JH, Rosenthal D, Clark M, *et al*. Transposed basilic vein versus polytetrafluoroethylene for brachial-axillary arteriovenous fistulas. *Am J Surg* 1998; 176: 219-216.

49 Khadra MH, Dwyer AJ, Thompson JF *et al*. Advantages of polytetrafluoroethylene arteriovenous loops in the thigh for haemodialysis access. *Am J Surg* 1997; 173: 280-283.

50 Hakaim AG, Scott TE. Durability of early prosthetic dialysis graft cannulation: Results of a prospective, nonrandomised clinical trial. *J Vasc Surg* 1997; 25: 1002-1006.

51 Burger H. Long-term outcome of different forms of vascular access. In: *Haemodialysis Vascular Access: Practice and Problems*. Conlon PJ, Schwab SJ, Nicholson ML, Eds. Oxford University Press, Oxford, 2000; 52-56.

52 **Ascher E, Gade P, Hingorani A, MazzarioIF, Gunduz Y, Fodera M, Yorkovich W. Changes in practice of angioaccess surgery: Impact of dialysis outcome and quality initiative recommendations. *J Vasc Surg* 2000; 31: 84-92.**

53 **Owens LV, Keagy BA, Marston WA. Management of the thrombosed dialysis-access graft. *Adv Vasc Surg* 2000, 8: 131-145.**

54 US Renal Data System: VI. Causes of death. *Am J Kidney Dis* 1995; 26: S93-S102.

55 US Renal Data System: *US Data System 1997 Annual Report*. Chapter X. Washington DC, 1997; 143-161.

56 Tordoir J. How does European practice compare with DOQI guidelines? *Proc 2nd International Congress Vascular Access Society* 2000; abstract IS2: 20.

57 Gibbons CP, Williams AJ, Donovan KL. Arteriovenous grafts are rarely necessary for haemodialysis access. *Proc 2nd International Congress Vascular Access Society* 2000; abstract 4.2: 29.

58 Glagov S, Giddens DP, Bassiouny H, White S, Zarins CK. Haemodynamic effects and tissue reactions at graft to vein anastomosis for vascular access. In: *Vascular Access for Haemodialysis - II*. Eds Sommer BG, Henry ML. Precept Press Inc., USA, 1991; 3-20.

59 Kinnaert P, Vereersraeten P, Toussain C, Van Geertruyden J. Nine years' experience with internal arteriovenous fistulas for haemodialysis: a study of some factors influencing the results. *Br J Surg*; 64: 242-246.

60 Miller PE, Carlton D, Deierhoi MH, Redden DT, Allon M. Natural history of arteriovenous grafts in hemodialysis patients. *Am J Kidney Dis* 2000; 36: 68-74.

61 Mason RA, Campbell R, Newton GB, Giron F. Synthetic graft angio-access in dialysis and nondialysis patients. In: *Vascular Access for Haemodialysis-II.* Sommer BG, Henry ML, Eds. WL Gore Inc and Precept Press Inc, USA, 1991; 158-165.

62 Fischer-Colbrie W, Clyne N, JogenstrandT, Takolander R. The effect of erythropoeitin treatment on arteriovenous haemodialysis fistula/graft: a prospective study with colour flow Doppler ultrasonography. *Eur J Vasc Surg* 1994; 8: 346-350.

63 Martino MA, Vogel KM, O'Brien SP *et al.* Erythropoeitin therapy improves graft patency with no increased incidence of thrombosis or thrombophlebitis. *J Am Coll Surg* 1998; 187: 616-619.

64 LeSar CJ, Merrick HW, Smith MR. Thrombotic complications resulting from hypercoagulable states in chronic haemodialysis vascular access. *J Am Coll Surg* 1999; 189: 73-79.

65 Biggers JA, Remmers AR Jr, Glassford DM, Sarles HE, Lindley JD, Fish JC. The risk of anticoagulation in haemodialysis patients. *Nephron* 1977; 18: 109-113.

66 Marston WA, Criado E, Jaques PF *et al.* Prospective randomised comparison of surgical versus endovascular management of thrombosed dialysis access grafts. *J Vasc Surg* 1997; 26: 373-381.

67 Wixon CL, Mills JL. Haemodynamic basis for the diagnosis and treatment of angioaccess-induced steal syndrome. *Advances in Vascular Surgery* 2000; 8: 147-159.

68 Schanzer H, Schwarz M, Harrington E, Haimov M. Treatment of ischaemia due to steal by arteriovenous fistula with distal artery ligation and revascularisation. *J Vasc Surg* 1988; 7: 770-773.

69 Goff CD, Sato DT, Bloch PHS, DeMasi RJ, Gregory RT, Gayle RG, Parent FN, Meier GH, Wheeler GR. Steal syndrome complicating haemodialysis access procedures: can it be predicted? *Ann Vasc Surg* 2000; 14: 138-144.

70 Duncan H, Ferguson L, Faris I. Incidence of the radial steal syndrome in patients with Brescia fistula for haemodialysis: its clinical significance. *J Vasc Surg* 1986; 4: 144-147.

71 Morsy AH, Kulbaski M, Chen C, Isiklar H, Lumsden AB. Incidence and characteristics of patients with hand ischaemia after a haemodialysis access procedure. *J Surg Res* 1998; 74: 8-10.

72 Bakran A, Singh UP, Ahmed A, How TV. Wrist/brachial pressure index - a simple method for assessing steal syndrome after proximal arm AV fistulae. Angioaccess for Haemodialysis. *Proceedings of the 2nd International Multidisciplinary Symposium, Tours.* 1999; 223.

73 TASC. Management of peripheral arterial disease (PAD) - TransAtlantic Inter-Society Consensus. *Eur J Vasc Endovasc Surg* 2000; 19 Suppl A: S153.

74 DeCaprio JD, Valentine RJ, Kakish HB, Awad R, Hagino RT, Claggett GP. Steal syndrome complicating hemodialysis access. *Cardiovascular Surgery* 1997; 5: 648-653.

75 Hye RJ, Wolf YG. Ischemic monomelic neuropathy: An under-recognised complication of hemodialysis access. *Ann Vasc Surg* 1994; 8: 578-582.

76 Deneuville M. Infection of PTFE grafts used to create arteriovenous fistulas for haemodialysis access. *Ann Vasc Surg* 2000; 14: 473-479.

77 Coyne DW, Lowell JA, Windus DW *et al.* Comparison of survival of an expanded polytetrafluoroethylene graft designed for early cannulation to standard wall polytetrafluoroethylene grafts. *J Am Coll Surg* 1996; 183: 401-405.

78 Ahern D, Maher J. Heart failure as a complication of haemodialysis arteriovenous fistula. *Ann Intern Med* 1972; 77: 201-204.

79 Levy J, Morgan J, Brown E. *Oxford Handbook of Dialysis.* Oxford University Press, London, 2001.

80 Smith T. *Renal Nursing.* Bailliere Tindall, London,1997.

81 Kronung G. Plastic Deformation of Cimino Fistula by Repeated Puncture. *Dial Transplant* 1984; 13: 635-638.

82 Back MR, Bandyk DF. Current status of surveillance of haemodialysis access grafts. *Ann Vasc Surg* 2001; 15: 491-502.

83 Andrew J. The Pre-dialysis Experience- Are individual needs being met? *EDTNA / ERCA J* 2001; XXV11: 72-74.

84 Bay WH, Cleef SV, Owens M. Haemodialysis Access: Preferences and Concerns of Patients, Dialysis Nurses and Technicians, and Physicians. *Am J Nephrol* 1998; 18: 379-383.

85 Diamond LH. Local Implementation of Clinical Practice Guidelines and Continuous Quality Improvement: Challenges and Opportunities. *Semin Dial* 2001; 13: 364-368.

86 Bagolan P, Spagnoli A, Ciprandi *et al.* A ten-year experience of Breschia-Cimino arteriovenous fistula in children: Technical evolution and refinements. *J Vasc Surg* 1998; 27: 640-644.

87 Bourquelot P, Stolba J, Macher MA, Loirat C. Vascular access in children. *Proc 2nd International Congress Vascular Access Society* 2000; abstract 11.1: 72.

88 Naiman G, Vogelfang H, D'angelis A, Lipsich J. Paediatrics hemodialysis vascular access. *Proc 2nd International Congress Vascular Access Society* 2000; abstract 11.3: 73.

Chapter 27

Chapter 28

Surgical management of varicose veins

Daryll Baker Consultant Vascular Surgeon [1]

Barrie Higgs Consultant Vascular Anaesthetist [1]

Jonathan Beard Consultant Vascular Surgeon [2]

[1] DEPARTMENT OF SURGERY, ROYAL FREE HOSPITAL, LONDON, UK
[2] SHEFFIELD VASCULAR INSTITUTE, THE NORTHERN GENERAL HOSPITAL, SHEFFIELD, UK

Introduction

Varicose vein operations are generally associated with a low surgical morbidity. The peri-operative management is similar for all cases and therefore ideally suited to an integrated care pathway, especially for day-case surgery. The integrated care pathway for varicose vein surgery is a proforma-based series of steps undertaken by all members of the health care team. It aims at ensuring a safe, rapid and "enjoyable" passage through the process of varicose vein surgery, and helps to empower patients to take an active part in their own management. This chapter focuses on the use of an integrated care pathway for patients undergoing primary saphenofemoral varicose vein surgery as a day-case procedure.

The Integrated Care Pathway

The integrated care pathway proforma is presented as a booklet separate from the hospital notes, often with some distinguishing mark such as a brightly coloured paper. The proforma is kept with the main hospital notes and all parts are completed even if this does involve some repetition of information, as it is important to gather all the information required in a structured format. The proforma used in our day-case unit can be found on the website.

There are three main parts to the integrated care pathway for varicose vein management (Figure 1):

◆ Pre-assessment clinic.

◆ Peri-operative management.

◆ Post-discharge care.

Pre-assessment clinic

The aim of the pre-assessment clinic is to ensure the patient is suitable and prepared (emotionally, physically and socially) to undergo the planned varicose vein procedure. This is usually performed under general or regional anaesthetic, but it is necessary to determine if they are suitable to have the procedure as a day-case or need to be admitted overnight because of medical problems e.g. asthma or angina. A trained nurse performing a proforma question-lead history and examination of the patient

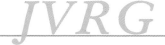

Figure 1 Algorithm for the surgical treatment of varicose veins in the day-case unit.

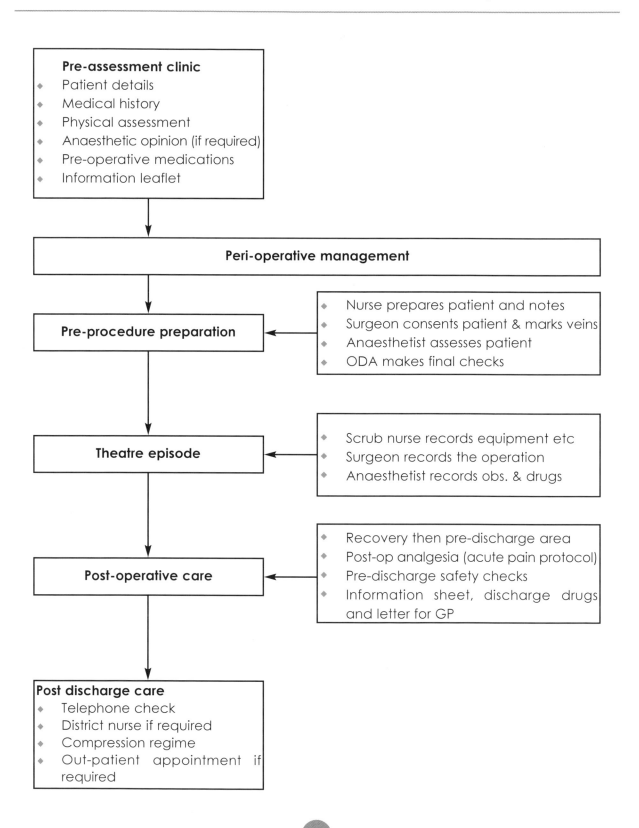

Pre-assessment clinic
- Patient details
- Medical history
- Physical assessment
- Anaesthetic opinion (if required)
- Pre-operative medications
- Information leaflet

Peri-operative management

Pre-procedure preparation
- Nurse prepares patient and notes
- Surgeon consents patient & marks veins
- Anaesthetist assesses patient
- ODA makes final checks

Theatre episode
- Scrub nurse records equipment etc
- Surgeon records the operation
- Anaesthetist records obs. & drugs

Post-operative care
- Recovery then pre-discharge area
- Post-op analgesia (acute pain protocol)
- Pre-discharge safety checks
- Information sheet, discharge drugs and letter for GP

Post discharge care
- Telephone check
- District nurse if required
- Compression regime
- Out-patient appointment if required

undertakes the assessment. The information gathered is divided into several sections:

Patient information and social assessment

This includes such information as address and telephone numbers of both the patient and the next of kin, whether an interpreter is needed, and if so, has this been arranged. If the patient is to be a day-case there needs to be an escort to take the patient home and their name and contact number as well as the supervision arrangements for the next 24 hours post-operatively have to be recorded.

It is important that the patient has a clear understanding of the planned procedure and will usually have received an information leaflet in the out-patient clinic (see chapter on medico-legal issues). This fact should be recorded in the proforma as this may prevent unjustified medico-legal claims relating to lack of informed consent [1] **(A)**. The patient should be asked if they understand the management plan and whether they have any questions about it.

Medical history

Problems arising from the anaesthetic are less likely if the patient has previously undergone successful anaesthesia. The nurse therefore needs to record any such events on the proforma.

A checklist of major diseases is then performed. This is aimed at identifying any problems that may result in complications during surgery. It is best to ask the patient about well-defined symptoms and simple diagnoses e.g. shortness of breath on lying flat and chest pain on exertion. Finally it is important to confirm that the patient is not pregnant, whether they smoke and how much alcohol do they drink.

Physical assessment

The nurse then checks the patient's height, weight and blood pressure.

Routine investigations including full blood count, serum urea and electrolytes, sickle cell status, chest x-ray and ECG are then ordered as required from a pre-determined checklist. Varicose vein surgery may require a pre-operative duplex scan [2] **(II)**. It is important at this stage to determine if this was considered necessary at the out-patient consultation and if so, that it has been undertaken (see chapter on the out-patient management of varicose veins).

Anaesthetic opinion

On the strength of the history, examination and investigations, an anaesthetic opinion may be requested to determine whether the patient is medically fit for day-case treatment. If the nurse has identified nothing untoward from the pre-assessment, then the anaesthetist does not need to review the patient until the day of surgery **(C)**.

Pre-operative requirements (including named drugs)

Any pre-operative medications are given to the patient with clear instructions on when to take them. Patients taking the oral contraceptive pill or hormone replacement therapy and those with other risk factors for DVT should be prescribed a single dose of low molecular weight heparin pre-operatively **(B)**. This is a better option than stopping oral contraceptive therapy and risking pregnancy [3].

Patient's acceptance and declaration

It is important that the patient is happy with the consultation and the plans for surgery and that they sign a declaration to this point. This is not the same as the consent form.

Peri-operative management

On the day of surgery several steps need to be successfully undertaken by the various members of the health care team, as well as the patient. Each person needs to follow and fill in his or her part of the proforma. This part of the integrated care pathway can be divided into several steps:

- Pre-procedure preparation.

- Theatre episode.

- Post-operative care.

Pre-procedure preparation

The patient writes in the proforma the time that they last ate, last drank, the name of their escort and their contact telephone number.

The nurse records the patient's vital observations (pulse, blood pressure, respiratory rate and temperature) and records the necessary blood results. The patient is prepared for theatre (including: identity bracelet attached, dentures removed, make-up and nail varnish removed as well as contact lenses, jewellery and hair grips).

The surgeon, with the aid of the full medical notes, confirms that the planned operation remains indicated and then consents the patient for the procedure **(A)**. It is important that the operation is discussed in detail and the potential risks, which were first discussed in the out-patient clinic and then re-discussed by the nurse in the pre-admission clinic are gone over one final time.

The surgeon also marks the sites for the varicose vein surgery. An arrow is drawn to indicate the site and side of the saphenofemoral or saphenopopliteal disconnection. The saphenopopliteal junction must be located with a duplex scan as the site of the junction can vary considerably **(B)**. The junction can be located in relation to the mid-point of the popliteal fossa or marked immediately before the operation. The varicose veins are identified with an indelible marker pen whilst the patient stands. It is best to draw two tramlines on either side of the varicose vein, in order to mark its course, with dots over the vein at the planned avulsion sites. The skin incisions are made next to the dots rather than through them to reduce the risk of tattooing **(B)**.

The anaesthetist, on the day of surgery, fills in the anaesthetic part of the proforma. This will include details about medical problems, allergies, drug therapy, teeth (caps and crowns) and the ASA rating.

The operating department practitioner, at the transfer bay, makes one final check just before the patient enters the operating theatre namely that the consent is signed, the dental status is known, the appropriate investigations are available and the varicose veins have been marked.

Theatre episode

As with all successful integrated care pathways, each member of the team plays a part and refers to and completes the appropriate part of the proforma.

The anaesthetist records the anaesthetic techniques used in the three stages of induction, maintenance and reversal. Intra-operative observation including pulse, blood pressure, oxygen saturation and end tidal carbon dioxide levels are recorded throughout the operation. Spinal anaesthesia seems a good alternative to general anaesthesia as it avoids post-operative nausea and vomiting. A saphenofemoral disconnection and stripping can be performed under a femoral nerve block but this inevitably leads to motor loss that prevents walking for several hours. Most surgeons infiltrate the groin wound with Marcaine 0.5% **(B)**. This reduces the need for post-operative opiates that may prevent same-day discharge due to nausea and vomiting [4] **(II)**.

The scrub nurse or ODA confirms that they have seen the consent form, records the position of the patient and the diathermy pad and that there has been no skin damage on removal. The use of a tourniquet and the duration of application are recorded as well as the swab, needle and instrument counts. A supine position is used for saphenofemoral disconnection. Saphenopopliteal disconnection can be performed in a lateral position. This allows the use of a laryngeal mask rather than a cuffed endotracheal tube that requires a deeper anaesthetic.

The surgeon records the operative note on a separate part of the proforma. This should include details of the procedure performed and an explanation for any deviation from the planned procedure (e.g. inability to pass the stripper). The following details should also be written down: use of an exsanguination tourniquet, type of compression bandage or stocking, duration of compression and the need for an out-patient appointment (see later).

Post-operative care

The nurse in recovery ensures that the patient safely recovers from the procedure. The blood pressure, pulse and oxygen saturation levels are observed regularly. The patient's pain score and level of consciousness is also recorded, as are regular observations of the wound sites. Any other medications including fluids can be prescribed and recorded in this part of the proforma. The nurse administers post-operative analgesia according to an acute pain protocol (Figure 2).

The nurse on the ward accompanies or takes over the care of the patient when the patient is sufficiently awake and stable enough to be moved back to the pre-discharge area. Many day units have trolleys that can be used for the operation, recovery and the ward area. These avoid the need for patient transfers. Other units use reclining chairs rather than beds in the pre-discharge area as these take up less space.

Prior to discharge the nurse confirms the patient is suitable to leave the hospital. This part of the proforma confirms that the patient is alert and orientated, the vital signs are within normal limits, the wound sites appear normal, the patient can walk unaided, has tolerated oral fluids and food and is pain-free. It is also important to check that the intravenous cannula, ECG leads and identity bracelets have been removed. The patients are given their discharge drugs, with written instructions on when to take them, a discharge information sheet and letter for the general practitioner. The information sheet should include a 24hr telephone number for patients to ring if they have any concerns after discharge **(B)**. An out-patient appointment is also made if requested by the surgeon (usually unnecessary). If untoward surgical or medical problems occur, then this fact should be recorded and a surgical or anaesthetic review requested. If it is not possible to discharge the patient then an inpatient bed

will have to be found and the on-call surgical staff informed.

Post-discharge care

The day after surgery the nurse telephones the patient to check they have no problems. This is recorded on the integrated care pathway proforma and the completed care episode is "signed off". The information sheet and the letter for the GP should specify whether there are any sutures that require removal by the practice nurse. Subcuticular Vicryl sutures in the groin and adhesive skin closures for the stab incisions improve cosmesis and avoid the need for a visit to the practice nurse **(III)**.

Protocols concerning post-operative compression vary. Some apply a non-adhesive compression bandage that is replaced by a stocking after 24hrs. This requires a visit by the community nurse. Cohesive acrylic bandages can be left in place for a week or more without loss of compression and avoids the need for a visit by the community nurse. There are many different regimes for post-operative compression but there seems no advantage of prolonging this for more than a week [5] **(I)**.

The discharge information sheet should advise frequent walks, elevation of the legs when not walking and avoidance of long-distance travel. It should also remind patients that bruising after VV surgery is very common and takes a few weeks to resolve.

Surgical considerations

There are some technical aspects of varicose vein surgery that contribute to a successful day-case episode and subsequent results. These include:

- Duration of the procedure.

- Saphenofemoral disconnection and stripping.

- Exsanguination tourniquets.

Chapter 28

Figure 2 Acute pain protocol used by the nursing staff in recovery after varicose vein surgery.

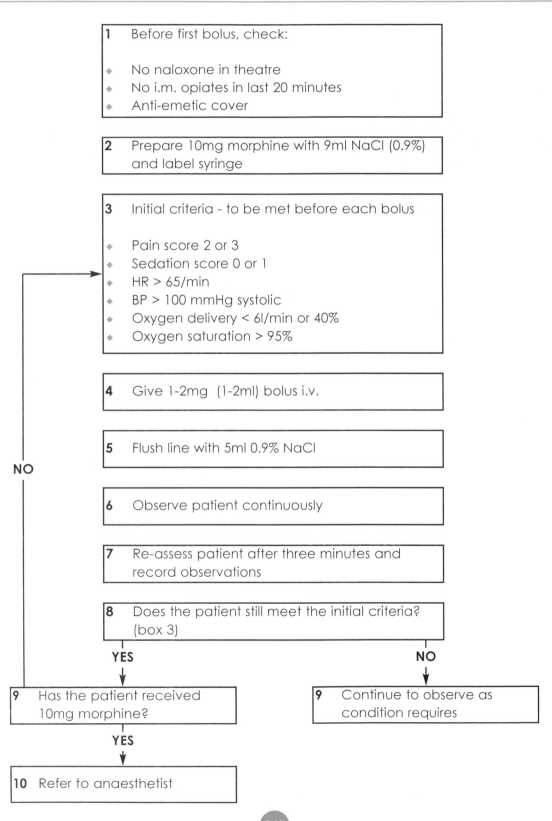

| 1 | Before first bolus, check:

◆ No naloxone in theatre
◆ No i.m. opiates in last 20 minutes
◆ Anti-emetic cover |

| 2 | Prepare 10mg morphine with 9ml NaCl (0.9%) and label syringe |

| 3 | Initial criteria - to be met before each bolus

◆ Pain score 2 or 3
◆ Sedation score 0 or 1
◆ HR > 65/min
◆ BP > 100 mmHg systolic
◆ Oxygen delivery < 6l/min or 40%
◆ Oxygen saturation > 95% |

| 4 | Give 1-2mg (1-2ml) bolus i.v. |

| 5 | Flush line with 5ml 0.9% NaCl |

| 6 | Observe patient continuously |

| 7 | Re-assess patient after three minutes and record observations |

| 8 | Does the patient still meet the initial criteria? (box 3) |

YES   NO

| 9 | Has the patient received 10mg morphine? |

| 9 | Continue to observe as condition requires |

YES

| 10 | Refer to anaesthetist |

NO

Figure 3 Boazul cuff rolled up to the thigh to provide an almost bloodless field. Note the tramlines and dots used to mark the varicose veins and the avulsion sites. The "landing zone" just below the knee for the stripper as it is passed down the LSV under the tourniquet from the groin is also marked. The phlebectomy hook seen on the table reduces the size of the skin incisions required for the avulsions.

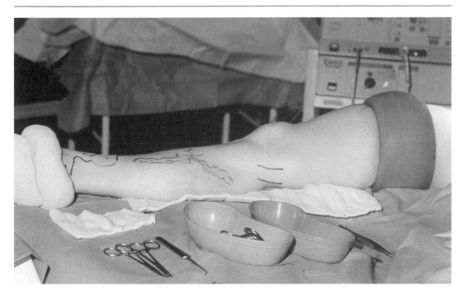

The long saphenous vein should be stripped to the knee to reduce the risk of recurrence [8] **(A)**. The Gloucester randomised trial showed the stripping reduced the reoperation rate from 20% to 6% at 6 years [9] **(A)**. Stripping to the knee reduces the risk of saphenous injury associated with full length stripping [10] **(A)**. The morbidity associated with stripping may be reduced by using a small stripper head or by an inversion technique although randomised trials have failed to show much advantage [11] **(III)**. The medial thigh tributary that joins the LSV just below the saphenofemoral junction should be ligated and divided before stripping to reduce the risk of a groin haematoma, as this tributary is too high to be compressed by the bandage **(III)**.

Duration of the procedure

Many anaesthetists feel that a day-case anaesthetic should not last more than one hour. Longer procedures increase the risk of post-operative nausea and vomiting that may prevent same-day discharge, and the risk of DVT is also increased **(II)**. This means that bilateral procedures should not be undertaken as a day-case unless there are two trained surgeons **(B)**. Many surgeons prefer to operate on one leg at a time. This virtually guarantees same-day discharge and ensures a more rapid post-discharge return to normal activity [6].

Saphenofemoral disconnection and stripping

Inadequate saphenofemoral disconnection is a cause of recurrence [7]. All tributaries beyond the secondary branches must be ligated and divided **(B)** to avoid leaving a network of veins that can connect the thigh veins with those on the abdominal wall and in the perineum. A segment of the lateral thigh tributary should be excised (or stripped if large) to prevent reconnection due to neovascularisation **(C)**.

Other minimally invasive techniques for ablation of the long saphenous vein include diathermy, sclerotherapy with large-volume microfoam and radiofrequency probes (VNUS) [12]. These all reduce the morbidity caused by stripping but other complications including burns and DVT have been described. The principle concern remains the increased risk of recurrence due to recanalisation. Randomised trials are required **(III)**.

Exsanguination tourniquets

Randomised trials have shown that tourniquets reduce blood loss significantly during varicose vein surgery [13,14] **(III)**. A sterile Esmarch bandage can be used but this is cumbersome and no match for modern Lofqvist or Boazul cuffs. These sterile "rubber doughnuts" are rolled up the leg and held in place with a wedge (Figure 3). The reduced blood loss benefits the patient, and results in a virtually bloodless operating field that aids avulsions, wound closure and bandaging **(A)**.

Chapter 28

Summary

- The surgical management of varicose veins is similar for all cases and therefore ideally suited to an integrated care pathway (II).

- Pre-assessment ensures appropriate selection of patients for day-case surgery (II).

- Information leaflets explaining the operation and possible complications reduces the risk of subsequent medico-legal claims (II).

- Thromboprophylaxis with subcutaneous heparin should be given to all those taking hormonal therapy (A).

- The surgeon should mark the veins and obtain the consent (A).

- Bilateral procedures should not be performed as a day-case unless there are two trained surgeons (B).

- The long saphenous vein should be stripped to the knee to reduce the risk of recurrence (A).

- Exsanguination tourniquets reduce blood loss during varicose vein surgery (I).

- Infiltration of the groin wound with Marcaine 0.5% reduces the need for post-operative opiate analgesia (II).

- On discharge, patients should be given a 24hr telephone number to phone if they have any problems (B).

- There seems no advantage in prolonging compression therapy for more than one week after the operation (A).

- Most patients do not require a post-operative out-patient appointment (C).

Further reading

1   Tibbs DJ, Sabiston DC, Davies MG, Mortimer PS, Scurr JH Eds. *Varicose veins, venous disorders and lymphatic problems in the lower limbs.* Oxford University Press, Oxford, 1997.

References (grade I evidence and grade A recommendations in bold)

1   **Ruckley CV, Bradbury AW. How do we prevent recurrence of varicose veins? In: *Venous disease*. Ruckley CV, Fowkes FGR, Bradbury AW, Eds. Springer, London, 1999; 239-245.**

2   Kent PJ, Weston MJ. Duplex scanning may be used selectively in patients with primary varicose veins. *Ann R Coll Surg Engl* 1993; 80: 388-389.

3   Drugs in the peri-operative period. Part 3 - Hormonal contraceptives and hormone replacement therapy. *Drug Ther Bull* 1999; 37: 78-80.

4   Onuma OC, Beam PE, Khan U, Malluci P, Adiseshiah M. The influence of effective analgesia and general anaesthesia on patients' acceptance of day case varicose vein surgery. *Phlebology* 1993; 8: 29-31.

5   **Raraty MGT, Greavey MG, Blair SD. There is no benefit from 6 weeks of compression after varicose vein surgery: a prospective randomised trial. *Br J Surg* 1997; 84: A574.**

6   Lees TA, Beard JD, Ridler BMF, Szymanska T. A survey of the current management of varicose veins by members of the Vascular Surgery Society. *Ann R Coll Surg Engl* 1999; 81: 407-417.

7   Darke SG. The morphology of recurrent varicose veins. *Eur J Vasc Surg* 1992; 6: 512-517.

8   **Sarin S, Scurr JH, Coleridge-Smith PR. Stripping of the long saphenous vein in the treatment of primary varicose veins. *Br J Surg* 1994; 81: 1455-1458.**

9   **Dwerryhouse S, Davies B, Harradine K, Earnshaw JJ. Stripping the long saphenous vein reduces the rate of reoperation for recurrent varicose veins: five-year results. *J Vasc Surg* 1999; 29: 589-592.**

10 **Docherty JG, Morrice JJ, Ben G. Saphenous neuritis following varicose vein surgery. *Br J Surg* 1994; 81: 695-698.**

11 Durkin MT, Turton EP, Scott DJ, Berridge DC. A prospective randomised controlled trial of PIN versus conventional stripping in varicose vein surgery. *Ann R Coll Surg Eng* 1999; 81: 171-174.

12 Chandler JG, Pichot O, Sessa C, Schuller-Petrovic S, Kabnick LS, Bergan JJ. Treatment of primary venous insufficiency by endovenous saphenous vein obliteration. *Vascular Surgery* 2000; 34: 201-214.

13 Sykes TCF, Brookes P, Hickey NC. A prospective randomised trial of tourniqets in varicose vein surgery. *Br J Surg* 1999; 86: A44.

14 Robinson J, Macierewicz J, Beard JD. Using the Boazul cuff to reduce blood loss in varicose vein surgery. *Eur J Vasc Endovasc Surg* 2000, 20: 390-393.

Chapter 29

Cardiac risk assessment for vascular patients

Colin J Ferguson Consultant Surgeon

Louis J Fligelstone Consultant Surgeon

DEPARTMENT OF SURGERY, MORRISTON HOSPITAL, SWANSEA, UK

Introduction

In almost every surgical situation there are options for operative and conservative treatment. The methods by which the surgeon assesses the suitability of a patient to undergo a particular operative procedure are complex and in the past ill-defined. There are a myriad of general considerations that must be taken into account relating to the patient's functional capacity, life expectancy, level of current suffering, the natural history of their condition, the morbidity and recovery time expected from the proposed treatment and the results for the procedure in the hands of the individual surgeon. All of these and many personal considerations of the patient and their family will have a bearing on the decisions made.

One major element that can be rationally assessed and to some extent quantified is the chance of the patient surviving the procedure, and the process of investigating this can result in measures being taken to improve this risk.

The "gut feeling" and "end of the bed assessment" have been legitimate tools of the experienced clinician but in the era of evidence-based medicine they may no longer be sufficient.

All patients undergoing surgery for aneurysmal disease, peripheral vascular disease and cerebro-vascular disease must be considered to have generalised arteriopathy until proven otherwise. Vascular surgery patients also have a high incidence of generalised co-morbidity and are being considered for procedures with amongst the highest morbidity and mortality rates, and lowest therapeutic index, within the entire surgical repertoire. In order to achieve satisfactory results we must take the greatest care, not only with our surgery but also with patient assessment.

We review current knowledge of cardiac assessment systems applicable to vascular patients.

Cardiac risk assessment

Cardiac status has been shown to be the most potent co-morbid factor relating to risk from non-cardiac surgery and therefore must be carefully assessed. Similarly of all non-cardiac procedures vascular surgery patients have the highest risk of cardiac complications.

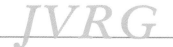

There is a high incidence of both overt and occult coronary artery disease (CAD) shown in studies of coronary angiography in vascular surgery patients (I). In a study of 1000 patients, there were normal angiographic findings in only 4% of those with clinical evidence of CAD. More alarmingly in those without clinical evidence of CAD only 14% had normal angiograms [1]. Starr *et al* [2] have shown a high prevalence of CAD in 471 patients who underwent coronary angiography prior to abdominal aortic aneurysm repair. They found that one in seven patients without clinical features of CAD had severe correctable disease. It can be argued that all vascular patients should undergo non-invasive assessment to reduce the risk of operating on patients with undiagnosed and untreated cardiac disease.

Clinical cardiac risk scoring systems

There are several clinical scoring systems available to assess cardiac risk [3,4,5]. The risk factors used and the scores attributable to them in these systems are shown in Table 1. These scoring systems are useful; however they require a level of cardiological expertise and attention to detail in clinical history recording and examination.

The American Heart Association and the American College of Cardiology have produced guidelines [6] for pre-operative cardiac risk assessment, which identifies low, intermediate and high-risk patients according to clinical criteria (II) (Table 2).

These criteria again require clinical skills to correctly elicit and interpret and the collaboration of a cardiologist is helpful. Clinical manifestations of CAD can often be occult in patients who are relatively immobile due to peripheral vascular disease, osteoarthritis, stroke, and also the elderly who constitute an increasing proportion of our patients.

Despite these confounding factors formalised clinical scoring systems are a good starting point in cardiac assessment and should be incorporated into the clinical care pathway documentation (B).

Special investigations for cardiac assessment

Echocardiography

In addition to clinical assessment and electrocardiography (ECG), echocardiography is commonly used as a predictor of peri-operative cardiac complications and is usually readily available. It can demonstrate unsuspected valvular pathology, measure left ventricular ejection fraction and give qualitative information regarding ventricular wall thickness, motion abnormalities and chamber dilatation. Bunt [7] has shown that detection of left ventricular dysfunction by echocardiography helps decision making regarding further investigation of CAD.

Ambulatory ECG

Twenty-four hour Holter monitoring can be used to show occult ischaemic events occurring during normal activity and this has been related to peri-operative cardiac complications [8]. However a review of the literature has shown a rather weak positive predictive value of 42% with sensitivity 93% and specificity 84% [9].

Exercise ECG

It seems sensible that a patient's response to exercise might predict their ability to withstand the insult of surgical intervention and indeed this would seem to be true. A variety of studies have shown that exercise ECG testing has a limited specificity for predicting peri-operative myocardial infarction (23-88%) [10,11]. However, when the exercise ECG is normal the likelihood of a cardiac complication is very low (0-1.5%) [10,12]. In addition to overt signs of myocardial ischaemia [13] on the ECG the patient's ability to achieve 85% of their maximum predicted heart rate is highly predictive of their ability to tolerate an operative procedure [12]. A normal exercise ECG is predictive of an acceptably low risk of cardiac complications following vascular surgery (II).

Exercise ECG testing unfortunately has a limited role in the patient population we deal with as their

Table 1 Clinical risk scoring systems.

Risk Factor	Goldman	Eagle	Detsky
Myocardial Infarct			
< 6 months	10	-	10
> 6 months	-	-	5
Q wave on ECG	-	1	-
CHC Angina			
Class 3	-	-	10
Class 4	-	-	20
History of angina	-	1	
Unstable angina < 3months	7	-	10
ECG rhythm			
Other than sinus	7	-	5
>5 PVCs/ minute	7	-	5
Ventricular ectopics			
requiring treatment	5	1	4
Suspected severe			
aortic valve disease	3	-	20
3rd Heart sound			
or gallop rhythm	3	-	-
Age > 70	5	1	5
Emergency surgery	4	-	10
Aortic, abdominal or			
thoracic surgery	3	-	-
Poor general status	3	-	5
Pulmonary oedema			
Within 1 week	-	-	10
Ever	11	1	5
Diabetes mellitus	-	1	-

Risk		Scores	
Low	0-12	0	0-15
Intermediate	13-25	1-2	16-30
High	>25	>2	>30

Table 2 American Heart Association and American College of Cardiology Task Force Report on peri-operative cardiovascular risk.

Major Risk
Unstable coronary artery disease
Decompensated heart failure
Significant arrhythmia
Severe valvular disease

Intermediate Risk
Mild angina pectoris
Myocardial infarction more than 30 days old
Compensated or prior heart failure
Diabetes mellitus

Minor Risk
Advanced age
Abnormal ECG
Rhythm other than sinus
Low functional capacity
History of stroke
Uncontrolled systemic hypertension

exercise tolerance is often limited by their vascular disease and other co-morbidities. Consequently a variety of alternative pharmacological stress tests have been devised.

Dipyridamole thallium scanning (DTS)

Thallium 201 is taken up by the myocardium in proportion to its blood flow. Dipyridamole acts via the potent coronary vasodilator adenosine to increase blood flow. If an area of myocardium is supplied by a stenotic vessel, blood flow will not increase in proportion to neighbouring areas following vasodilatation resulting in reduced uptake of Thallium 201. These areas of redistribution indicate viable myocardium that is at risk under stress. A defect present on the initial scan that persists indicates scarred myocardium.

Lette and co-workers [14] showed that 21% of patients with a reversible defect on DTS suffered a post-operative cardiac event. Other authors [15,16] have queried its routine use in low and high-risk patients as defined by clinical criteria. However, they have shown that intermediate risk patients have a low risk (3%) of a cardiac event if DTS shows no reversible defects and a high risk (30%) if it does. The main use of DTS is therefore to reclassify intermediate risk patients into either low or high risk groups [17].

Dobutamine stress echocardiography (DSE)

Dobutamine stimulates myocardial activity and produces coronary vasodilatation through increased heart rate and work, and therefore simulates the stress of surgery on the myocardium.

In this investigation dobutamine is infused until the patient achieves 85% of their predicted maximum heart rate. Transthoracic echocardiography is performed at rest and under stress and a positive result is indicated by the appearance of new wall motion defects or worsening of a resting wall motion abnormality (dyssynergy). The investigation is highly dependent on the skill and experience of the operator and is probably not suitable for occasional use. A meta-analysis of DTS and DSE demonstrated the predictive ability of the tests as shown in Table 3 [18]. As with the exercise ECG the ability of the patient to achieve their maximum predicted heart rate during DSE without ischaemia is predictive of risk [19].

Pharmacological stress testing can be used to sub-stratify patients found to be of intermediate risk on clinical scoring into groups of high and low risk of cardiac events during vascular surgery **(II)**.

Coronary angiography

The purpose of cardiac risk assessment is to aid decision making. It may be that, taken with other co-morbid factors and dependent on the indication for the vascular procedure being contemplated, a patient with excess cardiac risk according to the assessment so far described, will decide not to proceed any further.

Table 3 Predictive ability of Dipyridamole thallium scan and Dobutamine stress echocardiography.

Shaw et al 1996

DTS n=1994	%	Cardiac Events(%)
Normal	36	3
Fixed Defect	24	11
Reversible Defect	40	18
DSE n=445		
No Dyssynergy	48	0.4%
Dyssynergy	52	23%

If there is an imperative to proceed with surgery in a high-risk patient or when there is evidence of CAD from DTS or DSE, the patient should be offered percutaneous coronary angiography (PCA), with a view to performing coronary revascularisation if indicated. PCA itself carries the risk of serious complications and a mortality rate of 0.1% to 0.25% [20], which must be added to the risk of the coronary revascularisation procedure and the vascular surgery procedure. It must be noted that peripheral vascular disease is an independent risk factor for morbidity and mortality in patients undergoing coronary artery bypass grafting (CABG) [21].

The commonest finding at coronary angiography in vascular surgery patients is three-vessel disease [1,2]. This is frequently diffuse and not amenable to angioplasty or surgery. Patients with significant stenosis of the left main coronary artery or operable three-vessel disease would merit coronary revascularisation on prognostic grounds, providing that the myocardium that is to be revascularised is viable.

The results of CABG continue to improve. The operative mortality from elective coronary artery bypass grafting in an experienced institution should be 1 to 3% [22]. In the vast majority of cases this level of additional risk is acceptable, particularly for limb and life threatening conditions, if the procedure can be performed within a suitable timescale.

Which patients require cardiac investigation?

The investigation of cardiac risk has relative merits depending on the patient's vascular surgical diagnosis. Cardiac complications occur in infrainguinal procedures at least as frequently as in aortic procedures [23], as although an infrainguinal procedure may appear less stressful, this patient group is older and further down the arteriopathic pathway by the time they come to surgery.

Cardiac complications are the main source of mortality in carotid endarterectomy patients and these patients also merit investigation to assess their risk particularly as the therapeutic index of carotid endarterectomy is low.

There are circumstances when the urgency of the patient's condition precludes cardiac investigation, for instance acute limb threatening ischaemia and acutely symptomatic aortic aneurysms. Patients with severe ischaemic rest pain may also fall into this category. However in a unit with cardiology and cardiac surgery on site the basic investigations can often be performed on an urgent in-patient basis even in this circumstance. This may allow a cogent decision to be made regarding amputation rather than the uncertainty of revascularisation, with the possibility of graft failure and repeated procedures.

All elective patients with aortic aneurysms, carotid arterial disease and intermittent claudication should be investigated. We have suggested a protocol that allows the majority of patients to proceed to surgery with minimal delay from the investigations required but identifies those at highest risk from a cardiac event (Figure 1).

The selection of patients for sequential CABG or coronary angioplasty and vascular surgery depends

Figure 1 Pathway for cardiological risk assessment.

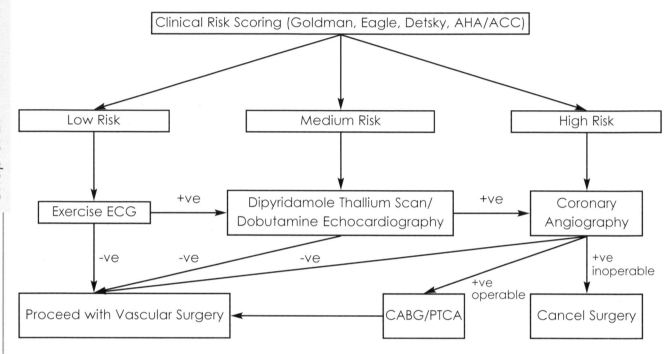

on a variety of factors, not least of which is the vascular surgery proposed and the natural history of the vascular condition.

All patients undergoing elective vascular surgery procedures, and patients undergoing urgent procedures in whom the timescale allows, should undergo formalised cardiac risk assessment to allow informed decision making **(B)**.

Does coronary artery revascularisation improve the outcome from vascular surgery?

We have identified clinical methods of stratifying vascular surgery patients according to their risk of peri-operative cardiac complications, and suggested techniques to further stratify the group at intermediate risk in order to identify those at highest risk. To date however, there have been no randomised controlled trials to evaluate the efficacy of coronary revascularisation in terms of outcome in these high-risk patients.

Coronary revascularisation is justified in its own right in patients with left main stem disease and three-vessel disease in terms of prognosis for subsequent myocardial infarction and death.

Studies from the Cleveland Clinic have demonstrated significant improvements in outcome as a consequence of a policy of submitting these patients to coronary revascularisation prior to vascular surgery (Table 4). Starr and colleagues [2] showed a 1.8% peri-operative mortality rate in aortic aneurysm patients who had previously undergone CABG and other studies have also alluded to improved results [24,25]. Coronary artery revascularisation prior to vascular surgery yields results similar to those in patients without coronary artery disease and superior to those with coronary artery disease treated medically **(II)**.

Table 4 Coronary artery revascularisation before vascular surgery.

Eagle *et al* 1997

N=314

Group	peri-operative MI %	Death %
No CAD	3	0
CAD Medical treatment	8.5	2.8
CAD Pre-operative CABG	0.6(p<0.01)	1.1 (N.S.)

Anecdotally there seems little doubt that patients who have undergone prior CABG are more robust in terms of their response to surgical stress, but there is clearly a need for prospective studies.

The pathway we have described is suitable for the vast majority of patients and is available on the JVRG website. There are categories of patients for whom such assessment is not helpful, i.e. those in whom a decision to operate would not be influenced by the results. These are however relatively few in number and even in this circumstance, clinical review by a cardiologist can help by optimising the patient's medical treatment. Recent evidence suggests that cardiac morbidity and mortality can be reduced in high-risk patients by beta-adrenergic blockade [26]. However this does not obviate investigation and surgical treatment of intermediate and high-risk patients [27].

Cardiology resources are undoubtedly stressed by the demands placed upon them by a systematised programme of cardiac investigation of vascular surgery patients. Close cooperation between the cardiology department and the vascular surgery team is important.

The pathway we have described is a philosophy of excellence that may not be instantly achievable and to what extent it is achieved will depend on individual circumstances. Although many surgeons will agree with the principles espoused it is clearly the case that in the midst of a busy practice, the delays that may be caused by cardiac assessment will be a disincentive to its implementation.

In the UK access to specialist investigations and cardiology services vary from hospital to hospital, but all vascular surgeons should have access to exercise ECG testing which will allow decisions to be made for most patients. Surgeons working in hospitals without specialist cardiology on site will need to collaborate with their local regional vascular surgery and cardiology services for more specialised investigations. Commissioning authorities are presently keen to resource initiatives that involve the establishment of clinical networks and this may be helpful in establishing working relationships between units.

Summary

- Cardiac disease is the major cause of morbidity and mortality in vascular surgery patients **(I)**.

- There is evidence that addressing this issue can result in improved outcomes in cases at high risk of adverse cardiac events **(II)**.

- Simple non-invasive testing and clinical scoring allows stratification of risk such that the majority of patients can proceed to surgery with minimal delay **(II)**.

- Patients at intermediate risk can be further assessed by DTS and DSE allowing selection of patients for coronary angiography with a view to cardiac intervention if appropriate **(II)**.

- We suggest that when clinical care pathways are being developed a protocol for cardiac investigation is incorporated **(A)**.

Chapter 29

References (grade I evidence and grade A recommendations in bold)

1   **Hertzer NR, Bevan EG, Young JR *et al*. Coronary Artery Disease in peripheral vascular patients: A classification of 1000 coronary angiograms. *Ann Surg* 1984; 199: 233.**

2   **Starr JE, Hertzer NR, Mascha EJ *et al*. Influence of gender on cardiac risk and survival in patients with infrarenal aortic aneurysms. *J Vasc Surg* 1996; 23: 870-880.**

3   Detsky AS, Abrams HB, McLaughlin JR *et al*. Predicting cardiac complications in patients undergoing non-cardiac surgery. *J Gen Intern Med* 1986; 1: 211.

4   Goldman L. Cardiac risks and complications of non-cardiac surgery. *Ann Intern Med* 1983; 98: 504.

5   Eagle KA, Rihal CS, Mickel MC *et al*. Cardiac risk of noncardiac surgery: influence of coronary disease and type of surgery in 3368 operations. *Circulation* 1997; 96: 1882-1887.

6   Guidelines for perioperative cardiovascular evaluation for noncardiac surgery. Report of the ACC/AHA task force on practice guidelines. *Circulation* 1996; 93: 1278-1317.

7   Bunt TJ. The role of a defined protocol for cardiac risk assessment in decreasing perioperative myocardial infarction in vascular surgery. *J Vasc Surg* 1992; 15: 626.

8   Raby KE, Selwyn AP. The role of ambulatory monitoring in assessing cardiac risk in peripheral vascular surgery. *Cardiol Clin* 1992;10(3): 467-73.

9   Haljamae H, Jivegard L. Cardiac risk factors: the effect of preoperative evaluation on outcome. *Perspect Vasc Surg* 1995; 8: 86-97.

10   Cutler BS, Wheeler HB, Paraskos JA, Cardullo PA. Applicability and interpretation of electrocardiographic stress testing in patients with peripheral vascular disease. *Am J Surg* 1981; 141: 501-506.

11   McPhail NV, Ruddy TD, Calvin JE *et al*. A comparison of dipyridamole thallium scanning and exercise testing in the prediction of post-operative cardiac complications in patients requiring arterial reconstruction. *J Vasc Surg* 1989; 10: 51.

12   McPhail N, Calvin JE, Shariatmadar A *et al*. The use of preoperative exercise testing to predict cardiac complications after arterial reconstruction. *J Vasc Surg* 1988; 7: 60-68.

13   Gauss A, Rohm HJ, Schauffelen A, *et al*. Electrocardiographic exercise stress testing for cardiac risk assessment in patients undergoing noncardiac surgery. *Anaesthesiology* 2001; 94(1): 38-46.

14   Lette J, Waters D, Lassonde J *et al*. Multivariate clinical models and quantitative Dipyridamole-thallium imaging to predict morbidity and death after vascular reconstruction. *J Vasc Surg* 1991; 14:160.

15   Eagle KA, Coley CM, Newell JB *et al*. Combining clinical and thallium data optimises preoperative assessment of cardiac risk before major vascular surgery. *Ann Intern Med* 1989; 110: 859.

16   Mangano DT, London MJ, Tubau JF. Dipyridamole thallium-201 scintigraphy as a preoperative screening test: A reexamination of its predictive potential. *Circulation* 1991; 84: 493.

17   L'Italien GL, Paul SD, Hendel RC *et al*. Development and validation of a Bayesian for perioperative cardiac risk assessment in 1081 vascular surgical candidates. *J Am Coll Cardiol* 1996; 27: 779-786.

18   Shaw LJ, Eagle KA, Gersh BJ, Miller DD. Meta-analysis of intravenous dipyridamole-thallium-201imaging (1985-1994) and dobutamine echocardiography (1991-1994) for risk stratification before vascular surgery. *J Am Coll Cardiol* 1996; 27: 469-475.

19   Das MK, Pellikka PA, Mahoney DW *et al*. Assessment of cardiac risk before nonvascular surgery: dobutamine stress echocardiography in 530 patients *J Am Coll Cardiol* 2000; 35(6): 1647-53.

20   Jansson K, Fransson SG. Mortality related to coronary angiography. *Clin Radiol* 1996 Dec; 51(12): 858-60.

21   Gersh BJ, Rihal CS, Rooke TW *et al*. Evaluation and Management of patients with both peripheral vascular and coronary artery disease. *J Am Coll Cardiol* 1991; 18: 203.

22   The Society of Cardiothoracic Surgeons of Great Britain and Ireland. National Adult Cardiac Surgery Database Report 2000.

23   Krupski WC, Layug EL, Reilly LM. Comparison of cardiac morbidity between aortic and infrainguinal procedures. *J Vasc Surg* 1992; 15: 354.

24   Lachapelle K, Graham AM, Symes JF. Does the clinical evaluation of the cardiac status predict outcome in patients with abdominal aortic aneurysms? *J Vasc Surg* 1992; 15: 964-971.

25   Erickson CA, Carbolla RE, Freischlag JA *et al*. Using Dipyridamole-thallium imaging to reduce cardiac risk in aortic reconstruction. *J Vasc Surg* 1996; 60: 422-428.

26   Poldermans D, Boersma E, Bax J *et al*. The effect of Bisoprolol on perioperative mortality and myocardial infarction in high risk patients undergoing vascular surgery. *N Eng J Med* 1999; 341 (24): 1789-1794.

27   Boersma E, Poldermans D, Bax JJ *et al*. Predictors of cardiac events after major vascular surgery: Role of clinical characteristics, Dobutamine echocardiography, and beta blocker therapy. *JAMA* 2001; 285 (14): 1865-73.

Chapter 30

Blood conservation in the vascular patient

Phil Dobson

Consultant Anaesthetist

SHEFFIELD VASCULAR INSTITUTE, THE NORTHERN GENERAL HOSPITAL, SHEFFIELD, UK

Introduction

Whilst donated, allogeneic, blood transfusion is undoubtedly very safe, there are potential adverse effects to the recipient and the cost to the health care system is high and increasing. In addition, the ability of the blood transfusion service to meet demand is proving to be increasingly difficult and the imminent introduction of vCJD testing of potential donors can only worsen the situation.

Although techniques for conserving blood have been used for many years, the current demand to reduce the requirement for allogeneic blood derives predominantly from the increasing fear of disease transmission, beginning in the late 1980s.

This chapter will aim to cover the literature relating to blood conservation, concentrating on vascular surgery where possible, and will propose guidelines that can be applied to vascular patients coming to surgery.

There are two elements to the conservation of blood products. Firstly, by using techniques which reduce the need for *any* blood transfusion and secondly, when transfusion is unavoidable by using autologous blood products.

To maximize the efficiency of blood conservation it is important that multiple techniques are considered for each patient.

Reduction in all transfusions

Pre-operative optimisation

Patients who have a low haematocrit prior to surgery are more likely to require transfusion [1-3] **(II)**. The use of iron preparations and erythropoietin therapy [4,5] have been shown to reduce the requirement for allogeneic blood transfusion in orthopaedic, urological and cardiac patients, especially when combined with other blood conservation measures. Erythropoietin therapy alone has been shown to save blood in cardiac [6] and orthopaedic patients [7,8] by increasing the pre-operative haematocrit. Also, haemodilution techniques for blood conservation can be used more effectively if the pre-operative haematocrit is raised [9].

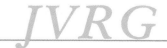

Aspirin therapy has been associated with increased blood loss during surgery [10]. Discontinuation of aspirin at least 7 days prior to surgery is necessary to allow normal platelet function. Patients taking anticoagulant medications should usually have these stopped prior to surgery and replaced if necessary by short acting agents whose effect can be readily terminated.

Patients with a history of bleeding disorder should have appropriate therapy to normalise coagulation pre-operatively.

Surgical technique

Operative blood loss can be difficult to predict and varies substantially between surgeons. There is no doubt that a surgical technique aimed at minimizing blood loss is crucial in any blood conservation strategy **(C)**. The details of surgical technique are beyond the scope of this chapter and the reader is referred to surgical texts.

The use of local haemostatic agents (oxidised cellulose, gelatin sponge, microfibrillar collagen haemostat, thrombin and fibrin glue) may aid surgical haemostasis.

Anaesthetic technique

In 1948 controlled hypotension produced by high spinal anaesthesia was shown to be associated with a dry surgical field [11] and further work using ganglion blocking agents to reduce blood pressure during anaesthesia also found a marked reduction in blood loss [12,13]. The consensus from subsequent studies is that well controlled deliberate hypotension can reduce blood loss by approximately 40% **(II)**.

In addition to hypotension, careful patient positioning during surgery may reduce blood loss by preventing venous congestion around the operative field [12].

Maintaining normothermia during surgery is associated with a reduction in allogeneic transfusion [14,15]. Hypothermia is associated with impaired blood coagulation and platelet function.

Permissive anaemia

Allowing the haematocrit to fall to lower than normal levels will lead to a reduction in blood transfusion requirements. The difficulty is deciding what is the minimum, critical haematocrit for an individual patient at any given time.

The physiological response to a fall in haematocrit is an increase in cardiac output due primarily to an increased stroke volume. This response maintains adequate tissue perfusion only if hypovolaemia is avoided at all times. It is also vital that haemoglobin oxygen saturation is high and hyper oxygenation can significantly increase oxygen delivery in patients with a low haematocrit [16,17].

In healthy subjects, tissue oxygenation is maintained down to a haematocrit of approximately 25%. There are reports of subjects tolerating a period with a very low haematocrit [18] and reviews of operations on Jehovah's Witnesses find that a poor outcome is associated only with haemoglobins less than 5 gm% [19,20]. However, many patients with coexisting disease, e.g. ischaemic heart disease, may not tolerate such low haematocrits. In addition, the increase in cerebral perfusion required to maintain tissue oxygenation during anaemia relies on cerebral vasodilatation, which may be limited and lead to cerebral ischaemia in patients with cerebrovascular disease. Also, in healthy volunteers an acute reduction in haemoglobin to below 7 gm% by normovolaemic haemodilution was found to impair cognitive function [21].

Thus, in patients with significant cardiac or cerebrovascular disease, the critical haematocrit may be relatively high. Published data, including recent guidelines from the Association of Anaesthetists of Great Britain and Ireland and a study of patients undergoing vascular surgery, support a minimum haemoglobin of 8 - 9 gm% [22-25] **(B)**.

Pharmacological techniques

Antifibrinolytic agents promote coagulation and tranexamic acid has been used safely in cardiac surgery to reduce blood requirements [26], as has aprotonin, a serine protease inhibitor [27-29]. Aprotonin and tranexamic acid have been used to reduce blood loss in liver resection and major orthopaedic surgery, with varying success [30-31].

A controlled trial using aprotonin for elective aortic reconstruction found no significant reduction in blood loss or requirements for blood products [32] and a double-blinded randomised trial studying the use of aprotonin during repair of ruptured abdominal aortic aneurysms had similar findings [33] **(I)**.

Thus, their use in non-cardiac surgery is equivocal and is not recommended at the present time **(III)**.

Desmopressin, which increases the levels of factor VIII; C and vWF and reduces bleeding time, may reduce blood loss related to aspirin therapy [34]. However, results of studies with cardiopulmonary bypass are equivocal [35,36] and a study of its role during aortic surgery found no benefit [37] and its routine use is not recommended **(III)**.

Autologous blood transfusion

The term autologous blood encompasses all blood products derived from the patient's own blood. This usually refers to red blood cells but may also include platelets and clotting factors. Autologous red cells may be obtained by pre-operative donation, acute normovolaemic haemodilution or by red cell salvage techniques.

Pre-operative autologous donation

Pre-operative autologous donation (PAD), the donation of several units of blood during the weeks prior to an operation, has been used extensively in the United States for more than 15 years, accounting for over 5% of all blood transfused in 1992. The drive for its use was predominantly a demand from patients due to the knowledge that HIV can be transmitted by allogeneic blood transfusion. Other advantages of pre-operative donation include avoidance of red cell sensitisation, augmentation of the blood supply, provision of blood for patients with alloantibodies and the prevention of some adverse transfusion reactions.

The ability of PAD to reduce the need for allogeneic blood has been established [38-40]. However, whether the use of PAD is efficacious is less certain for reasons of safety and cost.

Disadvantages of pre-operative donation include a relatively high incidence of complications during donation because the surgical patient considered for PAD may be less fit than an allogeneic blood donor and may donate blood weekly for up to 4 weeks [41-44]. Hypotension and significant dysrhythmias requiring treatment have been reported [41]. In one study the requirement for hospitalisation was 12 times greater for the PAD group compared with allogeneic donors [42]. For these reasons some recommend that patients with cardiovascular disease have close haemodynamic monitoring and medical supervision during predonation, which further adds to the cost.

Contraindications to donation include active infection, initial haematocrit below 34%, unstable angina, recent myocardial infarction, aortic stenosis, left main stem disease, uncontrolled hypertension, hypotension, epilepsy and significant respiratory disease [45].

Blood donation leads to a decreased haematocrit at the start of surgery despite measures to reduce this, including iron replacement [3,46] and erythropoietin therapy. This anaemia increases the chance of the patient requiring a blood transfusion of any kind [47] partly because of a lower pre-operative haemoglobin and also because if PAD blood is available there is a tendency to prescribe it even if there is no clinical need [48].

Predonated blood is more expensive than allogeneic blood because although the collection, testing and storage costs are similar, between half and two thirds of PAD blood is wasted [49].

Further limitations include the requirement for several weeks notice and guarantee of the operation date to allow efficient planning and use of the donated blood. In addition, the incidence of transfusion reactions due to clerical errors is not reduced.

Only patients undergoing operations that normally require blood transfusion should be considered, to reduce wastage of donated blood and the number of units donated should be equivalent to the hospital's maximum blood ordering schedule, MBOS, for that particular procedure [45,49]. Orthopaedic patients undergoing major joint arthroplasty are recognised as suitable candidates [50], where as general surgical, gynaecological and obstetric patients are less so [38].

The combination of erythropoietin and predonation in patients undergoing abdominal aortic surgery was found to be safe [51], but more evidence is needed; vascular surgical patients often have significant cardiovascular disease and may be at increased risk of complications during donation and thus the overall efficacy of predonation is less clear.

Acute normovolaemic haemodilution

Acute normovolaemic haemodilution (ANH) involves the removal of blood from the patient and replacement with an appropriate volume of clear intravenous fluid immediately prior to surgery. The blood is labelled and stored in theatre for retransfusion at the end of surgery or sooner if the blood loss is large or complications develop. Haemodilution may be classified as moderate (haematocit 25-30%) or extreme (<20%).

The reinfused autologous blood is fresh, contains functional platelets and has a relatively normal clotting profile. The technique is indicated in patients with malignancy or infection where cell salvage is currently contraindicated. Unlike PAD the technique is relatively cheap and does not require planning weeks in advance.

However, the removal of large volumes of blood immediately prior to surgery may lead to cardiovascular instability and this may lead to tissue ischaemia. During haemodilution, tissue oxygenation is maintained by an increase in tissue blood flow, secondary to vasodilatation and an increase in cardiac output. It is vital that hypovolaemia is avoided and careful patient selection and close monitoring of vital organ function is essential.

The effect of haemodilution on coagulation is variable. If crystalloid is used to maintain normovolaemia blood coagulability may actually be increased, whereas colloids, especially hydroxyethyl starch, may compromise coagulation [52].

Blood lost during surgery has a lower haematocrit and therefore contains fewer red blood cells, potentially reducing transfusion requirements [3]. Several studies have found a significant decrease in the requirement for allogeneic blood using the technique [53,54], although mathematical modelling [55,56] and a review [57] have questioned the ability of ANH to reduce allogeneic blood requirements significantly. A meta-analysis [58] and consensus conference [59] cast further doubt on the technique's efficacy **(III)**. Further trials employing better control of transfusion regimens are recommended.

Moderate ANH is less likely to produce cardiac complications but is less efficacious in conserving red blood cells. Extreme ANH has been used safely in young healthy patients [57] but is not recommended for the older, higher risk patient [61] who, even if they are asymptomatic may have silent coronary artery disease [62].

Studies comparing acute normovolaemic haemodilution and pre-operative autologous donation for patients undergoing radical prostatectomy [3] and hip arthroplasty [62] found both techniques to be equally efficacious in avoiding allogeneic blood requirement.

In addition, beneficial effects have been reported when acute normovolaemic haemodilution is used in combination with pre-operative erythropoietin therapy [3] or with the intra-operative use of artificial oxygen carriers [63].

The cardiovascular problems associated with ANH have lead to the suggestion that acute *hypervolaemic* haemodilution may provide similar benefits but with greater safety. Haemodilution, leading to reduced red cell loss, occurs due to the administration of volumes of clear fluid well in excess of fluid losses. There is evidence that ANH is well tolerated [64]. This may be helped by vasodilatation, which is associated with most forms of anaesthesia. This hypervolaemic state persists until fluid losses are allowed to exceed input, which usually occurs in the early post-operative period due to urine and third space losses, which lead to haemoconcentration.

Safety may be increased compared with ANH because the detrimental cardiovascular effects of hypovolaemia in association with haemodilution are less likely to occur, particularly around the time of induction of anaesthesia and periods of sudden blood loss.

Intra-operative cell salvage

The technique of human red blood cell salvage was first reported in Edinburgh in 1885. The procedure was used increasingly during the first part of the 20th century, but it was 1969 before the modern centrifugal separation technique was first used. The technique involves the collection, anticoagulation, filtering and washing of spilt blood. In order to reduce damage to red blood cells during collection suction pressure should not exceed 150 mmHg and if possible, blood should be allowed to pool before collection to reduce the blood air interface, which causes increased haemolysis.

Advantages of the technique include a lack of disease transmission, avoidance of transfusion reactions, safety in patients with multiple alloantibodies, avoidance of clerical errors, ready availability of blood during periods of rapid blood loss, a reduced demand on allogeneic blood supplies, acceptance of the technique by many Jehovah's Witnesses, reduced immunosuppression and psychological benefits to recipient.

The quality of processed, salvaged blood is high, with the red cells having a similar half life to allogeneic blood, normal 2, 3 DPG levels and a more favorable oxygen dissociation curve than allogeneic blood [65,66].

However, processed blood contains activated compliment and cytokines, reduced coagulation factors and free haemoglobin and platelets present in the processed blood are non-functional. Reports of fatal air embolus have been reported following the infusion of processed blood when a pressure infusor was used [67]. Hence it is imperative that the bag containing the processed blood does not contain air.

Indications for intra-operative red cell salvage include an anticipated blood loss >20% estimated blood volume, mean transfusion requirement >2 units, patients with rare blood groups, a shortage of allogeneic blood or religious beliefs which prevent the use of allogeneic blood.

Relative contraindications to the technique include surgery for malignancy, operations in non-sterile fields, contamination of shed blood by bowel contents, amniotic fluid, methylmacrylate cement, antiseptics, collagen haemostatic material or drugs not intended for systemic use and patients with viral antigen markers.

The processing of salvaged blood does not remove bacterial contamination [68], but reinfusion of blood in this situation has been reported without apparent problems [69]. Administration of broad spectrum antibiotics is recommended if it is felt that red cell salvage may be life saving in the presence of bacterial contamination.

There is controversy regarding the use of red cell salvage during cancer surgery, with some evidence suggesting its use does not lead to increased tumour recurrence, [70] but this is not an issue that is particularly relevant to vascular surgery. Filtering processed blood through a leucocyte depletion filter will *reduce* the proportion of tumour cells returned to the patient.

Whilst the use of red cell salvage during emergency aortic surgery may be life saving, there is conflicting evidence regarding the efficacy of intra-operative cell salvage for elective aortic surgery. Whilst a significant reduction in allogeneic blood requirements has been reported [71], other studies have not found any advantage of peri-operative cell salvage during infrarenal aortic surgery [72,73]. Several case reviews of vascular operations have shown a reduced need for allogeneic blood, both by using cell salvage alone [74,75] or combined with pre-operative donation [76], but none of these studies have been controlled.

The intra-operative use of passive collection systems has been shown to reduce blood requirements in aortic surgery [77], but this technique is limited because it is most efficient whilst the patient is anticoagulated. Also, blood is returned to the patient unwashed, which may lead to coagulation abnormalities if large quantities are re-infused [78]. A centrifugal, cell washing technique is preferable in these circumstances.

Post-operative red cell salvage has limited scope in vascular surgery because post-operative blood loss is (hopefully) low and wound drains are not routinely used.

In 1996 a consensus conference stated that "provided that a rigid standard operating procedure is in place and the equipment is easily available with appropriate staff training, the side-effects of intra-operative salvage are fewer than those associated with allogeneic transfusion." [79] Continuing audit, including the reporting of any adverse events, is required to support this statement in the setting of vascular surgery (III).

Artificial oxygen carriers

These preparations fall into two categories, perflurocarbon (PFC) emulsions and stroma-free haemoglobin solutions. Their use peri-operatively could reduce blood requirements by allowing a lower haematocrit to be tolerated. Unfortunately, current PFCs have decreased oxygen carrying potential and a higher viscosity compared with red blood cells, limiting their clinical efficacy and stroma-free haemoglobin solutions tend to have a short half life, high viscosity, a high affinity for oxygen and have side effects including nephrotoxicity, vasoconstriction and interference with phagocyte function.

Whilst studies have suggested that the use of a haemoglobin based oxygen carrier can reduce the need for allogeneic blood during elective aortic aneurysm surgery [80,81] further evidence of their efficacy is required before these preparations become part of standard clinical practice (III).

Summary

General principles

◆ It is important to question the prescribing of all blood.

◆ The aim is to implement the described techniques into widespread clinical practice and define the best combination of techniques for a given patient.

◆ This requires close co-operation between anaesthetists, surgeons and haematologists.

◆ Allogeneic blood is safe; some of the techniques of blood conservation are not without risk and should always be used with the patient's best interests in mind.

◆ In the context of vascular surgery there is a shortage of level I evidence.

Pre-operatively

◆ Aim; haemoglobin high normal range (B).
  • Optimise iron status (C).
  • Consider erythropoietin therapy (B).

◆ Normal coagulation?
  • Correct any haematological abnormalities (C).
  • Consider stopping antiplatelet therapy (C).
  • Careful timing of DVT prophylaxis (C).

◆ Co-existing disease - optimize, especially cardio-respiratory disease (C).

◆ Pre-operative autologous blood donation (C).
  • No contraindications, resources available locally, qualifying operation?
  • Predonate following local guidelines to obtain blood equal to maximum surgical blood ordering schedule (MSBOS).
  • Prescribe iron +/- erythropoietin, as per local guidelines.

Peri-operatively

- Use surgical technique to minimize blood loss and consider haemostatic agents **(C)**.

- Use controlled hypotension **(B)**.

- Maintain normothermia **(B)** and adequate arterial oxygen tension **(A)**, consider hyperoxia.

- Allow permissive anaemia, avoid hypovolaemia, use appropriate clinical monitoring **(B)**.

- Use *moderate* acute normovolaemic (or hypervolaemic) haemodilution following British Committee for Standards in Haematology guidelines [82] **(C)**.

- Use intra-operative cell salvage **(C)**.

- Monitor coagulation if blood loss is high (e.g. above 40% estimated blood volume) and treat abnormalities promptly. Carefully consider the use of intra-operative anticoagulation and the use of protamine **(C)**.

Post-operatively

- Use permissive anaemia with close attention to volume status and oxygenation **(B)**.

- Maintain normothermia **(B)**.

- Monitor coagulation and treat if appropriate **(C)**.

Further reading

1 Ramaz Salem M, Ed. *Blood Conservation in the Surgical Patient*. Williams and Wilkins, 1996.

References (grade I evidence and grade A recommendations in bold)

1 Goodnough LT, Brecher ME, Kanter MH, AuBuchon JP. Medical progress; transfusion medicine. Part II. Blood conservation. *N Engl J Med* 1999; 340: 525-533.

2 Bierbaum BE, Callaghan JJ, Galante JO, Rubash HE, Tooms RE, Welsh RB. An analysis of blood management in patients having total hip or knee arthroplasty. *J Bone Joint Surg* 1999; 81: 2-10.

3 Monk TG, Goodnough LT, Brecher ME, Colberg JW, Andriole GL, Catalona WJ. A prospective randomized comparison of three blood conservation strategies for radical prostatectomies. *Anesthesiology* 1999; 91: 24-33.

4 Goodnough LT, Marcus RE. Erythropoiesis in patients stimulated with erythropoietin; the relevance of storage iron. *Vox Sanguis* 1998; 75: 128-133.

5 Goodnough LT, Skikine B, Brugnora C. Erythropoietin, iron and erythropoiesis. *Blood* 2000; 96: 823-33.

6 Sowade O, Warnke H, Scigalla P, Sowade B, Franke W, Messinger D, Gross J. Avoidance of allogeneic blood transfusions by treatment with epoetin beta in patients undergoing open heart surgery. *Blood* 1997; 89: 411-418.

7 Stowell CP, Chandler H, Jove M, Guilfoyle M, Wacholtz MC. An open label randomized study to compare the safety and efficacy of perioperative epoetin alpha with preoperative autologous donation in total joint arthroplasty. *Orthopaedics* 1999; 22: S105-112.

8 Faris PM, Ritter MA, Abels RI. The effects of recombinant erythropoietin on peri-operative transfusion requirements inpatients undergoinig major orthopaedic surgery. *J Bone Joint Surg* 1996; 78A: 62-72.

9 Weiskopf RB. Mathematical analysis of isovolaemic haemodilution indicates that it can decrease the need for allogeneic blood transfusion. *Transfusion* 1995; 35: 37-41.

10 Ferraris VA, Ferraris SP, Lough FC *et al*. Preoperative aspirin ingestion increases operative blood loss after coronary artery bypass grafting. *Ann Thorac Surg* 1995; 59: 1036-7.

11 Griffiths HWC, Gillies J. Thoracolumbar splanchnicectomy and sympathectomy; anaesthetic procedure. *Anaesthesia* 1948; 3: 134-46.

12 Scurr CF. Reduction in haemorrhage in the operative field by the use of pentamethonium iodide. *Anesthesiology* 1951; 12: 253-7.

13 Enderby GEH, Pelmore JF. Controlled hypotension and postural ischaemia to reduce bleeding in surgery. *Lancet* 1951; 1: 663-6.

14 Kurz A, Sessler DI, Lenhardt R Perioperative normothermia to reduce the incidence of surgical wound infection and shorten hospitalization. *N Eng J Med* 1996; 334: 1209-1215.

15 Bock M, Muller J, Bach A, Bohrer H, Martin E, Motsch J. Effects of preinduction and intraoperative warming during laparotomy. *Br J Anaesth* 1998; 80: 159-163.

16 Habler OP, Kleen MS, Hutter JW, Podtschaske AH, Tiede M, Kemming GI, Welte MV, Corso CO, Batra S, Keipert PE, Faithful NS, Messmer KF. Effects of hyperoxic ventilation on haemodilution-induced changes in anaesthetized dogs. *Transfusion* 1998; 38: 135-144.

17 Zollinger A, Hager P, Singer T, Friedl HP, Pasch T, Spahn DR. Extreme haemodilution due to massive blood loss in tumour surgery. *Anesthesiology* 1997; 87:985- 7.

18 Weiskopf RB, Viele MK, Feiner J, Kelley S, Lieberman J, Noorani M, Leung JM, Fisher DM, Murray WR, Toy P, Moore MA. Human cardiovascular and metabolic response to acute, severe isovolaemic anemia. *JAMA* 1998; 279: 217-21.

19 Viele MK, Weiskopf RB. What can we learn about the need for transfusion from patients who refuse blood? The experience of Jehovah's Witnesses. *Transfusion* 1994; 34: 396-401.

20 Spence RK, Constabile JP, Young GS. Is haemoglobin level alone a reliable predictor of outcome in the severely anemic surgical patient? *Am J Surg* 1992; 58: 92-5.

21 Weiskopf RB, Kramer JH, Viele M, Neumann M, Feiner JR, Watson JJ, Hopf HW, Toy P. Acute severe isovolaemic haemodilution impairs cognitive function and memory in humans. *Anesthesiology* 2000; 92: 1646-52.

22 Blood transfusion and the anaesthetist; red cell transfusion The Association of Anaesthetists of Great Britain and Ireland September 2001.

23 Spahn Dr, Schmid ER, Seifert B, Pasch T. Haemodilution tolerance in patients with coronary heart disease who are receiving chronic beta-adrenergic blocking therapy. *Anesth Analg* 1996; 82: 687-94.

24 Spahn DR, Zollinger A, Schlumpf RB, Stohr S, Seifert B, Schmid ER, Pasch T. Haemodilution tolerance in elderly patients without known cardiac disease. *Anesth Analg* 1996; 82: 681-6.

25 Bush RL, Pevec WC, Holcroft JW. A prospective randomized trial limiting preoperative red blood cell transfusion in vascular patients. *Am J Surg* 1997; 174:143-8.

26 Van der Salm TJ, Ansell JE, Okike ON. The role of epsilon amino caproic acid in reducing bleeding after cardiac operations; a double blind randomized study. *J Thorac Cardiovasc Surg* 1988; 95: 538-540.

27 Royston D, Bidstrup BP, Taylor KM, Sapsford RN. Effects of aprotonin on need for blood transfusion after repeat open heart surgery. *Lancet* 1987; 2: 1289-91.

28 Munoz JJ, Birkmeyer NJ, Birkmeyer JD, O'Connor JT, Dacey LJ. Is epsilon aminocaproic acid as effective as aprotonin in reducing bleeding with cardiac surgery? A meta analysis. *Circulation* 1999; 99: 81-9.

29 Laupacis A, Ferguson D. Drugs to minimize perioperative blood loss in cardiac surgery; meta-analysis using perioperative blood transfusion as the outcome The International Study of perioperative Transfusion ISPOT investigators. *Anesth Analg* 1997; 85: 1258-67.

30 Hiippala ST, Strid LJ, Wennerstrand MI, Arvela JVV, Niemela HM, Mantyla SK, Kuisma RP, Ylinen JE. Tranexamic acid radically decreases blood loss and transfusions associated with total knee arthroplasty. *Anesth Analg* 1997; 84: 839-44.

31 Kasper M, Ramsay MA, Nguyen AT, Cogswell M, Hurst G, Ramsay KJ. Continuous small dose tranexamic acid reduces fibrinolysis but not transfusion requirements during orthoptic liver transplantation. *Anesth Analg* 1997; 85: 281-5.

32 **Ranaboldo CJ, Thompson JF, Davies JN, Shutt AM, Francis JN, Roath OS, Webster JH, Chant AD. Prospective randomized placebo controlled trial of aprotonin for elective aortic reconstruction. *Br J Surg* 1997; 84: 1110-3.**

33 **Robinson J, Nawaz S, Beard JD. Randomised, multicentre, double blind, placebo controlled trial of the use of aprotonin in the repair of ruptured abdominal aortic aneurysm. On behalf of the Joint Vascular Research Group. *Br J Surg* 2000; 87: 754-7.**

34 Flordal PA, Sahlin S. Use of desmopressin to prevent bleeding complications in patients treated with aspirin. *Br J Surg* 1993; 80: 723-24.

35 Woodman RC, Harker LA. Bleeding complications associated with cardiopulmonary bypass. *Blood* 1990; 76: 1680-97.

36 Hackmann T, Gascoyne RD, NaimanSC. A trial of desmopressin to reduce blood loss in uncomplicated cardiac surgery. *N Eng J Med* 1989; 321: 1437-43.

37 Clagett GP, Valentine RJ, Myers SL, Chervu A, Heller J. Does desmopressin improve haemostasis and reduce blood loss from aortic surgery? A randomized double blind study. *J Vasc Surg* 1995; 22: 223-30.

38 Kay LA. Predeposit autologous blood transfusion, logistics and costs in the public and private sector in Britain. *Haematology Review* 1992; 7: 17-25.

39 Bengtson A, Bengston JP. Autologous blood transfusion; Preoperative blood collection and blood salvage techniques. *Acta Anaesthesiol Scand* 1996; 40: 1041-56.

40 Thomas MJ, Gillon J, Desmond MJ. Consensus conference on autologous transfusion; Preoperative autologous donation. *Transfusion* 1996; 36: 633-9.

41 Speiss BD, Sassetti R, McCarthy RJ. Autologous blood donation; haemodynamics in a high risk patient population. *Transfusion* 1992; 32: 17-22.

42 Popovsky MA, Whitaker B, Arnold NL. Severe outcomes of allogeneic and autologous blood donation; frequency and characterisation. *Transfusion* 1995; 35: 734-7.

43 Goodnough LT, Monk TG. Evolving concepts in autologous blood procurement and transfusion; case reports of peri-surgical anaemia complicated by myocardial infarction. *Am J Med* 1996; 101: 33S-37S.

Chapter 30

44   McVay PA, Andrews A, Kaplan EB, Black DB, Stehling LC, Straus RG, Toy PT. Donation reactions among autologous donors. *Transfusion* 1990; 30: 249-52.

45   British Committee for Standards in Haematology Blood Transfusion Task Force. Guidelines for autologous transfusion; I Preoperative autologous donation. *Transfusion Med* 1993; 3: 307-16.

46   Kanter MH, van Maanan D, Anders KH, Castro F, Mya WW, Clark K. Perioperative autologous blood donations before elective hysterectomy. *JAMA* 1996; 276: 798-801.

47   Forgie MA, Wells PS, Laupacis. Preoperative autologous donation decreases allogeneic transfusion but increases exposure to all red blood cell transfusion: results of a meta analysis. International Study of Perioperative Transfusion Investigators. *Arch Intern Med* 1998; 158: 610-16.

48   Kanter MH, van Maanan D, Anders KH. Effect of decreasing preoperative autologous donations on subsequent transfusion rates. *Transfusion* 1997; 37supp: 4S.

49   Etchasen J, Petz L, Keeler E, Calhoun L, Kleiman S, Srider C, Fink A, Brook R. The cost effectiveness of preoperative autologous donation. *N Eng J Med* 1995; 332: 719-24.

50   Bierbaum BE, Callaghan JJ, Galanter JO, Rubash HE, Tooms RE, Welch RB. An analysis of blood management in patients having total hip or knee arthroplasty. *J Bone Joint Surgery* 1999; 81: 2-10.

51   Urayama H, Ohtake H, Tawaraya K, WatanabeY, Mills J. Autologous blood donation with erythropoietin in abdominal aortic aneurysm repair. *Vasc Surg* 2000; 34: 157-62.

52   Egli GA,. Zollinger A, Seifert B, Popovic D, Pasch T, Spahn DR. Effect of progressive haemodilution with hydroxyethyl starch, gelatin and albumin on blood coagulation. An in vitro thromboelastograph study. *Br J Anaesth* 1997; 78: 684-9.

53   Helm RE, Klemperer JD, Rosengart TK, Gold JP, Peterson P, De Bois W, Altorki NK, Lang S, Thomas S, Isom OW, Krieger KH. Intraoperative autologous blood donation preserves red cell mass but does not decrease postoperative bleeding. *Annals Thorac Surg* 1996; 62: 1431-41.

54   Kahraman S, Altunkaya KH, Celebioglu B, Kanbak M, Pasaoglu I, Erdem K. The effect of acute normovolaemic haemodilution on homologous blood requirements and total estimated red blood cell volume lost. *Acta Anaesthesiol Scand* 1997; 41: 614-7.

55   Feldman JM, Roth JV, Bjoraker DG. Maximum blood savings by acute normovolaemic haemodilution. *Anesth Analg* 1995; 80: 108-13.

56   Brecher ME, Rosenfeld M. Mathematical and computer modelling of acute normovolaemic haemodilution. *Transfusion.* 1994; 34: 176-9.

57   Goodnough LT, Grishaber JE, Monk TG. Acute preoperative haemodilution in patients undergoing radical prostatectomy; a case study analysis of efficacy. *Anesth Analg* 1994; 78: 932-7.

58   Bryson GL, Laupacis A, Wells GA. Does acute normovolaemic haemodilution reduce perioperative allogeneic transfusions? A meta-analysis. The international study of perioperative transfusion. *Anesth Analg* 1998; 86:9-15.

59   Desmond MJ, Thomas MJ, Gillon J, Fox MA. Consensus conference on autologous transfusion. *Transfusion* 1996; 36: 644-51.

60   Hogue CW, Goodnough LT, Monk TG Perioperative myocardial ischaemic episodes are related to haematocrit level in patients undergoing radical prostatectomy. *Transfusion* 1999; 39: 657-60.

61   Muir AD Reader MK Foex P Ormerod OJM Sear JW Johnston C. Preoperative silent myocardial ischaemia: incidence and prognosis in a general surgical population. *Br J Anaesth* 1991; 67: 373-7.

62   Goodnough LT, Despotis GJ, Merkel K, Monk TG. A randomized trial comparing acute normovolaemic haemodilution and preoperative autologous blood donation in total hip arthroplasty. *Transfusion* 2000; 40: 1054-7.

63   Spahn DR. Blood substitutes: artificial oxygen carriers: perfluorocarbon emulsions. *Critical care* 1999; 3: R93-7.

64   van Daele ME, Trouwborst A, van Woerkens LCSM, Tenbrinck R, Fraser AG, Roelandt JRTC. Transoesophageal echocardiographic monitoring of preoperative acute hypervolaemic haemodilution. *Anesthesiology* 1994; 81: 602-9.

65   O'Hara PJ, Hertzer NR, Santilli PH. Intraoperative autotransfusion during abdominal aortic reconstruction. *Am J Surg* 1983; 145: 215-20.

66   McShane AJ, Power C, Jackson JF. Autotransfusion, quality of blood prepared with a red cell processing device. *Br J Anaesth* 1987; 59: 1035-9.

67   Linden JV, Kaplan HS, Murphy MT. Fatal air embolism due to perioperative blood recovery. *Anesth Analg* 1997; 84: 422-6.

68   Boudreaux JP, Bornside GH, Cohn I. Emergency autotransfusion: partial cleansing of bacteria laden blood by cell washing. *J Trauma* 1983; 23: 31-5.

69   Timberlake GA, McSwain NE. Autotransfusion of blood contaminated by enteric contents: a potentially life saving measure in the massively haemorrhaging trauma patients. *J Trauma* 1988; 28: 855-7.

70   Hart OJ, Klimberg IW, Wajsman Z, Baker J. Intraoperative autotransfusion in radical cystectomy for carcinoma of the bladder. *Surg Gynaecol Obstet* 1989; 168: 302-6.

71 Thompson JF, Webster JHH, Chant ADB. Prospective randomized evaluation of a new cell saving device in elective aortic reconstruction. *Eur J Vasc Surg* 1990;4:507-12.

72 Clagett GP, Valentine RJ, Jackson MR, Mathison C, Kakish HB, Bengston TD. A randomized trial of intraoperative autotransfusion during aortic surgery. *J Vasc Surg* 1999; 29: 22-31.

73 Kelly-Patterson C, Awmar AD, Kelly H. Should the cell saver be used routinely in all infrarenal abdominal aortic bypass operations? *J Vasc Surg* 1993 ; 18: 261-65.

74 Patra P, Chaillou P, Bizouarn P. Intraoperative autotransfusion for repair of unruptured aneurysms of the infrarenal abdominal aorta. A multicentre study of 202 patients. *J Cardiovasc Surgery* 2000; 41: 407-13.

75 Szalay D, Wong D, Lindsay T. Impact of red cell salvage on transfusion requirements during elective abdominal aortic aneurysm repair. *Ann Vasc Surg* 1999; 13: 576-81.

76 Svensson LG How to obtain haemostasis after aortic surgery. *Annals of Thoracic Surgery* 1999; 67: 1981-2.

77 Thompson JF, Chant ADB Minimising blood transfusion in vascular surgery. *Hospital Update* 1991; 17: 700-14.

78 British committee for standards in haematology blood transfusion taskforce. II Perioperative haemodilution and cell salvage. *Br J Anaeth* 1997; 78: 768-71.

79 Desmond MJ, Thomas MJ, Gillon J, Fox MA. Consensus conference on autologous transfusion. Final consensus statement. *Transfusion* 1996; 36: 664-51.

80 LaMuraglia GM, O'Hara PJ, Baker WH, Naslund TC, Norris EJ, Li J, Vandermeersch E. The reduction of the allogeneic transfusion requirement in aortic surgery with a haemoglobin based solution. *J Vasc Surg* 2000; 31: 299-308.

81 Sprung JA, Popp H, O'Hara P, Woletz J. The successful use of haemoglobin based oxygen carrier as a primary blood substitute during abdominal aortic aneurysm repair with large blood loss. *Anesth Analg* 2001; 92: 1413-15.

82 British Committee for Standards in Haematology Blood Transfusion Task Force. Guidelines for autologous transfusion II. Perioperative haemodilution and cell salvage. *Br J Anaesth* 1997; 78: 768-771.

Chapter 30

Chapter 31

Critical care referral and outreach practice

Steve P Hutchinson

Consultant in Anaesthesia & Intensive Care

DEPARTMENT OF CRITICAL CARE, SHEFFIELD TEACHING HOSPITALS, SHEFFIELD, UK

Introduction

Vascular patients may be admitted to critical care facilities electively or in emergency circumstances. Elective patients may benefit from pre-optimisation within a critical care facility and/or have a period of planned post-operative care. Emergency critical care may be required post-operatively following urgent surgery, or for sick ward patients consequent on co-morbidity or peri-operative complications (Figure 1).

Guidelines on admission to and discharge from intensive care and high dependency units are described in a 1996 Department of Health document [1].

Intensive Care Unit (ICU) is appropriate for:

- Patients requiring advanced respiratory support alone.

- Patients requiring organ support of two or more organs.

The High Dependency Unit (HDU) is more appropriate for:

- Patients requiring support for a single failing organ system but excluding those needing advanced respiratory support.

- Patients who would benefit from more detailed observation or monitoring than can safely be provided on a general ward.

- Patients stepped down from intensive care.

- Post-operative patients who need close monitoring for longer than a few hours.

Consideration must always be given before referral to critical care, regarding the appropriateness of admission with respect to the reversibility of the current disease process, the impact of any associated co-morbidity and the wishes of the patient and their relatives.

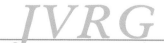

Figure 1 Critical care referral model.

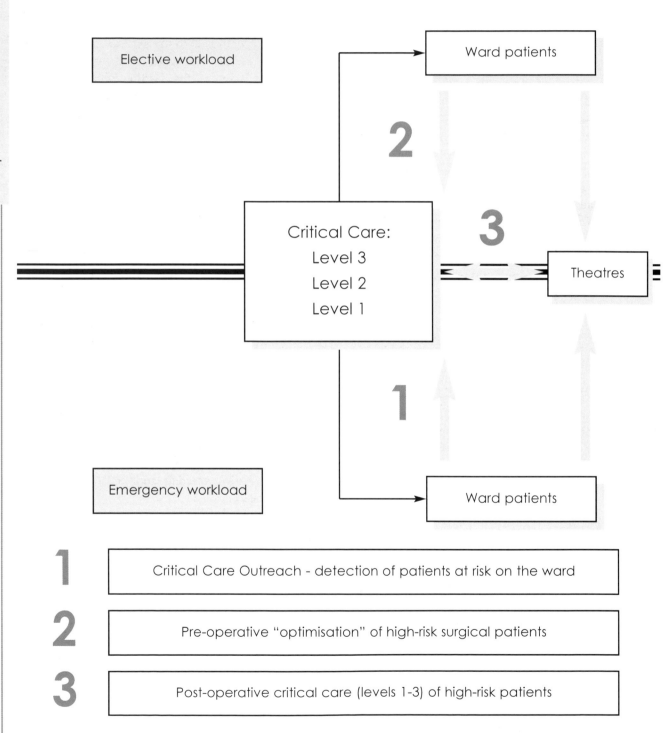

Critical care outreach

Healthcare moves forward with increasingly sophisticated treatments being made available to a population with ever growing expectations. Patients of advancing age and co-morbidity are now routinely offered procedures that previously would have been deemed too high risk. Unfortunately these increasing demands are not always married to increased resources at ward level and consequently, ward care can sometimes be substandard.

A quality agenda has put medical care increasingly under scrutiny in recent years. The 1993 national confidential enquiry into peri-operative deaths (NCEPOD) [2] **(I)** showed that two thirds of peri-operative deaths occurred three or more days after surgery, usually from cardiorespiratory complications, and in the ward environment. Approximately 20,000 deaths within 30 days of surgery are reported to NCEPOD each year. Increasingly, remediable factors associated with these deaths are being recognised.

The greatest number of deaths in intensive care and the highest percentage mortality, is in patients admitted to intensive care from hospital wards [3]. McQuillan found ward care prior to intensive care was frequently suboptimal and referrals to intensive care were made relatively late [4] **(I)**. Care was deficient in the management of airway, breathing and circulation, oxygen therapy and monitoring of severely ill ward patients prior to intensive care. McGloin [5] in a similar study found a lack of recognition of the severity of critical illness and inappropriate treatments **(I)**.

It has long been recognised that patients who deteriorate on the ward usually have abnormalities of simple physiological parameters that could have been detected prior to their critical illness [6-9]. Failure to recognise or take appropriate action in these critically ill patients may result in preventable deaths [5,10-12]. Interventions on the ward are beneficial and intensive care mortality was almost halved in McQuillan's study [4], if ward care prior to intensive care was good **(I)**.

The Audit Commission's examination of critical care provision in 1999 [13] **(I)**, acknowledged the increasing pressure the service is under and suggested a strategy that attempts to address the demand for critical care services, as well as the supply of service. Improvements in ward care prior to ICU may help address this demand.

In 2000 the Department of Health published its own review of critical care services, "Comprehensive Critical Care" [14] **(I)**, advocating "an integrated, hospital wide approach to the service.... that focuses on the level of care an individual patient needs rather than the location of the bed in which they find themselves". The existing divisions of patients into ward, high-dependency and intensive care patients should be replaced by an assessment of need:

Level 0   Patient whose needs can be met through normal ward care in an acute hospital.

Level 1   Patients at risk of their condition deteriorating, or those relocated from higher levels of care, whose needs can be met on an acute ward with additional advice and support from the critical care team.

Level 2   Patients requiring more detailed observation or intervention including support for a single organ failure or post-operative care and those stepping down from higher levels of care.

Level 3   Patients requiring advanced respiratory support alone or basic respiratory support together with support of at least two organ systems. This level includes all critically ill patients requiring support for multi-organ failure.

This philosophy has lead to the development of critical care outreach teams throughout the country. The primary aims of these teams are to share critical care skills hospital wide, identifying patients in need of increased levels of care. In doing so, some critical care admissions might be averted. Admissions that are not avoidable may be brought about in a more timely fashion, thereby reducing morbidity and mortality and the duration of critical care stay. With improvements in continuity of care and ward critical care skills, discharges to the ward from higher levels of care will also be facilitated.

Chapter 31

Critical care outreach services have developed largely without an evidence base for best practice. However, their instigation is recommended for the reasons discussed above **(C)**. The Intensive Care Society Standards Committee is currently preparing guidelines for this area [15]. Outreach activities have developed in four main areas:

- Education and support for ward staff in the recognition and basic management of patients developing critical illness.

- Detection of patients at risk of deterioration due to critical illness.

- At-risk critical care teams.

- ICU discharge ward follow-up.

Education

Medical and nursing training is deficient in the requirements to deal with patients at risk from critical illness [16,17]. Educational strategies are aimed at those delivering first line ward care and range from in-house training programs, through to national initiatives such as the ALERT [18] and CCrISP [19] programs. There is no evidence to validate these activities but they are recommended by national guidelines and fulfil clinical governance and risk management agendas **(C)**.

Detection of patients at risk

Identification of patients at risk of deterioration due to critical illness and those amenable to early intervention is fundamental to outreach care. A number of physiology based scoring systems have been developed for ward use, intended to aid the identification of patients at risk. All use the principle that patients deteriorating due to critical illness do so with easily identifiable physiological abnormalities. Many scoring variations exist because no system has been exhaustively validated. Attempts at validation of an early warning score by recruitment of huge patient numbers in a national multi-centre study has been suggested [20]. The currently most established types of scoring systems are the Early Warning Score [21] and the Modified Early Warning Score (MEWS) [22] (Figure 2). The latter has been subject to some limited validation and appears to result in earlier identification of critically ill patients and referral to ICU **(C)**.

Figure 2 Modified Early Warning Score.

Score	3	2	1	0	1	2	3
Pulse		<40	40-50	51-100	101-110	111-129	>130
B. P.	>40%↓	30%↓	15%↓	Normal	15%↑	30%↑	>45%↑
Resp. rate		≤8		9-14	15-20	21-29	≥30
Temp.		<35		35-38.4		>38.4	
CNS				A*	V	P	U
Urine	Nil	<1ml/kg/2h	<1ml/kg/h		>3ml/kg/2h		

* AVPU refers to conscious level;
Alert, responds to Verbal stimuli, Painful stimuli or Unresponsive.

The MEWS may be started on any patient causing concern, emergency admissions, stepped down patients from critical care, or specific diagnostic categories of patients such as pancreatitis. Scores are totalled according to the patient's observations. A score of 4 or more requires prompt review by medical staff and consideration for a "higher level" of care.

"Patient at risk" critical care teams

Identification of these patients must be associated with mechanisms to deliver appropriate care in a timely fashion. Medical Emergency Teams (MET) [23] and Patient At Risk Teams (PART) [24] have been developed in some institutions to replace cardiac arrest teams and try to provide more experienced medical care to these patients at an earlier stage of their illness. Although beneficial, a frequent criticism of this approach is that the result may be to further deskill the ward staff, producing short term benefit for some patients but exacerbating the longer term problems for many.

An educational approach allowing ward staff to provide better first line care and earlier and appropriate referral to higher levels of care might be a better strategy. Nevertheless Critical Care Outreach Teams to advise, support and facilitate these activities are recommended (C).

Intensive care discharge follow-up

Up to 10% of critical care admissions might be readmissions. Readmissions to critical care are associated with substantially increased mortality and length of stay [25]. One factor that may contribute to readmission is poor follow-up from critical care and formalisation of this process may reduce readmissions and the severity of illness at readmission [26]. Clearly a critical care follow-up service, in addition to any potential benefits on readmission activity, is also in an ideal position to share critical care skills with ward staff, one of the main objectives of an outreach service (C).

Peri-operative optimisation

It has been suggested that pre-operative admission of surgical patients to intensive care for cardiovascular optimisation may reduce post-operative mortality. Shoemaker [27] published a prospective trial of peri-operative "supra-normalisation" of cardiovascular indices in the management of high-risk surgical patients (Table 1). The rationale behind this study was the observation that in these surgical patients, spontaneous achievement of "supra-normal" cardiac index, oxygen delivery and consumption parameters, separated survivors from non-survivors. In the trial, pulmonary artery catheterisation, fluid loading and inotropes, were used to deliberately enhance cardiac index ($>4.5l/min/m^2$) and oxygen delivery (>600 ml/min/m^2) to "supra-normal" levels in the treatment group. This produced impressive reductions in morbidity and mortality over controls. The suggestion that limited cardiovascular reserve impacts on survival is supported by Older's work [28]. A series of surgical patients were divided into two groups by cardiopulmonary exercise testing. Patients with low anaerobic threshold had a mortality of 18% after major surgery, whereas those with a higher threshold had a mortality of only 0.8%.

Boyd [29] has since produced similar work in the UK using the same high-risk groups, reducing mortality from 23% to 5.7% and halving the complication rate. Vascular patients have also been shown to benefit from peri-operative optimisation in one study using a different protocol [30]. Other vascular studies however [31-33] failed to show benefit from optimisation practices in their surgical populations. It may be that the lack of benefit in these latter vascular studies was due to failure to produce "supra-normal" cardiovascular indices.

Another recent report has again shown benefit of pre-operative supra-normalisation in high risk patients [34], reducing mortality from 17% to 3% and shortening hospital length of stay in one treatment group. Adding further confusion however is a more recent large multicenter study [35] using dopexamine for optimisation, which failed to show benefits on mortality or length of stay. The authors and an associated editorial [36], suggest this difference from previous studies may be due to the already relatively low control group mortality at 13% compared to

Chapter 31

Table 1 Criteria for high-risk patients after Shoemaker.

- Previous severe cardio-respiratory illness (myocardial infarct, stroke, COAD)

- Extensive ablative surgery for carcinoma (oesophagectomy, gastrectomy etc)

- Severe multi-trauma (> 2 organs or 3 systems, or opening 2 body cavities)

- Massive acute blood loss (> 8 units), blood volume < 1.5l/m^2, haematocrit < 0.2

- Age > 70yrs or evidence of limited physiological reserve of one or more organs

- Septicaemia, positive blood culture, WCC >13 000/ml, Temp>38.3 $^\circ$C for 48hrs

- Shock, MAP < 60mmHg, CVP < 15cmH$_2$O, urine output < 20ml/hr

- Respiratory failure, PaO$_2$ <8 Kpa (FiO$_2$ > 0.4), mechanical ventilation > 48hrs

- Acute abdominal catastrophe (pancreatitis, ischaemic bowel, perforated viscus)

- Acute renal failure, urea > 17.9mmol/l, creatinine >265 mmol/l

- Late stage vascular disease involving aortic disease

earlier studies, a lower number of emergency surgical patients and a lower mean number of "high risk" (Table 1) criteria. A post hoc analysis of a higher risk subgroup within this study did show a reduction in mortality in one treatment group.

Benefits of peri-operative optimisation of cardiovascular parameters may be dependent on the patient population. Shoemaker's original supra-normal goals were derived from a relatively young surgical population. In the critically ill or septic intensive care populations, optimisation strategies have been generally disappointing [37] and may simply not be applicable. Within the surgical population it seems that sicker patients may benefit to a greater extent but benefit may only be seen if parameters are optimised before complications occur. Elective surgery with low mortality in well selected patients may well not be able to demonstrate sufficient outcome improvements to justify the extra intensive care resources that routine peri-operative optimisation would require.

These arguments are confused still further by the clear outcome benefits demonstrated by prophylactic beta blockade in vascular surgical patients [38,39]. Vascular surgical patients constitute a high-risk group particularly for peri-operative ischaemic heart disease. Beta blockade presumably reduces mortality by reducing myocardial work in the peri-operative period, protecting against myocardial ischaemia. This rationale is clearly at variance with the idea that survival benefit can arise from driving myocardial performance and tissue oxygen delivery.

There is some evidence for both treatment strategies but what remains unclear is exactly who benefits from which. It is possible that some patients with active ischaemic heart disease may benefit from beta blockade whereas others with limited cardio-respiratory reserve should perhaps have peri-operative cardiovascular optimisation. Alternatively a balanced approach, of maximising global oxygen delivery whilst limiting myocardial oxygen demand may be what is required.

A consensus group [40] recently stated that optimisation of oxygen delivery is indeed appropriate for a subgroup of surgical patients. Meta-analysis of 17 optimisation trials, over 2000 patients, suggests that for every 100 patients undergoing high risk surgery 11 lives might be saved by optimisation practices [40]. Unfortunately, despite this, it still remains unclear within this high-risk group, who will benefit, by how much, and what constitutes an optimum optimisation strategy **(III)**.

Planned post-operative intensive care

Vascular surgical patients frequently require post-operative critical care support. An individual patient's requirements will depend on their physiological status and operative category. Critical care support is most often required for mechanical ventilation, invasive monitoring, or the management of cardiovascular instability with vasoactive drugs. Often the requirement for critical care admission is clear because of the need for ventilation, or multi-organ support. Equally in many circumstances, when invasive monitoring, vasoactive drugs, or for example epidural management are the needs, peri-operative care might be provided in a number of locations such as the ICU, HDU, extended recovery area, specialist vascular unit or a normal ward. On the occasions, an objective risk assessment tool would be useful.

Scoring systems that allow triage of patients appropriate for admission to ICU, HDU, or ward care are not well developed [41]. Numerous scoring systems to assess peri-operative risk exist. The most established and widely used is the American Society of Anaesthetist physical status classification (ASA grade). There is a broad correlation with outcome, 84% of 20,000 NCEPOD deaths occur in patients of ASA grade 3 or more. However, there is a lack of specificity, and subjectivity occurs in application of the score. Scoring systems such as the Acute Physiology and Chronic Health Evaluation (APACHE) score [42], and its modifications, are applicable to critically ill populations but are not appropriate for pre-operative risk assessment. Goldman's Cardiac Risk Index [43] is a useful organ specific risk indicator but is not designed to take account of global patient peri-operative risk, or operative factors.

The Physiological and Operative Severity Score for enUmeration of Mortality and morbidity (POSSUM) [44], devised for comparative audit, is an effective tool in general surgical and vascular patients [45]. It takes into account both multi-system physiological variables and operative factors. Such a score, or a modified pre-operative score, could also be used for stratification of patients according to risk. However, it is not clear what risk should correspond to what level of care, or if this is the most effective method **(III)**.

Clinical judgement may be as effective [46] as scoring systems and in fact may stratify patients in a similar way [47] but frequently no formal calculation of risk is undertaken [48].

The notion of routine intensive care admission for post-operative care of vascular procedures in some centres has been questioned. With the implementation of clinical pathways and selective use of intensive care, more patients can be safely treated for carotid endarterectomy [49], aortic [50] and non-aortic [51] surgery with reduced use of intensive care resources. Extrapolation of such policies from one institution to another is not appropriate but guidelines to critical care usage, tailored to local circumstances, are feasible.

It should be noted that guidelines regarding critical care refer to categories of care, rather than geographical locations within a hospital. Clearly local circumstances in terms of equipment and staffing will determine what levels of care are available in different locations. Intermediate or level 1 care facilities (Comprehensive Critical Care), or extended stay post-anaesthetic recovery rooms might form a useful part of care pathways for some vascular patients.

Clear guidelines are not available but clinical pathways for post-operative support of vascular surgical patients can be devised to optimise critical care resource usage **(C)**. Pathways for the use of post-operative critical care must take into account:

◆ The patient's pre-operative physiological status.

◆ Operative risk and physiological insult.

◆ Intra-operative stability.

◆ Peri-operative risk consequent on the above variables.

Chapter 31

◆ Levels of monitoring, nursing staff, medical staff, and therapeutic interventions available in different locations.

Summary

◆ Critical care services in the UK are stretched **(I)**. Vascular surgery is a heavy user of these services. All aspects of critical care use need to be carefully evaluated to ensure maximum benefit.

◆ Critical care admissions from the ward do relatively badly **(II)**. Systems must be put in place to ensure the early recognition and appropriate timely management of patients "at risk" on the wards **(C)**.

◆ Peri-operative optimisation of oxygen delivery will benefit some patients. Although further work is needed to determine who will benefit and what is the best therapeutic approach **(III)**, clinicians must be willing to consider incorporating this into their practice.

◆ Critical care should be categorised as levels of care provision rather than traditional geographical locations within a hospital. Local care pathways for post-operative vascular patients should be developed, rationalising the use of critical care resources **(C)**. These will need to take into account a risk assessment of both patient and operation, but also local resources.

Further Reading

1   Vincent JL, Ed. Reducing Surgical Mortality and Complications. In: *Yearbook of Intensive Care and Emergency Medicine.* Springer-Verlag 2001; 57-67.

2   Vincent JL, Ed. Outreach: a Hospital-wide Approach to Critical Illness. In: *Yearbook of Intensive Care and Emergency Medicine.* Springer-Verlag 2001; 661-675.

References (grade I evidence and grade A recommendations in bold)

1   Guidelines on admission to and discharge from Intensive Care and High Dependency Units. Department of Health 1996.

2   **National Confidential Enquiry into Peri-operative Deaths 1991-2. London: HMSO.1993.**

3   Goldhill DR, Sumner A. Outcome of intensive care patients in a group of British intensive care units. *Crit Care Med* 1998; 26: 1337-45.

4   **McQuillan P, Pilkington S, Allan A, Taylor B, Short A, Morgan G, Neilsen M, Barrett D, Smith G. Confidential enquiry into the quality of care before admission to intensive care. *BMJ* 1998; 316: 1853-8.**

5   **McGloin H, Adam SK, Singer M. Unexpected deaths and referrals to intensive care of patients on general wards. Are some cases potentially avoidable? *J R Coll Physicians Lond* 1999; 33: 255-9.**

6   Frankin C, Mathews J. Developing strategies to prevent in-hospital cardiac arrest: analysing responses of physicians and nurses in hours before the event. *Crit Care Med* 1994; 22: 244-7.

7   Schein RMH, Hazday N, Pena M, Ruben BH, Sprung CL. Clinical antecedents to in hospital cardiopulmonary arrest. *Chest* 1990; 98: 1388-92.

8   Bedell SE. Incidence and characteristics of preventable cardiac arrest. *JAMA* 1991; 265: 2815-20.

9   Buist MD, Jarmolowski E, Burton PR, Bernard SA, Waxman BP, Anderson J. Recognising clinical instability in hospital patients before cardiac arrest or unplanned admission to intensive care. A pilot study in a tertiary-care hospital. *Med J Aust* 1999; 171: 22-5.

10   Dubois RW, Brook RH. Preventable deaths: who, how often and why? *Ann Intern Med* 1998; 109: 582-9.

11   Neale G. Risk management in the care of medical emergencies after referral to hospital. *J R Coll Physicians Lond* 1998; 32: 125-9.

12   Lawrence A, Havill JH. An audit of deaths occurring in hospital after discharge from the intensive care. *Anaesth Intensive Care* 1999; 27: 185-9.

13   **Critical to Success. The Audit Commission, London 1999.**

14   **Comprehensive Critical Care. A review of adult critical care services. Department of Health 2000. http://www.doh.gov.uk/pdfs/criticalcare.pdf**

15   Outreach. A guideline for the introduction of outreach services 2001 (draft). Intensive Care Society Standards Committee, London.

16 Harrison GA, Hillman KM, Fulde GWO, Jacques TC. The need for undergraduate education in critical care. *Anaesth Intens Care* 1999; 27: 53-58.

17 Daffurn K, Lee A, Hillman KM, Bishop GF, Bauman A. Do nurses know when to summon emergency assistance? *Intens and Crit Care Nursing* 1994; 10: 115-120.

18 ALERT. Acute Life threatening Events - Recognition and Treatment. Gary Smith. The University of Portsmouth. 1999.

19 CCrISP. Care of the Critically Ill Surgical Patient. The Royal College of Surgeons of England. 1999.

20 BEWSA. British Early Warning Score Assessment. A proposal.

21 Morgan RJM, Williams F, Wright MM. An early warning scoring system for detecting developing critical illness. *Clin Intensive Care* 1997; 8: 100.

22 Stenhouse C, Coates S, Tivey M, Allsop P, Parker T. Prospective evaluation of a modified early warning score to aid earlier detection of patients developing critical illness on a surgical ward. *BJA* 2000; 84: 663P.

23 Lee A, Bishop G, Hillman KM, Daffurn K. The Medical Emergency Team. *Anaesth Intens Care* 1995; 23: 183-186.

24 Goldhill DR, Worthington L, Mulcahy A, Tarling M, Summer A. The patient at risk team: identifying and managing seriously ill ward patients. *Anaesthesia* 1999; 54: 853-60.

25 Rosenberg AL, Hofer TP, Hayward RA, Strachan C, Watts CM. Who bounces back? Physiologic and other predictors of intensive care unit readmission. *Crit Care Med* 2001; 29: 511-518.

26 Russell S. Reducing readmissions to the intensive care unit. *Heart Lung* 1999; 28: 365-72.

27 Shoemaker WC, Appel PL, Kram HB, Waxman K, Lee TS. Prospective trial of supranormal values of survivors as therapeutic goals in high-risk surgical patients. *Chest* 1988; 94: 1176-86.

28 Older P, Smith R, Courtney P, Hone R. Preoperative evaluation of cardiac failure and ischaemia in elderly patients by cardiopulmonary exercise testing. *Chest* 1993; 104: 701-704.

29 Boyd O, Grounds MR, Bennett ED. A randomised clinical trial of the effect of deliberate peri-operative increase in oxygen delivery on the mortality in high-risk surgical patients. *JAMA* 1993; 270: 2699-707.

30 Berlauk JF, Abrams JH, Gilmour IJ, O'Connor SR, Knighton DR, Cerra FB. Pre-operative optimisation of cardiovascular haemodynamics improves outcome in peripheral vascular surgery. A prospective randomised trial. *Ann Surg* 1991; 214: 289-97.

31 Ziegler DW, Wright JG, Choban PS, Flancbaum L. A prospective randomised trial of preoperative optimisation of cardiac function in patients undergoing elective peripheral vascular surgery. *Surgery* 1997; 122: 584-92.

32 Valentine RJ, Duke ML, Inman MH, Grayburn PA, Hagino RT, Kakish HB, Clagett GP. Effectiveness of pulmonary artery catheters in aortic surgery; a randomised trial. *J Vasc Surg* 1998; 27: 203-11.

33 Bender JS, Smith-Meek MA, Jones CE. Routine pulmonary artery catheterisation does not reduce morbidity and mortality of elective vascular surgery: results of a prospective randomised trial. *Ann Surg* 1997; 226: 229-237.

34 Wilson J, Woods I, Fawcett J, Whall R, Dibb W, Morris C, McManus E. Reducing the risk of major elective surgery: randomised controlled trial of preoperative optimisation of oxygen delivery. *BMJ* 1999; 318: 1099-103.

35 Takala J, Meier-Hellmann A, Eddleston J, Hulstaert P, Sramek V. Effect of dopexamine on the outcome after major abdominal surgery: A prospective randomised controlled multicenter study. *Crit Care Med* 2000; 28: 3417-3423.

36 Bennett D, Boyd O. Oxygen delivery in surgical patients - Doesn't work, or does it? *Crit Care Med* 2000; 28: 3564-3565.

37 Poeze M, Greve JWM, Ramsay G. Goal orientated haemodynamic therapy: a plea for a closer look at using peri-operative oxygen transport optimisation. *Int Care Med* 2000; 26: 635-637.

38 Mangano DT, Layug EL, Wallace A, Tateo I. Effect of atenolol on mortality and cardiovascular morbidity after noncardiac surgery. Multicenter Study of Perioperative Ischaemia Research Group. *N Engl J Med* 1996; 335: 1713-1720.

39 Poldermans D, Boersma E, Bax JJ, Thomson IR, van der Ven LL, Blankensteijin JD, Baars HF, Yo TI, Trocino G, Vigna C, Roelandt JR, van Urk H. The effect of bisoprolol on peri-operative mortality and myocardial infarction in high-risk patients undergoing vascular surgery. Dutch Echocardiographic Cardiac Risk Evaluation Applying Stress Echocardiography Study Group. *N Engl J Med* 1999; 341: 1789-1794.

40 Grocott MPW, Ball JAS. Consensus Meeting: Management of the high-risk surgical patient. 13-14th April 2000, Christ's College, Cambridge, UK. *Clin Intensive Care* 2000; 11: 263-281.

41 Cuthbertson BH, Webster NR. The role of the intensive care unit in the management of the critically ill surgical patient. *J R Coll Surg Edinb* 1999; 44: 294-300.

42 Knaus WA, Zimmerman JE, Wagner DP, Draper EA, Lawrence DE. APACHE - acute physiology and chronic health evaluation: a physiological based classification system. *Crit Care Med* 1981; 9: 591-7.

43 Goldman L, Caldera DL, Nussbaum SR, Southwick FS, Krogstad D, Murray B, Burke DS, O'Malley TA, Goroll AH, Caplan CH, Nolan J, Carabello B, Slater EE. Multifactorial index of cardiac risk in non-cardiac surgical procedures. *N Engl J Med* 1977; 297: 845-50.

Chapter 31

Chapter 31

44 Copeland GP, Jones D, Waters M. POSSUM: a scoring system for surgical audit. *Br J Surg* 1991; 78:355-60.

45 Copeland GP, Jones DR, Wilcox A, Harris PL. Comparative vascular audit using the POSSUM scoring system. *Ann R Coll Surg Engl* 1993; 75: 175-7.

46 Hartley HM, Sagar PM. The surgeon's "gut feeling" as a predictor of post-operative outcome. *Ann R Coll Surg Engl* 1994; 76(suppl. 6): 277-8.

47 Curran JE, Grounds RM. Ward versus intensive care management of high-risk surgical patients. *Br J Surg* 1998; 85: 956-61.

48 Michaels JA, Payne SPK, Galland RB. A study of methods used for cardiac risk assessment prior to major vascular surgery. *Eur J Vasc Endovasc Surg* 1996; 11: 221-4.

49 Rigdon EE, Monajjem N, Rhodes RS. Criteria for selective utilisation of the intensive care unit following carotid endarterectomy. *Ann Vasc Surg* 1997; 11: 20-27.

50 Katz SG, Kohl RD. Selective use of the intensive care unit after non-aortic arterial surgery. *J Vasc Surg* 1996; 24: 235-9.

51 Bertges DJ, Rhee RY, Muluk SC, Trachtenberg JD, Steed DL, Webster MW, Makaroun MS. Is routine use of the intensive care unit after elective infra-renal abdominal aortic aneurysm repair necessary? *J Vasc Surg* 2000; 32: 634-42.

Chapter 32

Management of acute pain in vascular disease

Kate de Brett Pain Nurse

Peter MacIntyre Consultant Anaesthetist

DEPARTMENT OF ANAESTHETICS, ROYAL DEVON AND EXETER HOSPITAL, EXETER, UK

Introduction

The National Recommendations on the delivery of Pain Services [1] **(A)** underline the importance of timely and appropriate pain relief. Pain is a common feature of many vascular diseases and its management is not only essential for ethical and humanitarian reasons, but also to hasten recovery and reduce the incidence of post-operative complications. This chapter will examine the treatment strategies for patients with acute pre- and post-operative pain.

Basic principles of pain relief strategies

Although pain is a common symptom in vascular disease, its nature varies [2] **(I)**. It may be caused by inadequate tissue perfusion resulting in transient or continuous ischaemia, secondary changes such as skin ulceration, sudden changes in vascular dimension such as an expanding aortic aneurysm, rupture of the aorta or other intracavity organs, impairment of venous return resulting in oedema and pain from accompanying disease i.e. diabetic or ischaemic neuropathy. It is important to differentiate between nociceptive and neuropathic pain. Nociceptive pain results from injury to tissues with consequent release of biochemical substances that activate specialised receptors. Neuropathic pain is caused by a primary lesion or dysfunction in the peripheral or central nervous system. It is described as being a burning, stabbing or electrical feeling in the distribution of peripheral nerves or body dermatomes. It is often associated with abnormal paraesthesia, allodynia (pain as a result of a stimulus that does not normally provoke pain) and/or hyperalgesia (an increased response to a stimulus that is normally painful).

To distinguish between the different aetiologies and types of pain it is important to take a full pain history. This involves documenting the onset of the pain, the location, intensity, distribution, quality, and exacerbating and relieving factors. Treatment strategies vary depending into which category the patient fits. In difficult cases e.g. drug addicts, the hospital's specialist pain service should be involved as soon as possible. Having decided on the cause and type of pain a successful analgesic plan should include **(A)**:

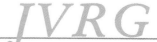

◆ Treating the cause of the pain if possible.

◆ Regular assessment of pain levels so that increasing or ongoing pain may be investigated and treated.

◆ Specific treatment for nociceptive pain using a multi-modal approach i.e. balanced analgesia.

◆ Specific treatment for neuropathic pain.

◆ Exclusion of contra-indications to analgesics in particular non-steroidal anti-inflammatory drugs (NSAIDs).

◆ Regular analgesia rather than "as required".

◆ Use of the oral route if possible.

◆ Plans to treat side effects in particular opioid related nausea, vomiting and constipation.

◆ Non-pharmacological techniques, such as positioning, limb elevation and education.

It is important to realise that patients presenting to vascular firms often have significant conditions that need to be taken into account when planning such regimes such as advanced age, renal impairment, coagulation abnormalities and extensive medication lists.

Pain scoring

Regular, accurate assessment of the degree of pain is essential to guide appropriate treatment and review, particularly when the pain intensity varies. The challenge of reliably quantifying pain remains as it is a personal experience that involves not only sensory input but modulation by physiological, psychological and environmental factors. There is no direct way of measuring pain apart from patient reporting. Although this is a subjective measure evidence points to pain scoring as being sensitive and consistent [3,4,5,6,7] (I). Several approaches may be used to assess pain:

◆ **Categorical scales** - such scales were the earliest pain measure [7]. Words are used to describe the magnitude of pain and the patient then picks the most appropriate word describing

their pain. The commonest is a four category scale using none, mild, moderate, severe. This approach has the advantage of being quick and simple but limits the number of descriptors.

◆ **Visual Analogue Scale** - using a simple 10cm "slide rule" the patient can measure the point on the rule that best describes their pain [8] (I).

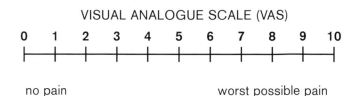

VISUAL ANALOGUE SCALE (VAS)

0 1 2 3 4 5 6 7 8 9 10

no pain   worst possible pain

This allows the patient an unlimited choice in describing their pain. The pain score is then obtained by measuring the distance from the no pain end to the patient's mark. A distance of 5 cm would represent a pain score of 5 out of 10. When categorical pain reports are compared to visual analogue scale distances moderate pain was found to correspond to a mean of 4.9 cm and severe pain a mean of 7.5 cm with 85% of severe pain scoring over 5.4 cm [9] (I).

◆ **Verbal Rating Scale** - the patient is asked to rate their pain on a scale of 0-10 (0=no pain and 10=worst imaginable pain). This approach is very easy, quick to use and correlates well with visual analogue scales [6] (I). It is probably the best to use in every day clinical use with a score of 6 or above equating to severe pain (B).

These methods of pain scoring are not suitable for all groups of patients e.g. the confused, those with learning difficulties, the unconscious, those with language difficulties. For these patients there are various recognized pain behaviours that can be used to guide treatment e.g. changes in facial expression, restlessness, distress, guarding.

Balanced analgesia for nociceptive pain

Having scored or rated pain it is important to treat it appropriately. It is widely accepted that in order to obtain maximum pain relief with minimal side effects it is necessary to combine different drugs such as paracetamol, a NSAID and a centrally acting drug such as an opioid **(A)**. This offers the potential for greater pain relief than when the agents are used separately as they act on different targets along the pain pathway. The evidence for this approach is well documented and discussed in "An Evidence-Based Resource for Pain Relief" by Henry McQuay and Andrew Moore [10] **(I)**. On the treatment of acute pain they conclude:

- Paracetamol, NSAIDs, tramadol and opiates are all effective analgesics either as sole agents or in combination.

- The old adage that if patients can swallow it is best to take drugs by mouth seems sensible. Certainly when they looked at NSAIDs there was no evidence that other routes of administration were superior.

- No one opioid was better than the other but there was good evidence that pethidine has a specific disadvantage [11] **(I)**. Our opiate of first choice is morphine.

- Traditional routes of administration for opiates were effective (PO, IV bolus, IM bolus, SC bolus, continuous IVI) but novel routes such as intra-nasal and transdermal though effective had no evidence to suggest they were superior in terms of reducing side effects.

Which NSAID drug to use and when, is still open to debate because of the number of different drugs available and lack of evidence as to cause and effect. The Royal College of Anaesthetists and the Cochrane and Bandolier Groups have tried to answer this question. The Royal College of Anaesthetists looked at NSAIDs as a whole and came up with guidelines for their use in the peri-operative period [12]. The working party produced recommendations according to the evidence available, the most important of which are summarised below.

Grade A

Based on the strongest evidence available, including at least one randomised trial as part of the body of literature of overall good quality.

- NSAIDs are not effective as the sole agent after major surgery in most patients.

- They are often effective after minor or moderate surgery.

- NSAIDs often decrease opioid requirement. Significant reduction in opioid side effects has been noted in a few studies only.

- NSAIDs increase bleeding time and some studies show increased blood loss.

Grade B

Based on availability of well conducted clinical studies but not randomised trials.

- The clinician should be aware that many drug interactions have been reported.

Grade C

Based on expert consensus of the group in the absence of studies of good quality.

- NSAIDs should not be given prior to surgery if there is an increased risk of intra-operative bleeding.

- NSAIDs should not be used in hypovolaemic patients.

- NSAIDs should be avoided in patients with impaired renal function.

- NSAIDs should be monitored regularly in all patients receiving NSAIDs after major surgery.

- NSAIDs should be used with caution in the elderly, patients with diabetes, vascular disease

Chapter 32

and after cardiac, hepatobiliary, renal or major vascular surgery.

♦ NSAIDs are contra-indicated in aspirin sensitive asthma and should be used with caution in other asthmatics.

The choice of NSAID in the peri-operative period is dictated by its analgesic efficacy and adverse effects. NSAIDs show much greater variability in their toxicity than in their efficacy and the largest difference demonstrated between the drugs relates to gastroduodenal ulceration. The different drugs have been classed into groups depending on the risk of GI ulceration [13,14] **(II)** e.g:

♦ High risk - ketoprofen, piroxicam, azapropazone.

♦ Intermediate risk - aspirin, naproxen, indomethacin.

♦ Low risk - ibuprofen, diclofenac.

In the peri-operative period it is sensible to use drugs in the low risk group. It is worth noting the use of selective cycloxygenase (COX) 2 inhibitors in the peri-operative period has not shown any advantages over current NSAIDs [15] **(III)**. Their role in this area of medicine remains undefined.

When the two drugs in the low risk group are compared in equianalgesic doses against placebo diclofenac seems to provide superior analgesia but in direct comparisons no significant difference has been shown between the two [16] **(II)**. Therefore the choice of drug is up to the individual prescriber. Many choose diclofenac over ibuprofen because it can be given by many routes e.g. IV, PO, PR and is therefore more versatile over the peri-operative period **(C)**.

Overall an indication of "what to use when" depending on the severity of pain is given in the Table 1 **(A)**.

Analgesics for neuropathic pain

Although most of the focus of the treatment of neuropathic pain is in the chronic pain setting,

neuropathic pain can occur acutely and anyone who has worked with a vascular firm will have seen patients with phantom limb pain on day 1 post-operatively. As with chronic pain first line treatment of neuropathic pain is with antidepressants or anticonvulsants. Both have been shown to be effective [17] **(I)** and which to use first usually depends on specific patient factors. If using an antidepressant amitriptyline is usually the drug of first choice. If effective but not tolerated because of side effects options include another tricyclic e.g. dothiepin or an SSRI antidepressant e.g. citalopram. Anticonvulsants commonly used are gabapentin, sodium valproate and carbamezepine. If either class of drug is only partially effective then they can be used in combination.

Alternatives that have proved useful are systemic local anaesthetic [17] **(I)** drugs or opioids [18] **(II)**. Opioids should not be used as a first line analgesic because their efficacy in neuropathic pain is variable though in some patients they can be beneficial. They should be tried if other classes of drugs have failed or are only partially effective **(B)**.

Advanced analgesic techniques

Some patients may be suitable for advanced analgesic techniques. These are usually patients undergoing major surgery or in severe pain requiring regular opioid analgesia. The two most common techniques are Patient Controlled and Epidural Analgesia.

Patient Controlled Analgesia (PCA)

Drug options: Morphine, Tramadol, Fentanyl.

Patient Controlled Analgesia can be a very effective method of delivering analgesia. Its use is largely confined to post-operative care but it can be used pre-operatively in appropriate patients. The technique uses an electronic infusion device and allows patients to self-administer analgesic drugs (usually opioids) intravenously or subcutaneously as required. A bolus dose is prescribed which is delivered when a patient pushes a button. A lockout time, during which no drug

Table 1 Recommendations for an analgesic ladder.

Treatment	Mild Pain (Pain score <3)	Moderate Pain (Pain score 3-6)	Severe Pain (Pain score >6)
Regular Paracetamol	Yes	Yes	Yes
As required NSAID	Yes	No	No
Regular NSAID	No	Yes	Yes
As required Tramadol	No	Yes	No
Regular Tramadol	No	Possibly	Possibly
As required Opiate	No	Possibly	No
Regular Opiate	No	No	Yes

can be delivered, is programmed into the device. A background infusion can be added if needed. Pain and sedation levels must be assessed and recorded hourly. A continuous background infusion can increase the potential for overdose and respiratory depression but maybe useful in difficult cases.

Suggested drug regimes for PCA are:

◆ Morphine 50 mg in 50 mls sodium chloride 0.9% @ 1mg/ml bolus dose with a 5-minute lockout.

◆ Fentanyl 500 mcg in 50 mls sodium chloride 0.9% @ 10-20 mcg bolus with a 5-minute lockout.

◆ Tramadol 500 mg in 50 mls sodium chloride 0.9% @ 10 mg bolus with a 5-minute lockout.

Studies comparing PCA with conventional methods of opioid analgesia e.g. intermittent IM/SC or continuous infusion have been contradictory. Some studies show no difference between the techniques while others show PCA as more efficacious [19] **(III)**. The evidence for its effect on post-operative morbidity is similarly contradictory and it may be no better than conventional methods [19] **(III)**. Where PCA may win is with patient and staff satisfaction. The patient is in

control of their analgesia delivery and therefore has less anxiety, does not have to wait for the delivery of analgesia, does not have to have injections and does not have to bother the nurses. It is not too difficult to see that these advantages apply as much to overworked nursing staff as to the patient [20,21,22] **(III)**. However this outcome is not universal as there are disadvantages to the technique particularly if the patient is unable to use or understand the equipment or while asleep does not push the button, wakes in pain and spends the next hour playing "catch up".

Epidural analgesia

Epidural blockade for the management of pain involves the injection and/or infusion of local anaesthetic +/- opioid into the epidural space. Continuous epidural analgesia is a common technique for managing patients with acute pre- and post-operative vascular pain. It is suitable for pain below the xiphisternum. It is safe to use at ward level, but staff need to be appropriately trained to care for and regularly monitor the patient. If not available, the patient should be managed in a high dependency unit **(A)**. More detail on what drugs to use, where to site the epidural and adverse events associated with

Table 2 Comparison of morbidity and mortality in patients having vascular surgery with or without regional anaesthesia.

Adverse Event	Neuroaxial Block % of patients suffering adverse event (number of patients).	No Neuroaxial block % of patients suffering adverse event (number of patients).
Death	2.5% (23)	3.8% (31)
Wound Infection	0.2% (2)	0.5% (4)
Pneumonia	2.4% (22)	6.8% (55)
Renal Failure	0.8% (7)	1.9% (15)
DVT	0	0
PE	0	0.1% (1)
MI	3.9% (35)	3.7% (30)
Cardiac Arrhythmia	2.1% (19)	3.8% (31)
Other Fatal Cardiac Event	3.3% (3)	0.1% (1)
Stroke	0.2% (2)	0.6% (5)
Peri-operative Transfusion >2 units	4.2% (38)	5.1% (41)

epidural analgesia are beyond the scope of this chapter but a good summary can be found in the July 2001, Educational Issue of the *British Journal of Anaesthesia* [23] **(I)**. What is of more relevance is the question "Does epidural analgesia affect surgical outcome?" This question has been addressed by Kehlet and Holte [24] **(II)**. They surmised that because epidural analgesia is the most effective method of pain relief after major procedures and is the most effective method in reducing surgical stress and autonomic responses that subsequent organ dysfunction and post-operative morbidity should be less. When they looked at the evidence for all types of surgery they found continuous epidural analgesia:

◆ Provided a significant reduction in post-operative pulmonary morbidity in major abdominal and vascular procedures from 16.7% to 10.4% and possibly in thoracic procedures. No benefit could be demonstrated for other types of surgery. They

concluded that more work is required to validate these findings as the number of patients studied was limited and there was considerable variation in pulmonary morbidity in the individual studies.

◆ May result in a clinically relevant reduction in cardiac morbidity but the reduction was not significant.

◆ Significantly reduces the risk of thromboembolic complications after lower body procedures from 62% to 28.7% but not after major abdominal surgery.

◆ Significantly reduces the duration of post-operative paralytic ileus.

A recent meta-analysis [25] **(II)** including 141 trials and a total of 9559 patients came to more expansive conclusions calculating central neuroaxial blockade (epidural and spinal anaesthesia) reduced the risk of DVT by 44%, PE by 55%, transfusion requirements by 50%, pneumonia by 39%, respiratory depression by 59% and myocardial infarction by 30%. Mortality was reduced by 30%. However most of the studies involved single dose regimes and the positive findings were obtained primarily after major orthopaedic operations. Twenty-two trials involved vascular surgery with 905 patients randomised to neuroaxial block and 806 to no neuroaxial block. The record of adverse events is summarised in the Table 2. This data seems to support the conclusions reached by Kehlet and Holte [24] **(II)**.

Summary

◆ It is essential that an accurate assessment of the nature and severity of the patient's pain is completed before prescribing an analgesic regime **(A)**.

◆ The type of pain present should dictate the analgesic regime **(A)**. The use of balanced, multi-modal analgesia, combined with regular assessment and review of pain levels, provides the best way to manage acute pain associated with vascular disease **(A)**. The evidence available supports this approach **(I)**.

◆ Debate still remains as to the best drugs, route of administration and techniques employed. This stems from conflicting data and poor quality trials. Intravenous PCA has not been shown to reduce morbidity or mortality compared with traditional delivery systems **(III)**.

◆ Epidural analgesia does seem to offer advantages over conventional regimes with better pain control and reduction in pulmonary and gastrointestinal complications. These advantages however seem to be confined to major abdominal and vascular procedures **(II)**.

◆ Epidural analgesia reduces the incidence of thrombo-embolic complications in lower limb surgery **(I)**.

References (grade I evidence and grade A recommendations in bold)

1 **Working Party on Pain National Recommendations on the Delivery of Pain Services. Royal College of Surgeons and Royal College of Anaesthetists 1990.**

2 Johansen KH. Pain due to Vascular Disease. In: *Management of Pain*. Bonica J. Lippincott, Williams and Wilkinson, 2001.

3 Wallenstein SL, Heidrich IIIG, Kaiko R, Houde RW. Clinical Evaluation of Mild Analgesics: the Measurement of Clinical pain. *Br J Clin Pharmacol* 1980; 10: 319S-27S.

4 Littman GS, Walker BR, Schneider BE. Reassessment of Verbal and Visual Analogue Ratings in Analgesic Studies. *Clin Pharmacol Ther* 985; 38:16-23.

5 Sriwatanakul K, Kelvie W, Lasagna L. The Quantification of Pain: an Analysis of Words Used to Describe Pain and Analgesia in Clinical Trials. *Clin Pharmacol Ther* 1982; 32: 141-8.

6 Murphy DE, McDonald A, Power C, Unwin A, MacSullivan R. Measurement of Pain: a Comparison of the Visual Analogue with a Non Visual Analogue Scale. *Clin J Pain* 1988; 3: 197-9.

7 Keele KD. The Pain Chart. *Lancet* 1948; ii: 6-8 [609].

8 Carr Eloise CJ, Mann Eileen M. *Pain: Creative Approaches to Effective Management.* MacMillan Press, 2000.

9 McQuay HJ, Carroll D, Poppletion P, Summerfield RJ, Moore RA. Fluradoline and Aspirin for Orthopedic Postoperative Pain. *Clinical Pharmacol Ther* 1987; 41: 531-6.

10 McQuay H, Moore A. *An Evidence-Based Resource for Pain Relief.* Acute Pain: conclusion. Oxford Medical Publications, 2000.

11 **Szeto HH, Inturrisi CE, Houde R, Saal S, Cheigh J, Reidenberg M. Accumulation of Norperidine, an Active Metabolite of Meperidine, in Patients with Renal Failure or Cancer. *Annals of Internal Medicine* 1977; 86: 738-41.**

12 The Royal College of Anaesthetists. Clinical Guidelines. Guidelines for the Use of Non-steroidal Anti-inflammatory Drugs in the Perioperative Period. March 1998.

13 Garcia Rodriguez LA. Nonsteroidal Anti-inflammatory Drugs, Ulcers and Risk: a Collaborative Meta-analysis. *Seminars in Arthritis and Rheumatism* 1997; 26(6 Supplement 1): 16-20.

14 Bandolier Library. More on NSAID Adverse Effects. Sept 2000; 79-6.

15 Langman MJ, Jensen DM, Watson DJ, Harper SE, Zhao P, Quan H, Bolognese JA, Simon TJ. Adverse Upper Gastrointestinal Effects of Rofecoxib Compared with NSAIDS. *JAMA* 1999; 282: 1929-33.

Chapter 32

Chapter 32

16 Collins SL, Moore RA, McQuay HJ, Wiffen PJ, Edwards JE. Single Dose Oral Ibuprofen and Diclofenac for Postoperative Pain. In: *The Cochrane Library*, Issue 1, 2002. Oxford: Update Software.

17 McQuay H, Moore RA, Eccleston C, Morley S, Williams ACdeC. Systematic Review of Outpatient Services for Chronic Pain Control. *Health Technology Assessment* 1997; Vol 1: No. 6.

18 Collett BJ. Chronic Opioid Therapy for Non-cancer Pain. *Br J Anaesth* 2001 87: 133-43.

19 MacIntyre PE. Safety and Efficacy of Patient Controlled Analgesia. *Br J Anaesth* 2001; 87: 36-46.

20 Chumbley GM, Hall GM, Salmon P. Patient Controlled Analgesia: an Assessment by 200 Patients. *Anaesthesia* 1998; 53: 216-21.

21 Kluger MT, Owen H. Patients' Expectations of Patient Controlled Analgesia. *Anaesthesia* 1990; 45: 1072-4.

22 Taylor NM, Hall GM, Salmon P. Patients' Experiences of Patient Controlled Analgesia. *Anaesthesia* 1996; 51: 525-8.

23 Rowbotham DJ. Advances in Pain. *Br J Anaesth* 2001; 87(1): 1-177.

24 Kehlet H, Holte K. Effect of Postoperative Analgesia on Surgical Outcome. *Br J Anaesth* 2001; 87: 62-72.

25 Rodgers A, Walker N, McKee A, Kehlet H, van Zundert A, Sage D, Futter M, Saville G, Clark T, MacMahon S. Reduction of Postoperative Mortality and Morbidity with Epidural or Spinal Anaesthesia: Results from Overview of Randomised Trials. *BMJ* 2000; 321: 1493.

Chapter 33

The chronic pain clinic

Neal Edwards Consultant in Pain Management

Andrea Wallbridge Clinical Nurse Specialist

CHRONIC PAIN CLINIC, THE NORTHERN GENERAL HOSPITAL, SHEFFIELD, UK

Introduction

The International Association for the Study of Pain defines pain as "an unpleasant, sensory and emotional experience associated with actual or potential tissue damage or described in terms of such damage". In other words, pain is subjective, is always an unpleasant sensation, and will have physical and non-physical components.

Types of pain

Pain can be described as either **nociceptive** or **neuropathic**.

Nociceptive

Nociceptive pain is an appropriate response to tissue damage via activation of the nociceptors. The pain is usually described as sharp or aching, and there is usually localised tenderness.

Neuropathic

Neuropathic pain is a consequence of damage to the nervous system either peripherally or centrally. The pain may be described as being lancinating, stabbing, burning, or electric shock like in quality, whilst deep tissue pain may be cramping or aching. The pain can be continuous or episodic, spontaneous or producible. A loss of normal sensation in the affected area is a common finding. Allodynia (pain produced by an innocuous stimulation), hyperalgesia (severe pain produced by normally easily tolerated discomfort) or hyperpathia (explosive pain following repetitive mild stimulation) may all be features.

Chronic pain is not easy to define but has been said to occur when the pain experience persists beyond the usual course of an acute disease, or beyond a reasonable time for an injury to heal or recurs at intervals for months or years [1] **(I)**. Whatever the underlying cause, chronic pain serves no useful biological function, but has profound physical, emotional and social and economical effects on the patient and their family. It is therefore logical that the management of chronic pain should consist of

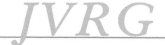

therapies aimed at all these areas and not focused to one particular area **(B)**.

In addition, inadequate management of chronic pain will inevitably have important consequences for patients, carers and for society as a whole. The increase in recognition of this has resulted in the development of increasing numbers of multi-disciplinary pain clinics.

Chronic pain may be seen in vascular surgical patients for a wide variety of reasons, including chronic ischaemic pain, venous ulceration, and peripheral neuropathic pain. Following surgery for vascular conditions, post-amputation pain is well described, however vascular surgery can also result in less well defined neuropathic pains and sympathetically mediated pain (complex regional pain syndrome).

The aim of this chapter is to suggest pathways of care for vascular patients with chronic pain conditions. However, for most patients with chronic non-cancer pain, the principles underlying their assessment and management are the same, whatever the underlying cause. These principles therefore represent the main focus of this chapter, although we do also discuss the treatment options available for phantom limb pains.

Assessment and treatment of chronic pain

Despite all the major technical advances in medicine, adequate management of patients with chronic pain remains a major challenge. Whilst more pain clinics are developing they almost invariably are under-resourced. Consequently patients with chronic pain which is either not amenable to surgery or indeed where surgery has been unsuccessful or has actually been the cause of the chronic pain, will often feel badly let down with nowhere to go. In addition, health professionals both in the primary and secondary care settings who are not experienced in managing chronic pain problems find these patients difficult to manage.

Patients with chronic pain will always have associated problems such as sleeping difficulties and general fatigue. Mobility, domestic duties, dietary intake and personal care may all be affected. In some patients the pain affects their ability to rationalise effectively resulting in over-evaluation of their condition, when their pain appears to be in excess of the underlying pathology. They may become somewhat isolated from society with a reduction in responsibility and social roles. Emotionally, patients often develop depression, poor concentration, poor memory and increasing inability to function. Patients often have unrealistic expectations as to what the medical profession can provide, becoming inappropriately reliant on social and medical support systems, continuing to seek and receive treatment from a wide variety of areas in a disorganised manner. Indeed, some patients show such desperation to relieve their pain that they manage to persuade health professionals to prescribe ineffective or even harmful treatments with their subsequent increased risks. Appropriate referral at an early stage to a multi-disciplinary pain clinic can often prevent such a scenario from occurring **(B)**.

Within chronic pain clinics a wide variety of different treatments are available and inevitably the availability of different treatments varies from clinic to clinic. These treatments can be classified into several broad areas:

◆ Education on the nature of the pain condition and effectiveness of treatment.

◆ Structured analgesic prescription.

◆ Psychological techniques e.g. cognitive behavioural therapy.

◆ Structured movement, mobility and rehabilitation programs (including physiotherapy and occupational therapy).

◆ Invasive treatments and nerve blocks.

◆ Complementary treatments e.g. acupuncture, hypnotherapy.

The specific treatment options offered to any particular patient would depend upon the patient's specific underlying pain problem, the consequences the pain has for the patient and the particular expertise available in the treating pain clinic.

Initial assessment

Initial assessment of a patient who presents with chronic pain should be constructed to assess three main areas:

- The presenting physical condition.

- Behavioural performance ability.

- Emotional cognitive state.

The presenting physical condition

This should include full medical history and full physical examination. In particular, there is a need for an accurate history of the underlying pain problem and of all previous treatments **(A)**.

Assessment of behaviour and performance ability

Evaluation of behaviour and performance should assess how appropriately the patient behaves and functions and in particular assess how the patient has adapted his behaviour to daily life. This would also look at the patient's existing coping strategies and styles. Disability and function should be assessed.

Cognitive emotional state

Evaluation of a patient's cognitive and emotional state should assess the presence of depression, anxiety, anger, guilt and any fears that the patient has, particularly fear of movement. It is essential to assess patients' social roles looking at their role within the family, their employment situation and also to specifically assess their behaviour in terms of reliance on visits to health professionals.

In broad terms, the aims of treatment of patients with chronic pain are to improve function and patient

self-reliance. The key step in treating the patient with chronic pain is to give the patient understanding as to the mechanisms underlying their chronic pain problem and the rationale behind the treatment approaches **(A)**. In particular, it is vital that the patient has realistic expectations of their treatments. Only then can specific treatment goals be set, and an individualised treatment plan formulated.

It is beyond the scope of this chapter to deal with all the treatments available within chronic pain clinics in detail. However, we will discuss analgesic prescribing and some aspects of cognitive behaviour therapy.

Analgesic prescribing

Patients with chronic pain will nearly always have been prescribed a wide variety of different medications. These drugs can be subdivided into those that have specific analgesic properties, and those whose primary indication is non-analgesic.

Analgesic preparations

Non-opioid analgesics: Aspirin, Paracetamol and non-steroidal anti-inflammatories (NSAIDs).

These drugs are extremely effective for the management of mild to moderate pain and are in widespread use for the treatment of headaches and musculoskeletal pain. Aspirin and NSAIDs inhibit the release of prostaglandins peripherally whereas paracetamol is thought to inhibit prostaglandin synthesis more centrally. Paracetamol has the advantage that it does not affect platelet function and does not harm the integrity of the stomach. However, it does not have any significant anti-inflammatory action. NSAIDs and aspirin on the other hand because of their effects in inhibiting synthesis and release of prostaglandins peripherally, have the side effects of the inhibition of platelet function, gastrointestinal toxicity, nephrotoxicity and the precipitation of asthma in susceptible individuals.

Combination analgesics

Because simple analgesic compounds have a ceiling effect they are often used in combination with narcotic analgesics. These combinations provide improved analgesia with the added affect of two drugs producing pain relief by different mechanisms. In addition, these combinations can reduce the potential for adverse reactions because each drug within the combination can be used at a reduced dose. There are a wide number of such analgesic combinations available. Whilst it is logical to combine weak opioids such as codeine with paracetamol or more peripherally acting non-steroidal anti-inflammatories, it is less logical to combine paracetamol with non-steroidal anti-inflammatories.

Opioid analgesics

Clinically, opioids can be classified as either weak or strong opiates. However, it is important to emphasise that even weak opiates can have very potent effects particularly when used in higher doses. There are a large number of clinically available opioids and differences in their effects can be explained in terms of their affinity to different sub-types of opioid receptor. However, the vast array of different types of opioid medications available tends to lead to more confusion and for most clinicians is not helpful. It is better that physicians become familiar with two or three different opioids for their patients rather than trying to use a wide variety of different opioids for different pain conditions.

In our own practice we limit these opioids to codeine compounds, tramadol, morphine, methadone, which has the advantage of a longer half life than morphine and is useful in neuropathic pain, and fentanyl which can be delivered through the transdermal route through the form of a patch. It is useful in patients with whom either absorption of morphine is poor or in whom morphine side effects, particularly constipation are proving a problem. However, it is generally agreed that strong opioids should only be prescribed for chronic non-cancer pain after all other reasonable attempts at analgesia have failed **(A)**. It is important that treatment goals are set. The primary purpose of their use should be recognised as improving quality of life for the patient. A single clinician should take primary responsibility for drug prescribing, and injectable opioids should not be used, particularly pethidine **(A)**.

Non-analgesic medications

Non-analgesic drugs can be defined as agents, which have "pain-relieving properties, unrelated to their primary clinical activity". Whilst a wide variety of non-analgesic medications are used within pain clinics, the commonest are the antidepressants and anticonvulsants.

Antidepressants

Despite the fact that none are licensed in the UK for use in chronic pain, antidepressants have been used for over 30 years, principally in the treatment of neuropathic pain. Most experience has been gained with tricyclic antidepressants, although monoamine oxidase inhibitors and selective serotonin reuptake inhibitors (SSRIs) have also been used.

Tricyclic antidepressants have an established role in the treatment of neuropathic pain [2] **(II)**. Non-selective tricyclic antidepressants such as amitriptyline, dothiepin and imipramine appear to be the most efficacious. Treatment should start with a low dose (25 mg amitriptyline, 10 mg in the elderly) and increased gradually. A trial of 6-8 weeks up to a minimum amitriptyline dose of 150 mg is needed to evaluate efficacy. Common side effects include sedation, and antimuscarinic effects (dry mouth, blurred vision, constipation and urinary hesitancy). Postural hypotension may also be a problem, especially in the diabetic patient with autonomic neuropathy. Due to their sedative effect, these drugs should be given at night. The role of selective serotonin re-uptake inhibitors (SSRIs) in chronic pain is less clear but paroxetine (40 mg daily) and citalopram (40 mg daily) have been shown to be effective compared with placebo in the treatment of painful diabetic neuropathy.

Anticonvulsants

Anticonvulsants have a definite role to play in the treatment of various chronic pain conditions [3] **(II)**, and are widely use in pain clinics. Carbamazepine and phenytoin are licensed for use only in trigeminal neuralgia whilst gabapentin is licensed for use in neuropathic pain of any cause. However, these drugs are widely used outside these specific conditions. The treatment of neuropathic pain is the principle indication for anticonvulsant use although they have also been used with varying degrees of success in many pain conditions.

Most antiepileptics have been used to treat chronic pain. The commonest now used are probably carbamazepine and gabapentin. Carbamazepine is the most studied of all the anticonvulsants used in chronic pain. Effective doses for analgesia are similar to those used to treat epilepsy. Carbamazepine is usually commenced at 100 mg to 200 mg twice daily. Adverse side effects include impaired mental or motor function, headache and gastrointestinal disturbances. Major side effects such as haematological disorders (leucopenia, aplastic anaemia, and thrombocytopenia) and severe cutaneous reactions (Steven Johnson syndrome) occur in approximately 5% of cases. Gabapentin is a newer antiepileptic and has recently been granted licence for use in all types of neuropathic pain. It is well tolerated by the majority of patients. However, 25% of patients do complain of drowsiness or dizziness whilst confusion ataxia, headache and peripheral oedema occur less frequently. Dosage regimes would normally start at 300 mg a day increasing gradually to a maximum of 1.8 g in three divided doses. The most frequently encountered complaint during longer-term use seen in our pain clinic is weight gain.

Cognitive behaviour therapy

The psychological treatment of choice for chronic pain patients with maladaptive behaviour is cognitive behaviour therapy. In such patients treatment is centred not on the specific pain problem but on the detrimental effects of that pain problem. Specifically cognitive behavioural therapy is aimed at reducing the influence of factors, which maintain patients' maladaptive behaviours and beliefs. Treatment strategies include:

- Reducing the influence of situations where behaviour leads to a positive re-enforcement of the pain behaviour.

- To encourage achievable goal setting with positive re-enforcement of successes when they are achieved.

- Re-enforcement of behaviours that demonstrate healthiness and well-being.

- To increase general fitness and function.

- To educate patients to have an insight into the benefit of the above treatment aims and to encourage positive thinking and deter negative thinking. In addition it is important that patients are educated to understand the needs for self-management of their pain problem and to reduce the often inappropriate reliance on health professionals.

It is important that to achieve these treatment aims that all staff clearly understand the aims and are consistent in their overall management of the patient. Unfortunately this can be a problem with chronic pain patients as they are often seeing many other health professionals in multiple specialties and it is therefore important that conflicting models of treatment are not employed simultaneously **(A)**. Also, other health professionals involved in their care should avoid the natural tendency to alter medications and treatments until the benefits of cognitive behaviour therapy have been ascertained. A recent systematic review and meta-analysis of randomised controlled trials of cognitive behaviour therapy for adults with chronic pain [4] concluded that "published randomised controlled trials provide good evidence for the effectiveness of cognitive behaviour therapy and behaviour therapy for chronic pain in adults". Effect sizes were also high compared with non-psychological treatments for chronic pain **(II)**.

A suggested pathway for the management of a patient with non-acute pain can be seen in Figure 1.

Post-amputation pain

Almost all amputees experience phantom sensations after amputation. The incidence of phantom pain is probably somewhere between 55% and 85% [5,6,7].

Phantom pain is usually intermittent primarily being localised in the distal parts of the missing limb. It is invariably described as being of a shooting, burning,

Chapter 33

Figure 1 Algorithm for the management of the patient with non-acute pain.

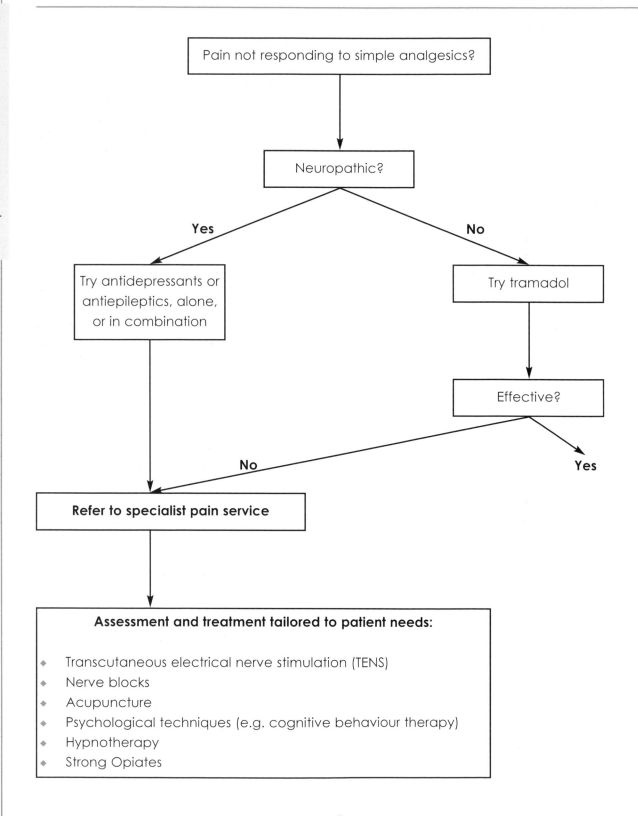

throbbing, stabbing nature. The onset of pain is usually within the first few days after surgery although it can occasionally be prolonged several months or years. The incidence of phantom limb pain does decrease a little with time, particularly in the first 6 months, as do the duration and frequency of attacks [8]. So far as risk factors for the development of phantom limb pain are concerned there is no known association with sex, site of amputation, reason for amputation or racial group. The incidence seems to be less in young children, but there is no association with age in older children or adults. Patients with pre-amputation pain may be at increased risk [8,9] **(III)**.

Stump pain is post-amputation pain, which is localised in the stump. It is quite common in the early post-amputation period, but usually subsides with healing. Before the diagnosis of stump pain is made, obvious local pathology such as infection, bone spurs and neuromas should be excluded. Stump pain persists in approximately 5%-10% of patients, is neuropathic in nature and is a particular problem as it interferes with prosthetic use. Examination of the stump often reveals hyperalgesia and allodynia.

Treatment

Treatment of phantom pain and stump pain following amputation are both difficult. Most studies looking into the treatment of phantom pain are methologically flawed and consequently clear evidence of effectiveness for differing treatment strategies is absent. Current treatment recommendations can only therefore be considered as guidelines based upon reported experiences rather than randomised controlled trials. Simple analgesics such as non-steroidal anti-inflammatories and paracetamol are usually ineffective. Treatments that have been reported as effective for phantom limb pain include tricyclic antidepressants [10], antiepileptic medications [11], opioid analgesics [12], TENS [13], acupuncture [14] and hypnotherapy [15] **(III)**. Surgical treatments such as sympathectomy, cordotomy and thalamotomy have been tried in the past. However, results have been disappointing and it is rare to find such treatments used today.

Treatment begins with vigilance and early recognition of the problem. Any patient with pain following amputation which is not responding to simple analgesics, should be considered as having phantom pain. It seems sensible to commence patients on tricyclic antidepressants and antiepileptics as soon as the diagnosis is made, and early referral to a pain specialist is recommended **(B)**. TENS and acupuncture should be tried early as they are inexpensive, simple and have no significant side effects **(B)**. Depending upon the patient's response to these simple treatments, strong opiate medication, psychological techniques and other therapies may be required.

Prevention

Studies have investigated whether the use of epidural analgesia prior to, during and following amputation can reduce the incidence of phantom limb pain. However, these studies have only been performed on small numbers of patients and the results are somewhat equivocal [16,17,18] **(III)**.

Summary

- Chronic pain may be seen in vascular surgical patients for a wide variety of reasons.

- Whatever the underlying cause it is very important that treating physicians and nurses recognise when pain is becoming chronic and understand the physical, emotional and social consequences to the patient and their family **(A)**.

- In particular, treatment should consist of multiple therapies aimed at helping the patient manage the consequences of their pain appropriately, in order to improve the quality of life for themselves and their family **(B)**.

- Early referral to multi-disciplinary pain clinics with expertise in this area is recommended **(A)**.

References (grade I evidence and grade A recommendations in bold)

1   **Bonica JJ. Importance of the problem. In: *Evaluation and treatment of Chronic Pain.* Aronhoff GM, Ed.   Baltimore.   Urban and Schwarzenburg, 1985.**

2   Sindrup SH, Jensen TS. Efficacy of pharmacological treatments of neuropathic pain: an update and effect related to mechanism of drug action. *Pain* 1999; 83: 227-230.

3   McQuay H, Carroll D, Jadad AR, Wifen P, Moore A. Anticonvulsant drugs for management of pain: A systematic review. *Br Med J* 1995; 311: 1047-1052.

4   Morley S, Eccleston C, Williams A. Systematic review and meta-analysis of randomised controlled trials of cognitive behaviour therapy and behaviour therapy for chronic pain in adults, excluding headache. *Pain* 1999; 80: 1-13.

5   Jensen TS, Krebs B, Neilson J, Rasmussen P. Phantom limb, phantom pain and stump pain in amputees during the first 6 months following limb amputation. *Pain* 1983; 17: 243-256.

6   Sherman RA, Sherman CJ. Prevalence and characteristics of chronic phantom limb pain among American veterans. Results of a trial survey. *Am J Phys Med* 1983; 62: 227-238.

7   Montoya P, Larbig W, Grulke N, Flor H, Taub E, Birbaumer N. The relationship of phantom limb pain to other phantom limb phenomena in upper extremity amputees. *Pain* 1997; 72: 87-93.

8   Jensen TS, Krebs B, Neilson J, Rasmussen P. Immediate and long-term phantom limb pain in amputees: Incidents, clinical characteristics and the relationship to pre-amputation limb pain. *Pain* 1985; 21: 267-278.

9   Nikolajsen L, Ilkjaer S, Kroner K, Christensen JH, Jensen TS. The influence of pre-amputation pain on post-amputation stump and phantom pain. *Pain* 1997; 72: 393-405.

10 Iacono RP, Sandyk R, Baumford CR, Awerbuch G, Malone JM. Post-amputation phantom pain and autonomous stump movements responsive to doxepin. *Function Neurol* 1987; 2: 343-348.

11 Elliott F, Little A, Milbrandt W. Carbamazepine for phantom limb phenomena. *N Engl J Med* 1976; 295: 678.

12 Urban BJ, France RD, Steinberger EK, Scoot DL, Maltbie AA. Long-term use of narcotics/anti-depressant medication in the management of phantom limb. *Pain* 1986; 24: 191-196.

13 Katz J, Melzack R. Auricular transcutaneous electrical nerve stimulation (TENS) reduces phantom limb pain. *J Pain Symptom Manage* 1991; 6: 73-83.

14 Ezzo J, Berman B, Hadhazy VA, Jadad AR, Lao L, Singh BB. Is acupuncture effective for the treatment of chronic pain? *Pain* 2000; 86: 217-225.

15 Siegel EF. Control of phantom limb pain by hypnosis. *Am J Clin Hypnosis* 1979; 21: 285-286.

16 Bach S, Noreng MF, Tjellden NU. Phantom limb pain in amputees during the first 12 months following limb amputation after pre-operative lumbar epidural blockade. *Pain* 1988; 33: 297-301.

17 Jahangiri M, Bradley JWP, Jayatunga AP, Dark CH. Prevention of phantom pain after major lower limb amputation by epidural infusion of diamorphine, clonidine and bupivicaine. *Ann R Coll Surg Engl* 1994; 76: 324-326.

18 Nikolajsen L, Ilkjaer S, Kroner K, Christensen JH, Jensen TS. Randomised trial of epidural bupivicaine and morphine in prevention of stump and phantom pain in lower limb amputation. *Lancet* 1997; 350: 1353-1357.

Chapter 33

Chapter 34

Surgical site infections

Nick JM London

Professor of Surgery & Honorary Consultant Vascular Surgeon

LEICESTER UNIVERSITY AND UNIVERSITY HOSPITALS OF LEICESTER TRUST, LEICESTER UK

Introduction

At any one time, 9% of patients in hospital are being treated for an infection that they acquired there and surgical site infections (SSIs) account for 11% of all hospital-acquired infections [1]. A recent survey of SSI in English hospitals [2] showed that the mean incidence of surgical site infection after vascular surgery and limb amputation was 8.1% and 14.5% respectively (I). However, it should be noted that the incidence of SSI after vascular surgery varied between 2.5% and 17% and for limb amputation between 7% and 22%, depending on the hospital surveyed. Seventy-eight percent of infections after vascular surgery were confined to the wound compared to 63% of infections after limb amputation [2].

It has been estimated that each patient with a SSI requires an additional hospital stay of 6.5 days, and hospital costs are doubled [3] (I). Deep SSIs involving organs, organ spaces or prostheses as compared to SSIs confined to the incision, are associated with an even greater increase in hospital stays and costs [4] (I). Although there is no definitive evidence that the incidence of SSIs has increased over the last 10 years, there seems little doubt that SSIs are increasingly difficult to treat. This may be partially explained by the emergence of anti-microbial resistant pathogens and the increased number of surgical patients who are elderly and/or have a wide variety of chronic debilitating or compromising underlying diseases. There has also been an increase in the number of patients receiving prosthetic implants [5] (I).

A survey of English hospitals revealed that the commonest organism to cause SSI was *Staphylococcus aureus* (38% of total infections) and of these staphylococcal infections, 61% were methicillin-resistant (MRSA) [2] (I). In the case of vascular surgery and limb amputation, 58% and 67% of all infections were caused by *Staphylococcus aureus*, of which 66% were methicillin-resistant [2] (I). MRSA is therefore the commonest cause of SSI after vascular surgery and amputation. These national data reflect our experience at the Leicester Royal Infirmary where we found that the overall SSI rate in vascular patients in 1994 and in 2000 were 5% and 4.6% respectively [6]. However, the proportion of SSIs caused by MRSA increased during the same period from 4% to 63%. In addition to the economic burden

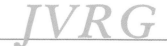

posed by all vascular SSIs, deep SSIs pose a particular threat with respect to limb loss or death. Thus in our experience, all patients with aortic graft infections died and all patients with infected prosthetic infrainguinal bypass grafts required an amputation [6].

Pathogenesis of surgical site infections

Microbial contamination of the surgical site is a necessary precursor of SSI. It has been shown that if a surgical site is contaminated with > 10^5 microorganisms per gram of tissue, the risk of SSI is markedly increased [7]. However, the dose of microorganisms required to produce SSI may be much lower when foreign material is present. This is because some bacteria that adhere to implanted medical devices, such as coagulase-negative *staphylococci*, produced a hydrated matrix of polysaccharide and protein and form a slimy layer known as a biofilm [8]. Bacteria in this biofilm are able to evade host defences and withstand antimicrobial therapy.

Source of infections

For most SSIs, the source of pathogens is the endogenous flora of the patient's skin, mucous membranes, or hollow viscera [9]. When mucous membranes or skin are incised the exposed tissues are at risk of contamination with endogenous flora. These organisms are usually aerobic gram-positive cocci (mostly *staphylococci*) but may include faecal flora (gram-negative aerobes or anaerobes) when an incision is made near the perineum or groin. Seeding of the operative site from a distant focus of infection can be another source of SSI pathogens, particularly in patients who have a prosthesis placed during the operation. Such devices provide a nidus for attachment of the organism [10]. Exogenous sources of SSI pathogens include surgical personnel, the operating room environment and all instruments and materials brought to the sterile field during an operation. Exogenous flora are primarily *staphylococci* and *streptococci* [11].

Risk factors for infections in vascular patients

There are certain recognised risk factors for SSIs that are particularly relevant to the patient undergoing vascular surgery. Thus, it is well established that patients with a coincident remote site infection are at increased risk of SSI [12] (I) and this is relevant to vascular patients with lower limb infections undergoing arterial reconstruction. Patients who are already colonised are at increased risk of SSI [13] (I) and many vascular patients are elderly and come from a nursing home environment where it has been shown that up to 17% of residents are colonised with MRSA [14]. Although there has been controversy concerning the contribution of diabetes to SSI risk, a recent study after coronary artery bypass grafting has shown a significant relationship between increasing levels of haemoglobin A_{1c} and SSI rate [15]. It has also been shown that raised glucose levels in the immediate post-operative period are associated with increased SSI risk [16] (II). A number of studies have shown that current cigarette smoking is an independent risk factor for SSI [17,18] (II). Again, this is of particular relevance to arterial surgery.

Prolonged pre-operative hospital stay is frequently cited as a risk factor patient for SSI risk [5] (I) and again many vascular patients do have a prolonged pre-operative hospital stay. Many vascular surgical procedures involve the groin and therefore require hair removal. It has been shown that pre-operative shaving of the surgical site the night before an operation is associated with a significantly higher SSI risk than either the use of depilatory agents or no hair removal [19] (II). This increased risk with shaving has been attributed to microscopic cuts in the skin that later serve as foci for bacterial multiplication. Shaving immediately before the operation compared to shaving within 24 hours pre-operatively is associated with a decreased SSI rate (3.1% versus 7.1%) [17]. Clipping hair immediately before an operation has been associated with a lower risk of SSI than shaving or clipping the night before an operation [20].

Other issues to specifically consider in the patient undergoing vascular surgery are that hypothermia (defined as a core body temperature below 36°C) increases SSI risk [21] (I) and this probably occurs because of vasoconstriction causing decreased delivery of oxygen to the wound space and subsequent impaired function of phagocytic leucocytes. A recent study has shown that in patients undergoing clean surgery that pre-operative warming reduced the SSI rate by two-thirds [22] (I) and certainly this paper taken with previous evidence suggests that hypothermia in patients undergoing vascular surgery should be minimised. Those operating on vascular patients are at increased risk of exposure to blood and although the wearing of surgical masks has not been specifically shown to reduce SSI rates [5] they should be worn in patients undergoing vascular surgery on the basis that they protect the wearer from inadvertent exposure. With respect to gowns and drapes, these should be impermeable to liquids [23].

Methods to reduce surgical site infections in vascular patients

Pre-operative measures

In view of the evidence presented above, it can be seen that whenever possible all infections remote to the surgical site should be treated prior to elective surgery (A). The pre-operative hospital stay should be kept as short as possible and tobacco cessation should be encouraged for at least 30 days prior to surgery (A). Glucose levels should be adequately controlled in diabetic patients and hyperglycaemia should be avoided peri-operatively (B). If hair removal is necessary, this should be performed immediately prior to surgery using electronic clippers (B). Although pre-operative antiseptic showers have been shown to reduce skin microbial colony counts [24], they have not been shown to reduce SSI rates [25]. Similarly, pre-operative eradication of nasal *Staphlococcus aureus* with mupirocin ointment has not been shown to reduce SSI rates [5].

Antibiotic prophylaxis

In general terms it is recommended that antibiotic prophylaxis in the context of clean operations is used whenever intravascular prosthetic material is inserted or for an operation in which a deep infection could pose a catastrophic risk [5] (A). Thus, although vascular procedures are usually clean, they frequently qualify for prophylaxis. The agent used for prophylaxis in vascular surgery should be active against *staphylococci*, should be administered intravenously and should be given at least 30 minutes prior to skin incision. Although there is no evidence to support a prolonged course of antibiotic prophylaxis in vascular patients, most surgeons continue prophylaxis for at least 24 hours and for longer in patients with indwelling central venous or arterial lines (B).

The routine use of vancomycin for prophylaxis is not recommended for any kind of surgery, because of the risk of promoting vancomycin resistance [26]. However, there may be certain clinical circumstances where vancomycin prophylaxis may be desirable. These include a cluster of SSIs due to MRSA or prophylaxis in patients known to be colonised with MRSA. These situations should always be discussed with the local infection control team [26].

Intra-operative measures

The most commonly used antiseptic agents for pre-operative skin preparation are the iodophores (e.g., povidone-iodine), alcohol-containing products or chlorhexidine gluconate. There are no well-controlled studies that have compared the effects of these agents on SSI rates [5]. One potential disadvantage of alcohol is its flammability. The antiseptic should be applied in concentric circles, starting at the site of the proposed incision. The surgeon should wear a face mask and gowns, and drapes that are effective barriers when wet should be used [5] (B). Surgical technique is thought to be important in the prevention of SSI. Haemostasis should be effective whilst preserving blood supply, devitalised tissue should be removed and dead space should be eradicated. If drains are used they should be closed suction and not be placed through the incision. Hypothermia should be avoided [21,22] (A).

Other techniques, that require further research before they could be recommended as being advantageous for prosthetic work include the use of separate "clean" theatres and laminar flow tents.

Post-operative measures

The majority of wounds in vascular surgery are closed primarily and covered with a dressing for 24 to 48 hours. There is no evidence of benefit from covering with a dressing beyond 48 hrs [5]. All drains pose an infection risk and should be removed as soon as they have stopped draining, usually within 24 hours [5] **(B)**.

Specific MRSA issues

Background

Methicillin-resistant strains of *Staphylococcus aureus* were first described in England in 1961 shortly after methicillin became available for clinical use [27]. Over the last 10 years MRSA has become an increasingly important pathogen and MRSA is now the commonest cause of SSIs in English hospitals [2] **(I)**. It is important to note that MRSA is not an additional infection burden, but instead is replacing methicillin-sensitive *Staphylococcus aureus*. Thus, in our own experience at the Leicester Royal Infirmary [6], the overall SSI rate in vascular patients did not change significantly between 1994 and 2000 (5.0% and 4.6% respectively), but the proportion caused by MRSA increased from 4% to 63%.

MRSA is proving a particularly difficult infection to treat and this may be for a number of reasons. First, the reason that most MRSA have not developed resistance to vancomycin is because its relatively low efficacy and high toxicity meant that it was only rarely used to treat *Staphylococcus aureus* infections. Thus *Staphylococci* were not exposed to vancomycin on a regular basis and have not become widely resistant to it. Paradoxically therefore, although most MRSA remain sensitive to vancomycin, this reflects the fact that vancomycin is a relatively ineffective antibiotic. In addition, because vancomycin is one of the few antibiotics to which MRSA remains sensitive, it has not been recommended for prophylaxis for fear of inducing resistance. It could be argued therefore that current antibiotic prophylaxis regimes "select out" MRSA because they are effective against the majority of bacteria apart from MRSA. It has been reported that

one of the unique features of MRSA is its ability to cause vein as well as prosthetic graft disruption [6,28]. Whether or not this is indeed a specific feature of MRSA or instead reflects our inability to treat the infection efficiently remains uncertain.

Prevention of MRSA infections

In addition to all of the measures discussed above, it has become apparent in recent years that handwashing by those looking after surgical patients is crucial in minimising MRSA infections [29] **(I)**. Indeed, it has been found that hand hygiene reduces the relative risk of MRSA transmission by 50% [29] **(I)**. Although formal handwashing with soap and water is required when there is soiling, alcohol-glycerol hand rubs cause less irritation than soap and decontaminates hands more effectively for a wide variety of organisms, including *S. aureus*, *Pseudomonas aeruginosa* and *Klebsiella* spp [29,30] **(I)**.

Alcohol glycerol hand rub dispensers should be located at each patient's bedside and used between each patient contact **(B)**.

Treatment of MRSA infection

Vancomycin is currently the drug of choice for treating MRSA infections caused by multi-drug resistant strains. Some strains are susceptible to rifampicin and adding this to vancomycin may improve outcome. Rifampicin should not be used alone to treat MRSA infections because *S. aureus* strains easily develop resistance to this agent. An alternative glycopeptide to vancomycin is teicoplanin. The advantages of teicoplanin are that it has low toxicity and can be given once daily, the disadvantage is its expense. There are no published studies that have addressed the duration of vancomycin therapy in patients with MRSA infections. It has been our policy to treat patients with vascular graft infections for a minimum of 6 weeks and for other infections (wound, pneumonia) to continue vancomycin for a week after clinical resolution of the infection. In order to minimise the psychological sequelae of prolonged patient isolation, we have managed some patients at home

Table 1 Treatment of MRSA carriers. Such treatment must be guided by an infection control physician.

Nasal carriage

♦ Apply mupirocin 2% in a paraffin base (Bactroban Nasal) to each nostril three times daily for 5 days.

♦ Culture nasal swab 2 days after treatment; if positive, repeat the treatment once and check also for throat carriage.

♦ If nasal swab remains positive, or the strain shows mupirocin resistance, consider alternative topical treatment (e.g. 0.5% neomycin + 0.1% chlorhexidine cream (Naseptin) or 1% chlorhexidine cream).

♦ Avoid repeated courses of mupirocin and the topical use of antibiotics that may be required for systemic use (e.g. fusidic acid, gentamicin).

Skin carriage

♦ Daily antiseptic bathing for 5 days (repeated if necessary) e.g. with 4% chlorhexidine, 2% triclosan, or 7.5% povidone-iodine.

♦ Wash hair twice weekly with an antiseptic shampoo/detergent.

♦ Hexachlorophane 0.33% powder for axillary or groin carriage.

Throat carriage

♦ Significance in relation to spread is unclear. May be difficult to eradicate.

♦ If there is clear evidence of transmission, consider a single 5-day course of oral treatment with either rifampicin plus fusidic acid or for susceptible organisms, ciprofloxacin.

after an initial period of in-patient treatment. This can be achieved by inserting a Hickman line and arranging for the District Nursing Service to administer teicoplanin once a day.

Two new antimicrobials that have activity against MRSA have recently become available. Quinupristin/daflopristin (Synercid) is a synergistic combination of two streptogramins [31]. However, it is only bacteriostatic and has to be given intravenously. The oxazolidones are a new class of antimicrobials with activity against MRSA. One of this group, oxazolidone (Linezolid) is orally active against *enterococci*, *pneumococci* and *S. aureus*, including MRSA. Resistance to both of these new agents has already been described and they should therefore only

Chapter 34

be used under the guidance of an infection expert [32] **(B)**. Both of these antibiotics are broad spectrum and this in itself may encourage the development of opportunistic resistance; for this reason future drug development must focus on targeted therapy.

Eradication of MRSA in known carriers

A recent study from our unit (in press) has shown that 4% of patients admitted for arterial surgery are colonised by MRSA. Presumably such patients are at a relatively higher risk for developing a MRSA surgical site infection. The management of such patients should first of all be a reconsideration of the risk/benefit ratios of reconstructive surgery and in the case of lower limb arterial occlusive disease, angioplasty, if possible, may be a lower risk alternative. If surgery is unavoidable then it would seem sensible to attempt eradication of MRSA prior to surgery and the methods for doing this are given in Table 1. The issue of vancomycin prophylaxis and its duration should be discussed with a consultant in communicable diseases.

Whether or not it is worthwhile or cost-effective to screen certain patients such as those previously known to have had MRSA or those who are transferred from nursing homes, has not been investigated in prospective studies.

Summary

General points

♦ The mean incidence of SSI after vascular surgery in English hospitals is 8% **(I)**. Each patient with a SSI requires an additional hospital stay of 6.5 days and hospital costs are doubled **(I)**.

♦ Vascular patients are at increased risk of SSI because many of the well recognised risk factors for SSI are prevalent amongst them **(I)**

♦ MRSA is the commonest cause of SSI after vascular surgery and amputation **(I)**. Hand-washing, particularly with alcohol-glycerol hand rubs reduces the risk of MRSA transmission by 50% **(I)**. Alcohol hand-rub should be available at every bedside and used prior to any contact with patients.**(B)**

Pre-operatively

♦ Encourage tobacco cessation for at least 30 days prior to surgery **(B)**.

♦ Identify and treat all infections remote to the surgical site before surgery **(A)**.

♦ Keep pre-operative hospital stay as short as possible **(A)**.

♦ Do not remove hair pre-operatively unless the hair around the incision site will interfere with the operation. If hair has to be removed, do this immediately prior to the operation, preferably with an electric clipper **(B)**.

Peri-operatively

♦ Prevent peri-operative hypothermia **(A)**.

♦ Glucose levels should be adequately controlled in diabetic patients and hyperglycaemia should be avoided **(B)**.

♦ Administer a prophylactic antimicrobial agent according to published recommendations **(A)**. Do not routinely use vancomycin for antimicrobial prophylaxis **(B)**.

♦ Use surgical gowns and drapes that are effective barriers when wet **(B)**. Thoroughly wash and clean around the incision site and use an appropriate antiseptic agent for skin preparation **(B)**.

♦ If drains are used they should be closed suction and should be removed as soon as they have stopped draining, usually within 24 hours **(B)**.

Further reading

1   London NJM, Nasim A. Management of methicillin-resistant *Staphylococcus aureus* infection in vascular patients. In: *The Evidence for Vascular Surgery*. JJ Earnshaw, JA Murie, Eds. tfm publishing Limited, Shropshire, 1999: 183-188.

2   Mangram AJ, Horan TC, Pearson ML, *et al*. Guideline for prevention of surgical site infection, 1999. *Am J Infect Control* 1999; 27: 97-134.

References (grade I evidence and grade A recommendations in bold)

1   Report by the Comptroller and Auditor General. The Management and Control of Hospital Acquired Infection in Acute NHS Trust in England. The Stationery Office, London, 2000.

2   **Surveillance of surgical site infection in English hospitals 1997-1999. Public Health Laboratory Service, London.**

3   **Plowman R, Graves N, Griffin M, *et al*. The socio-economic burden of hospital-acquired infection. Public Health Laboratory Service, London, 2000.**

4   **Vegas AA, Jodra VM, Garcia ML. Nosocomial infection in surgery wards: A controlled study of increased duration of hospital stays and direct cost of hospitalisation. *Eur J Epidemiol* 1993; 9(5): 504-510.**

5   **Mangram AJ, Horan TC, Pearson ML, *et al*. Guideline for prevention of surgical site infection, 1999. *Am J Infect Control* 1999; 27: 97-134.**

6   Nasim A, Thompson MM, Naylor AR, Bell PRF, London NJM. The impact of MRSA on vascular surgery. *Eur J Vasc Endovasc Surg* 2001; 22: 211-214.

7   Krizek TJ, Robson MC. Evolution of quantitative bacteriology in wound management. *Am J Surg* 1975; 130: 579-584.

8   Stewart PS, Costerton JW. Antibiotic resistance of bacteria in biofilms. *Lancet* 2001; 358: 135-138.

9   Altemeier WA, Culbertson WR, Hummel RP. Surgical considerations of endogenous infections - sources, types, and methods of control. *Surg Clin North Am* 1968; 48: 227-240.

10 Goeau-Brissonniere O, Leport C, Guidoin R, *et al*. Experimental colonization of an expanded polytetrafluoroethylene vascular graft with *Staphylococcus aureus*: A quantitative and morphologic study. *J Vasc Surg* 1987; 5(5): 743-748.

11 Calia FM, Wolinsky E, Mortimer EA Jr., *et al*. Importance of the carrier state as a source of *Staphylococcus aureus* in wound sepsis. *J Hyg* (Lond) 1969; 67: 49-57.

12 Valentine RJ, Weigelt JA, Dryer D, *et al*. Effect of remote infections on clean wound infection rates. *Am J Infect Control* 1986; 14: 64-67.

13 **Perl TM, Golub JE. New approaches to reduce *Staphylococcus aureus* nosocomial infection rates: Treating S. aureus nasal carriage. *Ann Pharmacother* 1998; 32: S7-S16.**

14 Fraise AP, Mitchell K, O'Brien SJ, *et al*. Methicillin-resistant *Staphylococcus aureus* (MRSA) in nursing homes in a major UK city; an anonymised point prevalence surgery. *Epidemiol Infect* 1997; 118: 1-5.

15 Gordon SM, Serkey JM, Barr C, *et al*. The relationship between glycosylated hemoglobin (HgA1C) levels and postoperative infections in patients undergoing primary coronary artery bypass surgery (CABG). *Infect Control Hosp Epidemiol* 1997; 19: 29.

16 Zerr KJ, Furnary AP, Grunkemcier GL, *et al*. Glucose control lowers the risk of wound infection in diabetics after open heart operations. *Ann Thorac Surg* 1997; 63: 356-361.

17 Bryan AJ, Lamarra M, Angelini GD, *et al*. Median sternotomy wound dehiscence: a retrospective case control study of risk factors and outcome. *J R Coll Surg Edin* 1992; 37: 305-308.

18 Vinton AL, Rraverso LW, Jolly PC. Wound complications after modified radical mastectomy compared with tylectomy with axillary lymph node dissection. *Am J Surg* 1991; 161: 584-588.

19 Seropian R, Reynolds BM. Wound infections after preoperative depilatory versus razor preparation. *Am J Surg* 1971; 121: 251-254.

20 Masterton TM, Rodeheaver GT, Morgan RF, *et al*. Bacteriologic evaluation of electric clippers for surgical hair removal. *Am J Surg* 1984; 148: 301-302.

21 **Kurz A, Sessler DI, Lenhardt R. Perioperative normothermia to reduce the incidence of surgical-wound infection and shorten hospitalisation. Study of Wound Infection and Temperature Group. *N Engl J Med* 1996; 334: 1209-1215.**

22 **Melling AC, Baqar A, Scott E, *et al*. Effects of preoperative warming on the incidence of wound infection after clean surgery: a randomised controlled trial. *Lancet* 2001; 358: 876-880.**

23 Granzow JW, Smith JW, Nichols RL, *et al*. Evaluation of the protective value of hospital gowns against blood strike-through and methicillin-resistant *Staphylococcus aureus* penetration. *Am J Infect Control* 1998; 26: 85-93.

24 Hayek LJ, Emerson JM, Gardner AM. A placebo-controlled trial of the effect of two pre-operative baths or showers with chlorhexidine detergent on postoperative wound infection rates. *J Hosp Infect* 1987; 10: 165-172.

25 Leigh DA, Stronge JL, Marriner J, Sedgwick J. Total body bathing with 'Hibiscrub' (chlorhexidine) in surgical patients: a controlled trial. *J Hosp Infect* 1983; 4: 229-235.

26 Hospital Infection Control Practices Advisory Committee. Recommendations for preventing the spread of vancomycin resistance. *Infect Control Hosp Epidemiol* 1995; 16: 105-113.

27 Michel M, Gutmann L. Methicillin-resistant *Staphylococcus aureus* and vancomycin-resistant *enterococci*: therapeutic realities and possibilities. *Lancet* 1997; 349: 1901-6.

28 Chalmers RTA, Wolfe JHN, Cheshire NJW *et al.* Improved management of infrainguinal bypass graft infection with methicillin-resistant *Staphylococcus aureus*. *Br J Surg* 1999; 86: 1433-1436.

29 Pittet D, Hugonnet S, Harbarth S, *et al.* Effectiveness of a hospital-wide programme to improve compliance with hand hygiene. *Lancet* 2000; 356: 1307-1312.

30 Teare L, Cookson B, Stone S. Hand hygiene. *BMJ* 2001; 323: 411-412.

31 Johnson AP, Livermore DM. Quinupristin/dalfopristin, a new addition to the antimicrobial arsenal. *Lancet* 1999; 354: 2012-13.

32 Linezolid for Gram-positive infections. *Drug and Therapeutic Bulletin* 2001; 39: 54-56.

Chapter 34

Chapter 35

Medico-legal and risk management issues

Bruce Campbell

Professor & Consultant Surgeon

DEPARTMENT OF SURGERY, ROYAL DEVON AND EXETER HOSPITAL, EXETER, UK

Introduction

The possibility of complaint or medico-legal action against surgeons has become an increasing threat in recent times. Combined with huge media coverage of "the Bristol affair" and other medical scandals there has been a demand for all those in the health services to monitor their performance, to learn from adverse events, and to seek ways of improving their practice [1,2]. This is part of the culture of "clinical governance" which has placed upon hospital chief executives and others a personal responsibility for these matters. Unlike most of the other areas in this book, there are no randomised trials on clinical governance or risk management. There is some published information on adverse events and medico-legal activity in vascular surgery, but measures to prevent or limit such problems have never reached the point of scientific study. This lack of "scientific evidence" does not, however, prevent recommendation of a whole succession of steps in the pathway of hospital care which will reduce the likelihood of medico-legal claims and complaints [3].

The Evidence

Vascular surgery has featured high on the list of specialities causing damage to patients in major studies of adverse events. In the Harvard Medical Practice Study [4] of 30,121 randomly selected hospital records, the percentage of adverse events was higher in vascular surgery (16%) than any other discipline, although interestingly the proportion judged to result from negligence was lower than other specialties (18%). Another major study from the United States (on 15,000 hospital admissions in Utah and Colorado) [5] found that the two operations most frequently associated with preventable adverse events involved the specialty of vascular surgery - lower limb bypass grafting (14% adverse event rate, with 11% judged preventable) and aortic aneurysm repair (19% and 8% respectively).

The Quality in Australian Health Care Study [6] (14,000 admissions) found an adverse event rate of 3% among vascular surgical patients, of which 49% were judged preventable, and 32% resulted in major permanent disability. This result needs to be viewed

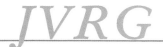

with caution because the adverse event rate in general surgery was higher than all other specialties (13%) and, like the studies from the United States [4-5] vascular surgery probably meant arterial surgery. This is important, because evidence from the UK shows that treatment of varicose veins (the commonest type of vascular surgical operation) is the most frequent cause of litigation against vascular and general surgeons [7].

In the UK, operations for varicose veins (properly the province of interested vascular surgeons) far outnumber all procedures for arterial disease, and these pose a special challenge in terms of information for patients, consent, and risk management. Records of medico-legal claims notified to the National Health Service Litigation Authority (NHSLA) and the Medical Defence Union (MDU) show that treatment of varicose veins is the commonest reason for medico-legal action against vascular and general surgeons (Table 1) [8] and they confirm that aortic and femorodistal work are high risk areas in arterial practice. Issues relating to inadequate counselling, information, and documentation are recurring themes. From a medico-legal standpoint this is all part of the process of consent (and documentation thereof). Therefore, it is worth making some general points about this process at the outset.

Table 1 Claims relating to the treatment of (a) varicose veins and (b) arterial disease, notified to the National Health Service Litigation Authority (NHSLA) since its inception in 1995 (totals - 84 for varicose veins and 80 for arterial disease) and to the Medical Defence Union (MDU) during the years 1990-9 (totals - 160 and 94 respectively). The NHSLA receives notification only about claims against NHS hospitals in excess of a certain value (about £5,000-10,000). The MDU figures are a reflection of private practice in the United Kingdom.

Varicose veins

Nerve damage	76
Incorrect/inadequate/unsatisfactory surgery	36
Discolouration/scarring after sclerotherapy	21
Femoral vein damage	16
Infection	15
Femoral artery damage	13
Deep vein thrombosis	11
Tourniquet damage	5
Miscellaneous	51

Arterial disease

Complications of aortic surgery	45
Failure to recognise/treat ischaemia	36
Bypass grafting problems	28
Nerve damage at operation	16
Failure to diagnose/treat aneurysms	10
Miscellaneous	39

Some general points about informed consent

The process of informed consent starts during the patient's first encounter with the surgeon, and continues right up to the moment that they submit to treatment. Some particular points to remember about informed consent are:

♦ Consent can either be implied (the patient undresses; allows application of a blood pressure cuff; arrives on the ward; gets on to operating theatre trolley) or express (the patient signs a consent form - but note that this is just one step in the process of informed consent).

♦ Patients only retain a small proportion of what they are told (and they may have misunderstood even this). Written information is essential in the setting of planned, elective treatment.

♦ From the medico-legal and governance standpoints no advice, counselling, giving of written information, or consent is likely to withstand analysis in retrospect unless it has been documented. If there are no written records, a court of law is likely to believe the patient's account of what they were told rather than the surgeon's.

Steps in the pathway of hospital care - medico-legal and risk management aspects

A summary of risk management considerations are outlined in Table 2.

Action on receiving the referral

Risk management starts here, because undue delay in seeing a patient with a condition which turns out to be urgent can result in a complaint or medico-legal claim. Vascular surgeons are fortunate compared with many other specialists because the degree of urgency is usually obvious (for example reference to suspected ischaemic rest pain makes the referral "urgent", while aching varicose veins are

never urgent: these referral cues contrast with "rectal bleeding" or "breast lump"). If in doubt about the nature of a referral contact the referring doctor - a delay in seeing genuine ischaemic rest pain may be a disaster, while wasting an urgent appointment on a patient with metatarsalgia is inefficient and annoying.

Some conditions may not require the patient to be seen at all - investigations can be arranged and the patient informed courteously by letter, without ever being seen in a busy NHS clinic. This results in a happy patient and savings to the service. One example is the "pulsatile lump in the neck" - almost always a tortuous carotid artery (write the patient a nice letter; arrange a scan; and then write to reassure them - a good medico-legal record of events).

A different kind of example is the referral of cosmetic varicose veins and/or thread veins, in areas of the country where these are not eligible for NHS treatment. Writing a polite letter to the general practitioner (I copy the letter to the patient) to clarify the situation is always preferable to meeting a patient in clinic and telling them then that they are not eligible for treatment - this simply invites dissatisfaction and complaint.

The out-patient clinic appointment - who sees the patient?

This chapter assumes competent, thorough assessment and treatment, and dwells on other aspects of risk management. It is, however, important to consider who does all these things. Always the consultant? A Specialist Registrar (how senior, and how experienced in vascular work?)? A Senior House Officer? Diagnostic and operative experience are always important considerations in allocating responsibility to trainees, but their skill in counselling patients is very variable. Many still regard talking to patients and documentation as unimportant compared with their operative ability (I always tell my trainees "You can teach a monkey to operate - I want you to look after my patients and talk to them!"). If trainees are to see and advise patients in clinic without substantial input from the consultant, risk management demands that they should:

Table 2 Risk management considerations in the pathway of vascular surgical care.

Steps in the pathway of care	Risk management matters to consider
Referral letter received	Degree of urgency? Is referral appropriate?
Out-patient clinic visit	Who sees the patient? Thorough counselling, including choices, expectations and risks. Involve family or friends Give written information Write explicit letter ? Deal with consent form
Pre-admission	?clinic with anaesthetist/surgical team/vascular nurse/ward nurse Check written information and consent Care pathway should specify when bloods/ECG/anaesthetic assessment are done
Admission	Check procedure: mark side Counsel patient again Sign consent (if not done before)
At operation	Adequate supervision of trainees Check all precautions (antibiotic and thromboembolism prophylaxis) Explicit operation note Consider written post-operative instructions Consider telephoning relatives (especially after major surgery or when prognosis is poor)
After operation	Tell patient (and relatives) - especially anything unexpected, and document Good records of any adverse events Clinical incident report if any disaster or dissatisfaction
Care after discharge	Clear advice to return if important deterioration occurs (document)

- Be allocated cases commensurate with their level of clinical experience (this does not always correlate with their seniority on the training programme).

- Avoid making definite decisions if they are uncertain, instead advising the patient as far as possible, explaining the situation, and subsequently discussing the case with the consultant.

- Recording in each letter that they are seeing the patient on behalf of a named consultant, ideally with a brief reason when they are seeing more complex cases (for example: "Thank you for your letter about Mr. Brown, whom I saw on behalf of Professor Campbell because he was in theatre with an emergency").

- Advise the patient thoroughly in the style of the consultant for whom they are working.

- Observe all the "risk management" points of letter writing described below.

Discussion with the patient

When a diagnosis is made which might require intervention the patient needs to be advised about a whole range of matters [9-10]: this is the first (and probably the most important) part of obtaining informed consent. Be certain that any relatives or friends attending with the patient are invited to be present - for high risk procedures such as major arterial surgery I insist on talking to the spouse (or any close, caring relative) as well, ideally at the clinic visit, but failing this at a later date. Fundamental among the points which need to be covered are:

- Details of the diagnosis and prognosis, including the prognosis without treatment.

- Different treatment options, including the option not to treat.

- Likely outcome of treatment, including the expected benefit and the risks of failure.

- Information about the recovery, including common side effects of the treatment.

- Risks of treatment - particularly those which are frequent or likely, and any which are very serious.

There are many other areas which may need to be covered, depending on the patient and the circumstances, and which are set out in the General Medical Council guidance on "Seeking patients' consent: the ethical considerations" [10]. This seems a formidable list, posing real problems in surgical specialties with high volume "minor" procedures. Vascular surgeons tend to deal electively with:

- Major arterial procedures - small in number and relatively high in risk - for which shared decision making and informed consent inevitably require a fair amount of time.

- Varicose veins - more difficult because of larger patient numbers and still a perception that they are "less important" (not a threat to life or limb, and many patients with comparatively trivial complaints). It is a frustrating paradox that treatment decisions and counselling often take longest for patients with the smallest varicose veins and the most trivial symptoms. However, these may well be the patients who pose the highest risk of complaint or medico-legal action - the surgical indications for treatment are marginal and the patient's expectations are high. Surgeons need to design and teach their own "systems" for advising these patients concisely but thoroughly.

Written patient information material

Most vascular surgeons now have written information about the procedures which they commonly undertake, but the requirements for advice booklets have advanced year upon year - especially with regard to the information they should contain about choices and risks. Producing good information booklets *de novo* does take time: they need to present a sensible balance between "welcome" information (what the operation involves; what happens afterwards; advice about the convalescence) and "unwelcome" information (chances of failure; expected problems like pain and bruising; and more serious complications). Information about complications ought nowadays to include some kind of reference to all serious recognised risks (including death). Succinct phraseology about many of these can be fairly "standard" for all booklets used in any surgical department: there is a huge potential for "reinventing the wheel" and existing information packages are available which can be amended in minor ways to suit each surgeon's practice. The package on "Varicose Veins" on the patient information website of the Vascular Surgical Society of Great Britain and Ireland [11] is an example of the detailed required by the NHS Direct.

When writing new patient information material, I always ensure that the draft has been read by all local consultant colleagues who may use it; nurses; a variety of patients and other lay people (for example hospital domestic staff). The comments made by these people may seem unnecessary and annoying, but they are important in crafting information packages which are thorough, understandable to all patients, and destined for use by all local clinicians. All written advice material must be dated, have an identifiable source (authorship), and it must be archived, so that a "master copy" can be produced in the event of a legal claim years later. Archiving must be done in a way which will make crystal clear which booklet a patient was given in any particular month or year.

If a claim arises, the patient can always assert that they did not read the information they were given. However, a robust defence can be mounted, provided a written record was made that a specific booklet was given, and an archived example is available. Additional measures which may assist in defending such a claim are an introductory paragraph in each booklet, specifically asking patients to read the sections on problems and risks, or a written record that the patient was advised to read these parts of the text.

It is now also necessary to consider whether patients should be given specific written information about blood transfusion (and its potential risks) and about anaesthesia (including the risks of epidurals, spinals, etc.). There may seem a risk of overburdening patients with information leaflets, but it is now probably appropriate to give such information to selected patient groups (for example about blood transfusion to those facing aortic surgery).

All the points made about booklets are equally applicable to videos, CDs, and other electronic means of giving patients information packages. However, printed booklets and sheets simply remain the easiest and most widely applicable means of giving detailed information at the present time. Information leaflets for common vascular conditions and procedures can be found on the website.

Answering patients' questions

Many patients nowadays have sought to become informed about their conditions and possible treatments before meeting a specialist (whether they are always well informed is another matter). They may ask searching questions about alternative treatments which must be respected and answered. Increasingly they will enquire about the outcomes of individual surgeons and hospitals. I advise proffering "benchmark" information (for example personal mortality figures for aortic aneurysm surgery, or personal stroke rates after carotid endarterectomy) as a matter of routine, and recording that the patient has been informed about these in the out-patient clinic letter.

Letters to referring doctors and to patients

These are a cornerstone of risk management. Apart from a description of the clinical problems and findings, copies of letters in the healthcare record offer the quickest way of recording what the patient was told in terms of treatment choices, pros and cons of treatment, risks, and information about the recovery.

When patients are unsure about treatment, or when they have difficult choices to make, then sending them a copy of any letter may be both helpful to them, and an additional step in risk management. I do this frequently, saying to patients ".......... some of the letter will be in technical language, but the choices will be clear". Always ensure that letters make clear that a copy has been sent to the patient: the referring doctor needs to know, and the copy in the healthcare record provides medico-legal evidence.

Quite apart from copying "medical" letters to patients, writing directly to them (usually with a copy to the family doctor) offers major potential benefits.

♦ Letters allow patients time to digest information at home and to consider points with their family and friends.

♦ Copies of such letters provide tangible evidence of the information given to the patient if medico-legal action ensues. There can be no reasonable argument that the patient "was not told" anything written in a letter to them.

♦ If a provisional plan has already been made in clinic, writing to the patient after investigations have been done (for example after a duplex scan or arteriogram) may save another clinic visit, as well as providing good evidence of a further step in the process of informed consent.

♦ Following a complex inpatient referral, an immediate letter to the patient is hugely appreciated; it saves endless writing in the notes (I may simply write "For conservative treatment. Discussed. Will dictate letter".) and provides a high level of "risk management" record keeping without great expenditure of time.

Admission to hospital and pre-operative preparation

Admission to hospital now often occurs very shortly before planned procedures, either as part of hospital strategy; for day case operations; or increasingly because of unexpected lack of inpatient beds. For planned admissions shortly before operation all counselling about the procedures should already have been done: advice ought simply to be repetition (concentrating on the practicalities rather than the risks at this stage) although the patient may have concerns or questions which need to be handled

sympathetically - both for pastoral and for medico-legal reasons. This may, however, be the first time that many patients meet the anaesthetist: it is therefore important that concerns about anaesthesia have been dealt with in advance. Last minute changes of plan present special risks of complaint or litigation.

Unexpected lack of inpatient beds for major procedures worries most surgeons, and it may be that care pathways have to be revised in ways which allow for comprehensive preparation of patients without the expectation of admission the day before surgery. This may not only mean preadmission clinics (involving anaesthetists) but also new patterns of working on surgical wards (for example nursing shifts which allow admission very early in the morning).

At the time of admission to hospital it is essential that the relevant investigations are reviewed (for example the arteriogram before bypass surgery or the duplex scan before carotid endarterectomy). The "side" must be marked - amputation of the wrong digit or even the wrong limb still occurs (less of a risk in vascular practice, when there is usually obvious ischaemic damage, but still a disaster waiting to happen). Any changes in the patient's clinical state must be recorded and considered, especially if there has been a long interval between investigation and admission. (Has a tight carotid stenosis occluded? Has the femoral pulse vanished prior to femorodistal bypass? Has their ischaemic rest pain resolved?). The consent form needs to be dealt with if it has not been signed before, and this deserves some special comments.

The consent form

All hospitals require consent forms to be signed before surgical operations. In vascular practice signed consent is also necessary for endovascular treatments (angioplasty, stenting, lysis) and is generally used prior to arteriograms (which rarely can cause serious complications). Traditionally, signing of the consent form is done after admission to hospital - often in hurried circumstances. This practice, and a number of widespread misunderstandings about consent forms need to be considered when designing care pathways:

The legal status of the consent form

The patient's signature on a consent form is one important piece of evidence that consent was given, but it is no more than a part of the evidence, and from the legal standpoint the consent form is essentially "hearsay". Other pieces of documented evidence relating to information given and consent (for example letters and notes) are just as important, and are often more explicit.

When the form is signed

Patients should have the opportunity to study and consider the consent form, and expecting them to sign under any pressure of time just before the operation risks censure, in the event of any medico-legal claim regarding consent. It is entirely reasonable for consent forms to be signed at some time before admission to hospital (for example in clinic). There is an ill-defined legal requirement to reaffirm the patient's consent shortly before the operation if much time (for example more than a month or two) has elapsed since the initial form was signed.

Which doctor should sign the form

Ideally this should be either the consultant or one of the surgical team who is capable both of doing the procedure and answering any questions about it. This is understandably regarded as a chore by many consultants, and can pose logistic difficulties for them (the patient may need time to digest information after the clinic visit, and then be admitted to hospital very shortly before operation - often at an unpredictable time). Local agreements about when forms can be signed (for example in clinic) may facilitate their signing by senior clinicians.

If there is explicit information in the health record about what the patient has been told, then signing of the consent form by a more junior doctor may be reasonable, provided that the patient does not ask that doctor questions which he cannot answer competently (when a more senior member of the team must become involved).

Handling of the consent form

This is the subject of huge misunderstandings, resolution of which could improve matters greatly for both doctors and patients. When dealing with consent forms in the design of care pathways it is important to understand that:

♦   Signing of the consent form does *not* need to be witnessed. It is entirely reasonable for the patient to consider and sign the form in private.

♦   The form does *not* need to be handed to the patient by the doctor who has signed it, nor retrieved from the patient by that doctor. Failure to understand this is one of the biggest obstacles in the efficient handling of consent forms. There is no reason why a signed form should not be handed to the patient and retrieved from them by any designated member of the hospital staff, provided that they are not called upon to answer any queries which may arise. Delegating the "handling" of consent forms to others facilitates the signing of forms by senior doctors who have advised patients. (I have never understood why consent forms cannot be dealt with by post - like other admission details - the patient being advised not to sign if they have any remaining queries).

The operation

Advice about the safe conduct of vascular operations could be expanded to fill a book, but particular considerations from a medico-legal standpoint include:

♦   The side and site of the operation should be checked again before starting the procedure.

♦   Adequate supervision of trainees.

♦   Prophylactic measures should always be checked by the operating surgeon - specifically the appropriate administration of prophylactic antibiotics and antithrombotic prophylaxis.

At the end of the operation:

◆ An adequate operation note should be written immediately in the healthcare record (preferably in a distinctive way - such as in red ink - this should be agreed locally). This may be very brief for straightforward operations if a typed note is to follow, but it must contain adequate information for others who might be called to see the patient - especially after emergency, complex or unusual procedures.

◆ Adequate post-operative instructions must be written. In other countries (for example the United States) these are very comprehensive, and it is likely that practice in the United Kingdom will move in this direction. Nevertheless, it is prudent to write down any instructions which are particularly important (for example: "Must continue Dextran 40 by IV pump. Foot pulses not palpable. Observe that foot is pink: if colour changes call me"). If this is not done and nurses do not alert the surgical team to an important change, then needless acrimony can occur, especially if a medico-legal claim ensues.

◆ Dictate an explicit operation note. This is an ideal opportunity to record the reasons for decisions; what the patient and relatives were told immediately before the operation; special difficulties; and concerns about prognosis. Details of important prophylactic measures can also be placed on record in the operation note, to emphasize a high standard of care.

◆ Consider telephoning or talking to close relatives immediately, especially if an operation has been complex; if the findings or procedure were unexpected; or if the prognosis is poor. This indicates a high level of concern and care; it prepares relatives for the possibility of an adverse outcome; and it helps to create a relationship between the surgeon and the family which makes inappropriate complaint or medico-legal action much less likely.

After the operation

Be sure that the patient and their relatives know what was found and what was done (again a brief written record "Fully explained to patient" is invaluable). If any kind of complication, mishap, or adverse event has occurred (or if one occurs subsequently) explain this clearly to the patient, and to appropriate relatives (yet again, record this - "Discussed with Mr. Brown and his wife"). If any mishap has been a result of accident, then there is no harm in being open to the patient about this, and apologising, in a careful and appropriate way. Such explanation and apology should always be done at a senior level. It is far better to have an open rapport with the patient about adverse events than later to be accused of any kind of "cover up".

Clinical incident reporting

Clinical incident reports are aimed at "damage limitation" if any adverse event occurs [12]. Nurses and other professions allied to medicine have long regarded "Incident Reports" as a normal aspect of practice [13], but many doctors still seem to have difficulty with the concept and practicalities of submitting reports on clinical incidents. These difficulties are related to:

◆ Concern about the way reports might be used by hospital managers, and possible disciplinary action.

◆ Fear that a report will be seen as admission of negligence (especially when they believe that they have not been negligent).

◆ Concern that if they submit incident reports regularly, they will appear to be having more bad outcomes than their colleagues.

◆ A belief that submitting reports is a waste of time.

◆ Lack of time in a busy life.

All surgeons need to understand that the prime purpose of clinical incident reporting is to protect them and their hospital, and not to apportion blame or to damage reputations. Indeed, a surgeon who has not submitted a clinical incident report for a situation which was, in retrospect, likely to lead to a medico-legal claim may be subject to justifiable castigation by hospital managers. The aim of such reports is to allow a coordinated approach to:

Medico-legal and risk management issues

◆ Ensuring the very best clinical care in the light of the problem.

◆ Thorough counselling of the patient and their relatives.

◆ Ensuring good documentation.

◆ Getting statements from relevant staff, while events are still fresh in their minds.

◆ Alerting the hospital's legal team to a potential problem at the earliest possible stage.

A clinical incident report should be submitted for any situation in which the surgeon sees a likelihood of complaint or litigation. This may range from the most serious disaster (for example: amputating the wrong leg); through complications causing serious disability - even if treatment has been of high standard (for example: paraplegia after aortic grafting); to concern about a patient or their relatives complaining unreasonably about their care on the ward.

Care and advice after discharge from hospital

The patient should be told clearly how to and where to return if there is a risk of early deterioration or important change in their clinical condition (for example: concern about possible infection in a diabetic foot or near a bypass graft; or a critically ischaemic foot awaiting surgery). This advice must be documented, and patients must be clear about exactly whom they should contact or where they should report. Failure to do this can result in accusations that they were "not told what to do" or "just pushed out, and look what happened". Explicit advice about the signs of graft occlusion, and what to do if they occur, is also necessary in the longer term for patients with bypass grafts.

If the patient has had problems or complication, ensure good follow-up, and easy access if the situation worsens. Failure to offer good follow-up risks the accusation that the medical staff "didn't care/weren't interested", which can help to fuel a medico-legal claim.

Summary

◆ There are increasing numbers of complaints and medico-legal claims relating to vascular services.

◆ These demand a high level of attention to all the details of communication, documentation and other risk management activities set out in this chapter.

◆ A vascular team with a culture of good, thorough, and sympathetic communication with their patients at all times is an unlikely target for frequent litigation.

◆ Information leaflets should be used for common vascular conditions and procedures **(A)**.

References

1 A first class service: quality in the new NHS. Department of Health. 1998.

2 An organisation with a memory. Department of Health. 2000.

3 Campbell B, Callum K, Peacock NA. *Operating within the law.* tfm Publishing, Shropshire, UK, 2001.

4 Brennan TA, Leape LL, Laird NM, *et al.* Incidence of adverse events and negligence in hospitalized patients. *New Engl J Med* 1991; 324: 370-6.

5 Gawande AA, Thomas EJ, Zinner MJ, Brennan TA. The incidence and nature of surgical adverse events in Colorado and Utah in 1992. *Surgery* 1999; 126: 66-75.

6 Wilson RM, Runciman WB, Gibberd RW, Harrison BT, Newby L, Hamilton JD. The Quality in Australian Health Care Study. *Med J Aust* 1995; 163: 458-71.

7 Goodwin H. Litigation and surgical practice in the UK. *Br J Surg* 2000; 87: 977-9.

8 Medico-legal claims in vascular surgery. Campbell B, France F, Goodwin H. *Ann R Coll Surg Engl* 2002 (in press).

9 Seeking patients' consent: the ethical considerations. General Medical Council, London W1N 6JE. 1998.

10 Reference guide to consent for examination or treatment. Department of Health, London SE1 6HX. 2001.

11 http://www.vssgbi.org

12 Clinical Negligence Scheme for Trusts. Risk management standards. London. National Health Service Litigation Authority. 2000.

13 Lindgren O. Clinical incident reporting in NHS Trusts. *Health Care Risk Report* 1996 (May): 15-17.

Chapter 36

Data collection and audit

Biddy Ridler Vascular Research Associate

Bruce Campbell Professor & Consultant Surgeon

VASCULAR SURGICAL SOCIETY OF GREAT BRITAIN AND IRELAND AND
DEPARTMENT OF SURGERY, ROYAL DEVON AND EXETER HOSPITAL, EXETER, UK

Introduction

The need for consistent and accurate data collection is crucial given the demands of clinical audit, governance and accreditation [1,2], quite apart from the motives of personal curiosity and service planning. The after effects of the Bristol affair and other high profile medical scandals have prompted a demand for accurate figures by which the performances of different hospitals and surgeons can be compared. At a national level vascular surgery is near the forefront of clinical audit in the UK. Vascular surgeons need to demonstrate their fitness to practise by providing evidence of a high standard of medical care. They are accountable not only to their patients but also to managers and to politicians - this is the essence of clinical governance.

Data collection is defined as the systematic gathering of data (information as a series of observations, measurements or facts) for a particular purpose from questionnaires, interviews, observation, existing records, electronic devices and other sources. It is usually followed by statistical analysis of the data [1].

Audit has many definitions (the Oxford English Dictionary lists six, dating from 1435), but perhaps the most relevant in a medical context is a "detailed review and evaluation of selected clinical records by qualified professional personnel for evaluating quality of medical care" [2].

Data collection and audit are inter-related, forming the so-called "audit loop" for assessing outcomes and implementing change where appropriate, and then seeing if real changes have resulted, by re-auditing. This process may be performed by an individual vascular surgeon, by the surgical team, by a multi-disciplinary group or by a professional organisation such as the Vascular Surgical Society of Great Britain and Ireland (VSSGBI). Audit can take the form of planned projects with collection of data over a limited period or continuous monitoring of outcomes. The information generated can be used at local level for departmental or hospital Trust reports; or nationally by specialist societies and by government departments.

It is often difficult to carry out thorough clinical audit in the "real world" of medical practice with its heavy workload, time restraints and limited resources. Some

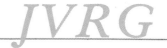

surgeons have designed their own systems - often dependent on personal efforts or adhoc arrangements for both data collection and input, and frequently incapable of easy interaction with other local or national databases. At the same time hospitals have introduced their own new information systems, but with similar deficiencies - they may fail to fulfil the requirements of clinicians and there are often insufficient staff for adequate collection of data for good comparative audit.

This chapter addresses the problems of data collection for clinical audit and offers some suggestions and solutions.

Data collection

What data to collect

The first problem in data collection is deciding what information to collect. It must be sufficient to provide meaningful outcome analysis, but there is always a risk of collecting excess data which wastes time. All the people involved need to meet to discuss the purpose and scope of data collection and to agree a minimum dataset. It is sensible to run a pilot study to check that the items agreed are straightforward and practical to collect and to see whether they withstand subsequent analysis [3].

Important words and terms should be defined in a data definitions list [4].

Methods of data collection

The way the data are collected will depend on the resources available (personnel and money) and also on personal choice and convenience.

- **On paper** The simplest method, which may not be particularly time-efficient, is on paper forms printed out and accurately copied as needed. The data can then be transferred manually or via a scanning software/analysis package such as snap (Mercator Research Groups Ltd, 5 Mead Court, Thornbury, Bristol, BS12 2UW) onto an electronic database. This method has been used

by the VSSGBI for audits such as National Outcome Audit 1999 [5].

- **Direct electronic transfer** Data may be transferred directly onto a general database, such as Excel or Access (Microsoft Corporation, One Microsoft Way, Redmond, Washington, 98052-6399, USA) or to a clinical tracking/integration system such as the Patient Analysis and Tracking System PATS (Dendrite Clinical Systems Limited, 5th Floor, 63-66 Hatton Garden, London, EC1N 3LE). The PATS system is currently in use for the National Vascular Database, collecting data from the three "key" or "index" operations which are abdominal aortic aneurysm repair (emergency and elective), carotid endarterectomy and infra-inguinal bypass grafting.

- **Local computer databases** Data may be entered onto an existing hospital or an individually designed "bespoke" system. This process can be done in "real time" - for example in the operating theatre, or retrospectively from the patients' hospital notes. Information such as the pathology reports may be viewed on the hospital computer system and integrated electronically or added in manually to the database.

Whichever method is used, some form of electronic data collection is recommended, and support will be required from the local Information Technology (IT) department. The level and quality of this support varies from hospital to hospital.

Data entry and personal responsibilities

Data may be entered by a variety of people such as data entry clerks, vascular nurses, research assistants, clinical audit staff or surgeons and their teams. Vascular surgeons, and those working closely with them, should ensure they collect as relevant and complete data as possible. It is important that the following principles are observed:

◆ Whoever enters data is responsible for accuracy and completeness.

◆ Data collection should be organised by a local coordinator who acts as the "keeper" of the data.

◆ Clinical information is confidential and for medico-legal reasons must be kept in a secure area.

◆ There must always be "back up" (for example to a server in the IT department) in case of computer failure.

◆ There must be safe means of transmission of data away from the place where it is entered to regional or national databases. Increasingly this is done electronically via "e-mail" on the World Wide Web. Most National Health Service (NHS) hospitals now have an electronic "firewall" set up using passwords and protecting the data by encryption (concealment). This process converts the data to cipher or code in order to prevent unauthorised access.

The Data Protection Act and patient identities

Patients' confidentiality must be protected by removing as much personal identification as possible to comply with the Data Protection Act 1998 [6] which came into force in 2000. This sets out rules for processing information and applies to paper records as well as those held on computers.

◆ Ideally only personal NHS numbers should be used in place of the patient's name - these are nationally recognised numbers but they are not available in every hospital at present.

◆ The current local hospital number and date of birth/age are the most commonly used patient identifiers to check for missing or erroneous data at present.

◆ Some departments provide their own patient codes relating to each specific audit and/or provide a user password to their database.

Protecting surgeons' confidentiality

Surgeons must also be protected if they are willing to contribute to comparative outcome audits. They should be asked to sign consent forms agreeing to release of their anonymised data for analysis, clinical presentations and future publications. An individual confidential code should be issued for each surgeon and for each hospital.

Hospitals must be prepared to provide evidence for verification of data, as at least 10% ought to be reviewed periodically for accuracy and completeness.

Practical tips for data collection

Accurate and accessible information is fundamental for good data collection, but the process depends on the conscientiousness and reliability of those who enter the data. The following tips may be useful, especially if data are being entered retrospectively or if data entry is being carried out away from the clinical area and from any regular contact with the clinicians:

◆ Ask the clinical secretary for copies of the relevant operation notes - this helps to track down emergency as well as the elective cases. Keep these copies for cross checking.

◆ Request direct computer access to the hospital information system - this makes it easier to find where any patient's notes/health records are located on the tracer system. They can then be "tagged" with a brightly coloured label, so that they are returned for data entry after the clinical episode has been completed.

◆ Check with the Medical Records Department that they agree to the placing of conspicuous adhesive labels stating the database name on the front covers of the notes. These labels will identify the patient should they return to the hospital and/or be readmitted. Follow-up data may then be obtained.

Chapter 36

Optimum working conditions for data entry

Occupational Health departments should provide advice [7], but the following are important practical tips for staff who spend many hours entering data:

- Use a good quality, height-adjustable supporting chair which has lumbar support and arm rests.

- Take care with your posture by sitting upright, elbows at 90 degrees to the horizontal, and wrists resting on the keyboard.

- Use as large a monitor screen as is efficient and affordable and ensure the screen is in front of you, not to the side.

- Clean your screen frequently.

- Inform your optician if you are spending the majority of your working day in front of a computer screen.

- Make sure you take occasional breaks away from the screen - five to ten minutes in any hour is recommended.

- Music from compact disks/tapes may aid concentration.

Explanation, evidence and process of audit

Standard outcome audit

This method looks at simple outcomes such as deaths and also complications, for example post-operative wound infections.

- It works for low-risk/simple procedures such as varicose vein surgery or hernia repair.

- It does not take into account the patient comorbidity, which may well influence the success or failure of more major surgery.

Comparative outcome audit

This method gives a more accurate and relevant result as it takes into account the casemix of a particular group of patients [8]. It uses those factors which are known from previous studies to influence outcome. The method by which adjustment for casemix is calculated is known as *Risk stratification*:

- This is a way of comparing groups within a given population (for example patients undergoing aortic aneurysm repair) who have different potential risk factors influencing a particular outcome.

- Agreed standards are established against which comparisons of individual surgeons (or individual hospitals) can be made.

There are various types of risk stratification. One of the simplest relates outcomes to separate risk factors in a table using the *Bayes theorem*. This involves a mathematical probability process which can be used to determine a particular outcome based on any combination of risk factors for a particular patient, building and re-defining the risk model as the data increase [9]. The process is known as *Bayesian analysis*. It is a set of mathematical rules for integrated evaluation of prior knowledge and new information. It revises the probability of a particular event happening based on the fact that some other event has already happened and is expressed in the form of *Bayes statistics* as the equation:

$P(H/d)=P(d/H) \times P(H)/P(d)$, where H is a hypothesis and d is experimental data.

The Bayesian meaning of the different terms is:

$P(H/d)$ is the degree of belief in the hypothesis H, after production of the data d

$P(H)$ is the prior probability of H being true

$P(d/H)$ is the ordinary likelihood function

$P(d)$ is the prior probability of obtaining data d

- The assessment of the level of risk, or complication rate, may depend on and be governed by many factors, for example - the patient characteristics such as age, gender, concurrent disease (such as diabetes), the timing of the admission and surgery, the grade of the operator and the urgency of the operation.

An example of a selection of potential risk factors relevant to vascular surgery is set out below:

1. Age	0-49, 50-59, 60-69, 70-79, 80-89, >89 years
2. Build	Normal, Obese or Cachectic
3. Diabetes	Yes or No
4. Gender	Male or Female
5. Number of Procedures	One, Two or >Two
6. Redo	Yes or No
7. Dyspnoea	None, On exertion or Limiting/at rest
8. Smoking	Never or Yes
9. Timing	Elective, Urgent or Emergency

These factors are used to produce a level of risk, or what is known as prior probability or odds [10].

The records are checked for consistency of data to exclude any errors. Then the cases are divided into sets, each set matched, for example, by hospital, surgeon and operative procedure. A risk model (see below) can then be applied, by a mathematical process known as logistic regression, to the first or training set and then tested against each subsequent or test set.

The *risk score* indicates the chance of a procedure-specific complication for an individual patient by a particular surgeon. It works best for selected "hard" or definite end points such as myocardial infarction or death, although as the data volume increases, risk scoring may be able to be applied to other outcomes such as graft occlusion or renal failure.

This process is used to produce a *risk model* which can be used to determine outcome for a particular

procedure. Individual surgeons can then compare their actual results against the national predicted outcomes to audit their performance.

As the volume of data grows, the more accurate will be the risk score and the risk model, provided the data are as complete and free of errors as possible.

The National Vascular Database

This database monitors the outcomes of the three index vascular procedures - abdominal aortic aneurysm repair (emergency and elective), carotid endarterectomy and infra-inguinal bypass grafting.

- The datasets (which can be viewed on the JVRG website) were based on a previous national audit carried out by the VSSGBI for two months in 1998, and reported in 1999. Vascular surgeons were invited to submit data for *all* operative vascular procedures during that interval [5].

- The data were subjected to risk stratification using the POSSUM (Physiological and Operative Severity Score for the enUmeration of Morbidity and Mortality) system, which had previously been applied to general surgical procedures [11].

- This produced a risk score specifically related to vascular procedures, and eliminated some irrelevant factors previously thought to affect outcomes.

- In addition, risk models were obtained from POSSUM physiology scoring alone which accurately predicted morbidity and mortality.

- Building on these results, it is now possible to provide increasingly accurate figures comparing the performance of an individual surgeon against the national standard. The reliability of the system will increase further still with the volume of data accumulated.

- Provided the surgeon carries out a reasonable number of cases (at least 10) each year then it is possible to produce accurate risk scored

Chapter 36

outcomes as time progresses. These are known as *cumulative risk scores* which provide an overall picture of performance and allow for both "bad times" (such as learning curves for new procedures or especially difficult cases) and "good times". The results produced may well become part of professional revalidation and reaccreditation in the future.

As an example Figure 1 illustrates the risk adjusted results of a hypothetical surgeon for hospital deaths (in theatre, ITU/Recovery or ward) from 1999 to mid - 2001.

demonstrate the pattern of occurrences over the same time interval.

When sufficient data have been entered, it should be possible to predict the outcome of a particular procedure for each surgeon, given the risk factors for each individual patient.

This may be demonstrated in a one-page report for an individual surgeon. Figure 2 shows the risk adjusted mortalities over 2 years for the index vascular procedures: carotid endarterectomy, infrainguinal bypass graft (IIB) and ruptured and unruptured

Figure 1 Cumulative mortality (risk adjusted) 368 cases - results of a hypothetical surgeon.

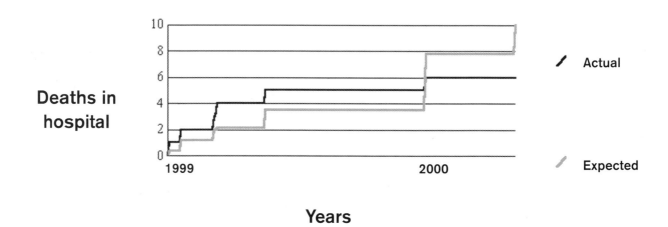

When collection of the surgeon's data first began, there were one then two more actual deaths (as shown by the black line) than expected deaths (as shown by the grey line). This levelled out to one more death during mid-1999 and 2000, after which the surgeon can be seen to have performed a little better than expected.

This example could equally apply to a group of surgeons within a vascular unit. It is important to note that these are cumulative figures, demonstrating outcome over time, and that they can be continued for subsequent years.

A simple ("crude") non-risk adjusted calculation of the number of deaths is "static" at the moment of calculation, does not allow for casemix, and does not

abdominal aortic aneurysms (AAA). The standardised mortality ratio (SMR) is the ratio of observed to predicted mortality, and the confidence interval (CI) expresses the possible range of results in which the true value lies. The results from each procedure for that particular surgeon can thus be compared with the national figures. The surgeon's results for unruptured AAA and carotid endarterectomy were within the expected limits while the outcome for ruptured AAA were better than expected. However, an observed mortality rate of 32.14% for IIB puts that surgeon's results below the predicted rate of 14.18%. This may be a warning marker, but it should be recognised that these are small numbers and, as demonstrated previously may be a period of "bad times", so caution should be exercised and subsequent results awaited and analysed.

Figure 2 Summary report by Consultant.

This report contains information on the four index procedures for Consultant code 1 in the period 1 Jan 1999 - 31 Dec 2001. Negative outcomes were defined as Died in theatre or Died in hospital.

	Carotid	IIB	Ruptured AAA	Unruptured AAA
Count	39	28	12	31
Observed mortality rate	0.00	32.14	8.33	6.45
SMR	0.00	2.27	0.19	0.69

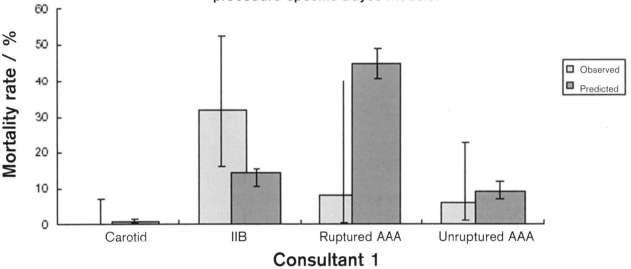

Observed and predicted mortality rates by procedure according to the procedure-specific Bayes models.

Consultant 1

Ruptured AAA
Recorded number of deaths = 1 out of a total of 12
Observed rate = 8.33% (95% CI: 0.44-40.25%) versus Predicted rate = 44.95% (95% CI: 41.02-48.95%)
SMR = 0.19 (95% CI: 0.00-1.03)

Unruptured AAA
Recorded number of deaths = 2 out of a total of 31
Observed rate = 6.45% (95% CI: 1.13-22.84%) versus Predicted rate = 9.30% (95% CI: 7.19-11.92%)
SMR = 0.69 (95% CI: 0.08-2.51)

Carotid
Recorded number of deaths = 0 out of a total of 39
Observed rate = 0.00% (95% CI: 0.00-7.39%) versus Predicted rate = 0.86% (95% CI: 0.41-1.42%)
SMR = 0.00 (95% CI: 0.00-10.89)

IIB
Recorded number of deaths = 9 out of a total of 28
Observed rate = 32.14% (95% CI: 16.58-52.43%) versus Predicted rate = 14.18% (95% CI: 10.74-15.83%)
SMR = 2.27 (95% CI: 1.03-4.30)

The more rapidly all vascular surgeons contribute to the National Vascular Database the more robust and helpful the data will become.

The vascular surgery dataset will be appraised periodically and amended as necessary and in the future may be integrated into patient care plans. These provide a concise multi-disciplinary approach to patient care and already contain some of the required fields for risk scoring. It is hoped that integration in this way would provide a more time-effective way of collecting data and improving its completeness.

Other specialties linked to vascular surgery have shown an interest in similar systems of data collection and audit. Vascular radiologists have developed their own datasets based on the vascular surgery parameters and vascular anaesthetists are evaluating a supplementary dataset.

Summary

♦ The demands of clinical governance make good data collection and audit a fundamental part of clinical practice **(A)**.

♦ National databases for comparative outcome audit will assume increasing importance as a means of auditing outcomes for individual surgeons and will come to form part of the process of reaccreditation.

♦ Accurate information produced in this way will provide a means of protecting both the surgeons and their patients in the future.

Further reading

1   The Vascular Surgical Society of Great Britain and Ireland. National Outcome Audit Report 2001 (in press).

Acknowledgement

We are grateful to Dr Robin Kinsman, Data Analyst, Dendrite Clinical Systems, for producing the charts for the National Vascular Database.

References

1   National Library of Medicine, PubMed MeSH Browser http://www.ncbi.nlm.nih.gov/PubMed/

2   National Library of Medicine, PubMed MeSH Browser http://www.ncbi.nlm.nih.gov/PubMed/

3   Prytherch DR, Ridler BMF, Beard JD, Earnshaw JJ. A model for national outcome audit in vascular surgery. *Eur J Vasc Endovasc Surg* 2001; 21: 477- 483.

4   The definitions associated with the Adult Cardiac Surgical minimum dataset of the Society of Cardiothoracic Surgeons GBI Database Report 1999-2000 Appx12 p154.

5   Earnshaw JJ, Ridler BMF, Kinsman R. The Vascular Surgical Society of Great Britain and Ireland National Outcome Audit Report 1999.

6   Data Protection Act 1998. Crown Copyright 1998. The Stationery Office Limited. ISBN 0 10 542998 8.

7   Croner's display screen equipment. Croner Publications Ltd 1992. ISBN 1 85524 1765.

8   Copeland GP, Jones D, Walters M. POSSUM: a scoring system for surgical audit. *Br J Surg* 1991; 78: 356-360.

9   http://www.bayes.com/theorem.

10   L'Italien GJ, Paul SD, Hendel RC *et al*. Development and validation of a Bayesian model for perioperative cardiac risk assessment in a cohort of 1,081 vascular surgical candidates. *JACC* 1996; 27(4): 779 - 786.

11   Prytherch DR, Whiteley MS, Higgins B *et al*. POSSUM and Portsmouth POSSUM for predicting mortality. *Br J Surg* 1998; 85: 1217 - 1220.

12   Campbell WB, Earnshaw JJ. Getting governance to work in surgery. *Ann R Coll Surg Engl* (Suppl) 2001; 83: 56-57.

Chapter 37

Clinical networks for vascular surgery

Martin Thomas Consultant Vascular Surgeon [1]

Jonathan Michaels Consultant Vascular Surgeon [2]

[1] DEPARTMENT OF VASCULAR SURGERY, ST. PETERS HOSPITAL, CHERTSEY, SURREY, UK
[2] SHEFFIELD VASCULAR INSTITUTE, THE NORTHERN GENERAL HOSPITAL, SHEFFIELD, UK

Introduction

Vascular operations are better performed by vascular surgeons with vascular anaesthetists [1] **(II)**. This has been generally accepted for elective vascular procedures but less so for emergencies. Many hospital trusts are now searching for ways of establishing emergency cover for patients with vascular disease in the belief that outcomes will be improved. Emergency vascular operations require a consultant surgeon but the lack of enough appropriately trained consultants in each hospital has made the provision of a consultant based emergency service difficult.

Specialisation in surgery

For centuries, surgery has been evolving specialties and over the past 100 years the process has accelerated. Orthopaedic and paediatric surgery, urology and thoracic surgery, to name but a few, have separated from general surgery. While this process is well advanced for elective surgery it has been slower to develop for emergencies. In bygone years I have operated urgently on patients with such diverse conditions as perforated colon, bleeding oesophageal varices, stab injury to the heart, infantile pyloric stenosis and of course ruptured abdominal aortic aneurysm. In the circumstances of elective surgery such cases would be treated by five different specialist surgeons (colorectal, upper GI, thoracic, paediatric and vascular) but for emergency cases this is often not so. The enlarging body of surgical knowledge has made it impossible for one person to practise all aspects of surgery. This, together with patient expectations and increasing litigation, is forcing ever more specialisation that now must also include emergency procedures.

Although exceptionally gifted surgeons may be able to turn their hands to many different operations, there is nevertheless evidence that a specialist who performs often a certain operation, such as resection of abdominal aortic aneurysm (AAA), will obtain better results. Surgeons who regularly perform an operation electively are likely to obtain better results when dealing with related emergencies.

Specialisation has not been driven by surgeons alone, but also by patient demand, by clinical governance and litigation, and by NHS guidelines.

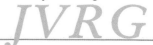

Recent reviews on cancer services have highlighted these trends and the same principles apply to emergency surgery.

Providing such specialist emergency rotas has proved very difficult as there are usually not enough surgeons in one hospital to work more than a single general surgical rota. A lone vascular surgeon cannot offer a seven day a week service. If vascular surgeons, breast surgeons and urologists no longer participate in the general emergency rota, then those that remain carry an unacceptably onerous commitment. The answer to this problem in vascular surgery is for a group of hospitals to co-operate in manning a vascular emergency rota.

In many parts of the country vascular services have grown without effective strategic planning. A number of reviews have been published concerning the problems of vascular services and emergency cover [2,3,4]. The Vascular Surgical Society of Great Britain and Ireland (VSSGBI) is currently tackling this problem. However it has become very clear that a solution cannot be imposed from above or by management.

Only clinicians can effect lasting changes in clinical practice that work. Although there are common principles in providing emergency cover, often arrangements reflect local circumstances [5,6]. It must be remembered, when making plans for vascular surgical services, that a significant workload involves venous disease, limb ulceration, amputation and varicose veins. Major arterial surgery is only a part of the service to be provided and it is easy to upset the balance.

Requirements for emergency vascular cover

Both the Surrey Vascular Group and the Avon Vascular Group have reported that over 95% of emergency vascular procedures are done by consultants [7,8].

A vascular emergency rota therefore requires a consultant vascular surgeon on call all the time. This surgeon should be supported by a vascular radiologist, as CT scans and angiography are required, an appropriately trained anaesthetist and have access to ITU beds. Ideally the vascular surgical rota should be separate from the general surgical rota. Only surgeons regularly involved in elective vascular surgery should provide an out-of-hours service **(A)**. According to a recent audit reported in 2000 by the VSSGBI, 40% of vascular surgeons have no fixed rota and only 18% rotate with another hospital [9]. Emergency arrangements remain ad hoc. Trusts have recognised the need for emergency vascular cover and a number of independent reviews have been commissioned such as a recent one in West London. It has been suggested that a group of four vascular surgeons should cover a population of 600,000 to provide an efficient service [10,11] **(B)**. A population of a million would require six surgeons. We have found that, for both the Surrey Vascular Group and the North Trent Vascular Network, a million people provide ample work, but without the surgeons becoming overwhelmed.

Models for provision of vascular services

There are a number of potential models for the organisation of vascular services, and each of these has its relative advantages and disadvantages. The difficulty that arises is in balancing the conflicting demands. On one side is the need for a large unit that creates the critical mass necessary to provide full emergency cover in both vascular surgery and vascular radiology, provides potential economies of scale and allows a degree of sub-specialisation. Against this are the needs to provide support to local services, equity of access, and to meet the clear public preference for local provisional services [12]. Essentially the possible models fall into three broad plans:

- The provision of large centralised units.

- "Hub and Spoke" arrangements.

- Collaboration between neighbouring hospitals.

Large centralised units

A potential model for the provision of vascular services would be to have large centralised units, similar to regional cardio-thoracic centres. This would allow the concentration of expertise, a critical mass of staff providing acceptable on-call rotas and economies of scale with potential for sub-specialisation, and the provision of specialist equipment. There are two main disadvantages with such an arrangement. The first and most significant is that vascular services cannot easily be isolated, and as long as there are smaller hospitals that provide a range of other acute services, there will be a need for some degree of local vascular support. In addition to this the centralised unit is the least effective in providing local access to services.

"Hub and spoke" arrangements

"Hub and spoke" arrangements are an intermediate arrangement in which there is a large unit at the "hub" hospital, with a planned network of surrounding "spoke" hospitals providing an agreed range of services. Such services need to be provided in an integrated way between the "hub and spoke" hospitals, and may have a combination of "out-reach" (in which specialist staff from the "hub" travel to the "spoke" hospitals), or in-reach (in which specialists from the "spoke" hospitals carry out some activities in the "hub"). In such an arrangement the emergency and much of the more specialist facilities are provided in the "hub", with out-patient facilities, day case operating, and a range of other services (depending upon the local facilities) being carried out in the "spokes".

The North Trent Vascular Network

In North Trent, a large vascular centre was set up in Sheffield in 1995 with the amalgamation of the vascular services at the Northern General and Royal Hallamshire Hospitals. In 1999 further re-organisation set up a North Trent Vascular Network in which there are two "hub" hospitals, those in Sheffield and Doncaster, with Doncaster providing support to a "spoke" in Worksop, and Sheffield providing support to Rotherham and Barnsley.

The "hub and spoke" arrangement around Sheffield provides a full range of emergency vascular surgical and radiological services on a continuous basis in Sheffield at the Northern General Hospital site. Out-reach vascular clinics and day-case operating are carried out at the other site within Sheffield and at hospitals in Barnsley and Rotherham. The "spoke" hospitals carry a range of other diagnostic and treatment procedures depending upon the available resources at each hospital. Such procedures include some diagnostic and interventional radiology, and a range of elective in-patient operating. The "hub" provides all emergency cover, usually with the transfer of patients, although it is occasionally necessary for the on-call surgeon to travel for an emergency, e.g. for a problem that arises in the operating theatre when there is no vascular surgeon on site. The out-reach service also provides support to other specialities, including such areas as joint diabetic clinics and ward referrals.

Major elective in-patient vascular operating represents a relatively small number of patient episodes compared with out-patient, diagnostic services and varicose vein surgery. The "hub and spoke" arrangement can provide a satisfactory solution in terms of access to local services, for both patients and other clinicians.

Equitable cooperation

This model works well for similar sized hospitals located within a reasonable distance of each other. Travelling time between hospitals should probably be no more than an hour although this has not been formally tested **(B)**. In more remote parts of the country longer travelling times do not seem necessarily to affect results [13]. If colleagues can agree on a format this system can be set up quickly and at minimal cost. The benefits of such a system to patients and clinicians alike can more than compensate for any potential problems many of which are illusory. One example covering a million people is to be found in Bristol. The clinical results of the Avon Vascular Group, which were reported to the Association of Surgeons of Great Britain & Ireland in April 2001, were excellent. In one year the group saw 86 patients with a ruptured aneurysm of which 69

Chapter 37

underwent surgery with a mortality of one third [8]. Another example of equitable co-operation is the Surrey Vascular Group which has been providing full-time consultant vascular cover for 4 years.

Surrey Vascular Group

The Surrey Vascular Group (SVG) was set up in 1997. Six surgeons from three trusts serve one million people. Hospitals accept their own vascular emergencies during the day, but from 5pm - 8am during the week and from 5pm Friday to 8am Monday, the on-call surgeon treats any urgent case. The Health Authority is 30 miles across at its widest point and the longest distance between hospitals, all of which are connected by dual carriageway, is 18 miles. Travelling time by road is therefore under an hour. Each surgeon is on call one night in six and every sixth weekend. Radiological colleagues try to mesh their own on-call with the surgical rota [14].

Who travels - patient or surgeon?

There has been much debate as to whether it is better for the surgeon to travel to the patient or vice versa. We have found that both are necessary depending on circumstance. It is often easier and quicker for the surgeon to travel (Table 1) especially for an opinion. Immediate travel by the surgeon is required for on-table vascular disasters which occur during operations on patients with orthopaedic, urological, gynaecological or other conditions (Table 2). Similarly patients with acute hypotension following a vascular catastrophe such as a ruptured aortic aneurysm may also be best treated without transfer.

Transfer of such patients can lose precious time. Once a patient has had a successful operation then they can be moved out to an ITU bed if none is available in-house. It is our policy to operate first and then seek an ITU bed for the survivors.

Frequently the junior surgeon on call will have little vascular experience and we have found it necessary in such cases to go and inspect any doubtful limb. To transfer an elderly and infirm patient 18 miles or more to another hospital on a Sunday, just for an opinion, is disruptive for the patient and family and is a burden on scarce resources. These patients require an ambulance often with a junior doctor and nurse escort to effect a safe transfer. Patients under the care of other clinical specialties who have had a secondary ischaemic event, such as limb ischaemia following myocardial infarction, are best visited. Similarly desperately ill immovable patients, usually on ITU, must stay put. I recently travelled to a neighbouring ITU to examine a 19 year old girl with meningococcal septicaemia and bilateral lower limb ischaemia. A dying patient who develops a dead leg for which no treatment is indicated should also be seen and the relatives interviewed. Transfer of such patients is inappropriate.

Some patients may be better off moved to the on call base hospital. If angiography, angioplasty, stenting or thrombolysis is being considered for acute limb ischaemia then this is best done in the base hospital (B). A close eye can be kept on progress without excessive travelling for the clinician. Furthermore we have arrangements that the hospital on call should provide radiological services including angiography. This allows the vascular radiologists as well as the surgeons in the other two hospitals to be off duty. A patient who requires a procedure or operation urgently that day, rather than immediately, can be transferred. A requirement for an ITU bed may need transfer within the group as available ITU beds can be scarce.

Workload

Workload has been audited and is summarised in Table 3. This shows that in a typical on-call weekend the surgeon will perform one major procedure such as repair of an abdominal aortic aneurysm and be involved in one lesser problem, such as instituting intravenous heparin therapy. At least one of the other two hospitals will be visited at least once as well as the base hospital. Two other significant phone calls for advice will be fielded. The busiest weekends to date have required repair of four abdominal aortic aneurysms in three different hospitals while occasionally no calls occur at all. An anxiety has been the risk of being called to two separate emergencies in different places at the same time. This has only

Table 1 Surrey Vascular Group - circumstances in which surgeon or patient travels.

SURGEON TRAVELS	PATIENT TRAVELS
OPERATION	Urgent Operation
Hypotensive vascular catastrophe (AAA)	Angiography/plasty/stent
On table disasters	Thrombolysis
Trauma	ITU bed
Acutely ischaemic limb	
OPINION	
Chronic ischaemic limb	
Dead leg	
Secondary ischaemic event	
Immovable patient	
Inexperienced juniors	

Table 2 On table disasters to which the author has been called urgently over the past ten years.

Ischaemic leg following fracture/dislocation	3 orthopaedic
Ischaemic arm following fracture/dislocation	2 orthopaedic
Damaged popliteal artery and vein (knee)	2 orthopaedic
Bleeding false aneurysm (femoral)	1 orthopaedic
Bleeding subclavian artery (trauma)	1 orthopaedic
Bleeding iliac and pelvic veins (hip)	1 orthopaedic
Bleeding iliac and pelvic veins (bladder)	1 urology
Bleeding iliac vein (laparoscopy)	1 gynae
Damaged aorta (laparoscopy)	1 gynae

Table 3 Surrey Vascular Group - weekend workload.

CAN ONE SURGEON COVER 1 MILLION PEOPLE?	
AVERAGE	One major procedure
	One minor procedure
	One other hospital visited
	Two other phone calls
MOST	Four ruptured AAA
LEAST	Zero calls
DOUBLE CALL	Twice in 3 years
DISTANCE	0 - 200 miles

occurred twice in three years. The on-call surgeon may have to drive up to 200 miles in a weekend visiting patients, although usually the distance is less than this. Once operated on, the patient is handed over to the home team the next day or on Monday for post-operative care. Easy and direct contact between surgical colleagues, by home or hospital phone and via e-mail, helps to insure seamless continued care. Such communication promotes mutual trust and is a stimulus to develop agreed treatment protocols and guidelines. Our experience demonstrates that a single vascular surgeon with adequate support can cover a million people for emergencies over a weekend.

Clinical forum and audit

The Surrey Vascular Group meets regularly to discuss clinical matters as well as management and policy. Clinical meetings include all members of the teams, vascular nurses and technologists, junior and senior surgeons, radiologists and others.

Cooperation between hospitals covering a million people can produce useful data and provides a powerful tool, not yet fully realised, for audit. Protocols

and guidelines for the management of patients can be developed. We have agreed antibiotic prophylaxis regimens for example. Although there is very much more to be done, we have achieved infinitely more than would have been possible as three separate centres.

Concept of a single department

Traditionally consultants have been appointed to a particular hospital and develop a fierce loyalty. For an equitable cooperative rota to succeed well such allegiances need to be mollified. In both Surrey and North Trent the concept of a single department of vascular surgery spread over several hospital sites has been developed. We believe that the primary allegiance of the doctors is to the clinical vascular service they provide and to its patients rather than to the bricks and mortar of a hospital building (Figure 1). This enlarged single clinical service will allow improvements in practice, agreed protocols, good audit and a comprehensive and co-ordinated training programme [15]. In many parts of the UK it is only by co-operating across old boundaries that new clinical services, that offer radical improvements for the patients, can be established.

The future

Health Authorities recognise that proper provision for emergency vascular patients is needed. Yet five out of six surgeons performing vascular surgery still do not have complete and reliable cover. The precise model depends on local circumstance. In an ideal world most surgeons would prefer to work in a single large centre.

Without a complete change in the pattern of health provision across the country, with fewer but larger hospitals, this is simply not an option in most areas today. A hub and spoke model or an equitable co-operation between hospitals can be instituted with minimal disruption. Surgeons need to look further than just arranging rotas. The establishment of a single vascular department with common policies, practices and training programmes is needed (A). Even if such a department is spread over more than one hospital site, more can be achieved for our patients than by disparate individual surgeons.

There are two main ways in which a satisfactory networked vascular service can be delivered, "hub and spoke" or collaborative arrangements. Examples have been given of areas in which such arrangements are already working. Each of these has different advantages and disadvantages, and will be appropriate to different geographical areas. In particular the "hub and spoke" arrangement is most suited to areas where there is a large single centre with one or more smaller surrounding centres of population, which are not individually sufficiently large to justify a fully equipped vascular unit. The collaborative arrangement will be more suited to areas in which there are hospitals that are placed closely enough together to allow collaborative emergency rotas, but in which each hospital is large enough to allow the development of a fully equipped vascular service.

Whatever the local arrangement, it is clear that the development of high quality vascular services requires an integrated network approach ensuring that existing evidence is used in providing formal arrangements for the management of vascular disease [16] (A).

Figure 1 The clinical network for vascular services.

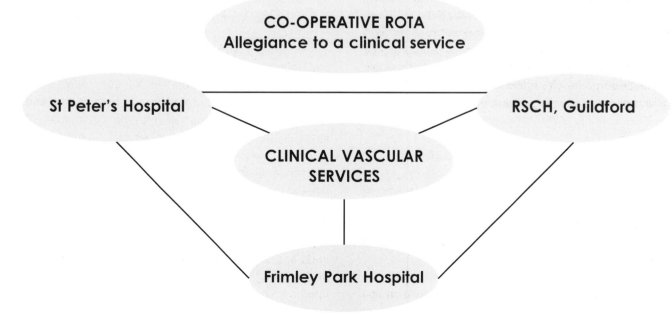

Chapter 37

Summary

♦ Health Authorities require proper provision of emergency vascular cover **(A)**.

♦ Nearly half the surgeons performing vascular surgery have no reliable rota.

♦ Different models will suit different circumstances.

♦ Hub and spoke or equitable co-operative rotas can be set up with minimal disruption.

♦ The single centre is an attractive concept but not feasible in most areas.

♦ Single cohesive departments serving half to one million people should be created **(B)**.

References (grade I evidence and grade A recommendations in bold)

1   Michaels J, Brazier J, Palfreyman S, Shackley P, Slack R. Cost and outcome implications of the organisation of vascular services. *Health Technology Assessment* 2000; 4 (11) 26-45.

2   **The Provision of Emergency Vascular Services. Vascular Surgical Society of Great Britain & Ireland at the Royal College of Surgeons, London. November 2001.**

3   Cook SJ *et al.* Patient outcome alone does not justify the centralisation of vascular services. *Ann R Coll Surg Eng* 2000; 82; 268-71.

4   Michaels JA, Galland RB, Morris PJ. Organisation of vascular surgical services: evolution or revolution? *BMJ* 1997; 309; 387-88.

5   Michaels JA *et al.* Provision of vascular services in the Oxford region. *Br J Surg* 1994; 81; 377-81.

6   Campbell WB, Ridler BMF, Thompson JF. Providing an acute vascular service: two years experience in a district general hospital. *Ann R Coll Surg Eng* 1996; 78(suppl), 185-89.

7   Dawson K, McFarland R, Thomas M. Shared emergency vascular cover between two district general hospitals: implications for a consultant service. Annual Meeting Vascular Surgical Society of Great Britain & Ireland, London, November 1997.

8   Baird RN, Baker AR, Hine C *et al.* Inter-hospital provision of emergency vascular services for a large population: Early outcomes and clinical results. *Br J Surg* 2001; 88 suppl 1; 50.

9   Earnshaw JJ. Audit of vascular surgical activity. Vascular Surgical Society of Great Britain and Ireland. November 2000.

10 Wolfe JHN. The future of vascular services: the need for a strategy. *BMJ* 1997; 315; 695-96.

11 Arora S, Wolfe J, Maheeswaran R *et al.* A strategy for vascular services - testing the 600,000 population model. *Ann R Coll Surg Eng* 2000; 82 ;176-81.

12 Shackley P, Slack R, Michaels J. Vascular patients' preferences for local treatment: an application of conjoint analysis. *J Health Serv Res Policy* 2001; 6: 151-7.

13 Shackley P, Slack R, Booth A, Michaels J. Is there a positive volume-outcome relationship in peripheral vascular surgery? Results of a systematic review. *Eur J Vasc Endovasc Surg* 2000; 20(4): 326-35.

14 **The provision of Vascular Radiological Services. Vascular Surgical Society of Great Britain & Ireland at the Royal College of Surgeons, London Nov. 2001**

15 Wolfe J, Wood R, de Cossart L. Inextricably linked: training and service in peripheral vascular surgery. *Ann R Coll Surg Eng* 1997; 79; 321-23.

16 **Michaels J, Palfreyman S, Wood R. Evidence-based guidelines for the configuration of vascular services. *J Clin Excellence* 2001; 3: 145-53.**

Chapter 38

Transfer protocols for vascular emergencies

Peter M Lamont Consultant Vascular Surgeon

Frank CT Smith Consultant Senior Lecturer in Vascular Surgery

VASCULAR SURGERY UNIT, BRISTOL ROYAL INFIRMARY, BRISTOL, UK

Introduction

Hospitals serving a population of 250,000 to 400,000 people find that two or three vascular surgeons are sufficient to cover the elective vascular surgery workload. As onerous emergency rotas become less acceptable in the modern era, so a conflict develops between the provision of elective services and the provision of an equitable emergency rota. The days of the pluripotential general surgeon, able to cope with every emergency from bleeding oesophageal varices to ruptured aortic aneurysm, are rapidly ending. Patients are demanding specialist expertise as evidence accumulates that surgical outcomes are better in the hands of specialist surgeons, especially in vascular surgery [1,2,3]. At the same time, newly appointed consultant surgeons who undertake no elective vascular surgery are understandably reluctant to manage emergency cases outside their own specialist field of interest.

Vascular surgeons can no longer depend on their general surgical colleagues to assist in the provision of a local vascular emergency service. Equally they do not wish to commit to a 1 in 2 or a 1 in 3 vascular emergency rota and cannot justify the appointment of additional vascular colleagues to expand the rota as there would not then be enough elective vascular work to go round.

One solution proposes that the elective vascular services from adjacent hospitals should coalesce on a single site [4]. Such a site would have sufficient numbers of vascular surgeons to provide an acceptable emergency rota and might continue to provide a vascular presence at the adjacent hospitals through out-patient clinics and day surgery lists. In practice this ideal has proved very difficult to achieve, except in a few large city conurbations. No hospital would willingly lose its elective vascular service and few settled and established vascular surgeons would wish to move to an alternative site. Nevertheless, in such a model, it is implicit that vascular emergency patients would need to be transferred to the emergency site from hospitals with no vascular emergency service.

Given that such centralisation is proving difficult to achieve, vascular surgeons are increasingly looking to provide collaborative emergency vascular rotas with neighbouring vascular units. Each unit provides an elective vascular service to its local population, but transfers patients or surgeons between participating

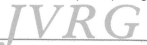

hospitals for emergency care. Audit studies to date show no adverse effects on patient outcomes by such collaborative arrangements **(II)** [5,6,7]. This collaborative model is discussed in more detail in the chapter on the provision of vascular services.

There are other variations offering combinations of the above centralist or collaborative models, but in most models patient transfers from the receiving hospital to the hospital on-call for vascular surgery are required, especially if a participating hospital has no elective vascular surgery service. There are some circumstances, such as a haemodynamically unstable patient or a patient who is already in the operating theatre after trauma, when the on-call vascular surgeon will have to travel to the receiving hospital. Given that the majority of vascular emergency cases will require transfer to the hospital on-call, the first question to ask is whether such transfers will compromise patient outcomes.

The safety of patient transfers

Much of the evidence for the safety of patient transfers relates to ruptured abdominal aortic aneurysm (RAAA). These patients are often elderly with significant co-morbidity and may be haemodynamically unstable. Time would appear to be of the essence if good outcomes are to be obtained.

There is good evidence that outcomes for elective surgery are better in the hands of specialist vascular surgeons **(II)** [3,8,9]. Paradoxically there is often no difference in the outcomes for emergency RAAA repair between vascular and general surgeons provided the hospital undertakes a significant amount of elective vascular surgery **(II)** [10,11].

While at first sight this lack of significant difference in RAAA mortality may argue the case against a vascular emergency rota, it must be remembered that these outcomes relate to operative mortality. When the overall mortality of RAAA presenting to a hospital is taken into account, a very different picture emerges **(II)**. A recent survey in Wales showed no difference in operative mortality between vascular and non vascular surgeons for RAAA (61% *versus* 69%) [11]. Conversely the overall mortality of patients presenting to hospital, including non-operated patients, was 65% for vascular surgeons but 89% for non vascular

surgeons (P<0.0001). This was because vascular surgeons operated on 89% of the patients who presented to hospital, whereas non vascular surgeons operated on only 36% (P<0.0001). A similar picture emerges in Scotland, where out of 372 patients with RAAA who were not transferred to a vascular unit from their presenting hospital in a 7 year period, only 24 (6.4%) underwent surgery and only 14 (3.8%) survived [12].

The risk of misadventure during transfer must therefore be balanced against the very low (4% - 11%) chance of survival by staying at the receiving hospital where it seems that non vascular surgeons are much less likely to offer an opportunity of surgical repair **(B)**. In fact it is extremely difficult to show that transferring patients with RAAA to a vascular surgeon offers any disadvantage. In units which receive cases from large geographical areas, the distance travelled by the patient to hospital has not affected outcome [12-16]. Likewise the time from onset of symptoms to surgery has no effect on outcome [16,17,18] and one study from America has shown no difference in survival provided the knife to skin time in haemodynamically stable patients is less than 6 hours from initial presentation to hospital **(III)** [19].

The most significant factors affecting survival from RAAA are signs of haemodynamic instability, either hypotension or cardiac arrest **(II)**. Patients who require cardiopulmonary resuscitation prior to surgery have very poor outcomes and fewer than 10% survive, even when presenting directly to vascular surgeons [17]. Many patients present with initial hypotension which responds rapidly to colloid infusion. The patient then stabilises and can be transferred. Difficulty arises when hypotension is sustained, but better than average results can be obtained even with hypotension lasting up to one hour before surgery. Mortality increases with duration of hypotension, being 30%, 58%, 63% and 65% respectively with durations of 1, 2, 3 and 4 hours [16]. Even after 4 hours duration of hypotension the outcome is better than in some hospitals without a vascular surgeon, as noted previously. Such patients can be transferred with active medical attendance if local arrangements preclude travel of the vascular surgeon to the patient **(B)**.

The Vascular Surgical Society of Great Britain and Ireland consider it safe to allow transfer times of up to one hour for RAAA and two or more hours for acute limb ischaemia [4]. The risk of clinical deterioration in transit is more than outweighed by the benefit of access to a fully equipped vascular service.

Which patients need transfer

The three main vascular emergencies are ruptured aneurysm, acute limb ischaemia and vascular trauma. When designing a protocol to suit local circumstances, the vascular surgeons involved need to decide whether they are just covering patients from the community needing emergency treatment that day, or all vascular emergencies whether they present in house or from the community. Most in house vascular emergencies arise during normal working hours and might be most easily dealt with by the local vascular team, even if they are not on-call. Indeed it may suit some units to provide emergency cover to collaborating hospitals only between 5pm and 8am, with local teams providing cover during normal working hours. Other units may choose to provide 24 hour emergency cover, so as not to disrupt the elective activities of the local unit when it is not on-call. Whatever the local choices, some clear agreement will be needed on who is responsible for emergencies arising in house **(A)**.

Likewise some patients with symptomatic but non leaking aneurysms or with acute on chronic lower limb ischaemia may not need emergency treatment on the day of presentation. Such patients can be kept under the care of the general surgeons at their admitting hospital and handed over to the local vascular team the next day. Where doubt exists in such cases, telephone advice from the vascular surgeon on-call may be more appropriate than an unnecessary patient transfer.

No patient would wish to undergo an uncomfortable transfer unless it was definitely required. Not all patients with an acute abdomen and hypotension have a ruptured aneurysm and further investigation with CT may be required to confirm the diagnosis. Up to 60% of patients may be misdiagnosed by the referring practitioner [18]. Patients with acute onset of symptoms and a tender pulsatile abdominal mass require no further investigation [20], but a mass is not always easy to feel in the acute, distended abdomen. In such cases the accuracy of CT at 92% [21] is preferable to the use of ultrasound, which

may only detect 51% of patients with a rupture **(II)** [18]. Thus where doubt exists a CT should be performed before arranging a transfer. Patients without a ruptured aneurysm are spared an unnecessary journey and the CT scans can be transferred with the patient when a leaking aneurysm is found.

In some haemodynamically unstable or unfit patients, the decision to transfer may be a difficult one and it may be better to transfer the surgeon if the hospitals are in close proximity. Likewise in acute limb ischaemia, the decision to transfer requires a suitable level of experience to discriminate between viable and non viable limbs. These decisions need to be made at a relatively senior level and require a degree of experience not normally found at the PRHO or SHO level. The protocol must therefore specify what grade of staff should be empowered to initiate the transfer and this will most likely be at SpR or Consultant level **(A)**. It is also essential to have some arrangements for alerting the on-call hospital's vascular team that a transfer is proposed, such as a direct SpR to SpR phone call. Figure 1 outlines an algorithm for the transfer of patients with a suspected ruptured AAA.

Other disciplines may be affected by the patient transfer. There should be clear local agreements on how to handle the transfer of a patient when no vascular radiology services or intensive care beds are available at the on-call hospital. It may be better to undertake radiology at the presenting hospital before transferring the patient to avoid the later return of the patient back to the presenting hospital because no vascular radiology service is available at the receiving hospital. Although it is ideal to run vascular surgery and vascular radiology rotas in parallel, the shortage of vascular radiologists and the demands of general radiology rotas may prevent this arrangement from being universally available at the present time. It is perfectly possible to run a successful vascular surgery rota even though a vascular radiologist is not always available at the receiving hospital, but vascular radiology is such an important part of emergency vascular services that vascular radiologists should be fully involved in the design of local transfer protocols **(A)**.

Likewise ITU consultants need to be fully involved in local discussions. There is often an anxiety that being on-call for a catchment population of over one million people will put excessive demands on the local ITU. In practice these anxieties prove groundless, but it may be useful to look at the total volumes of cases anticipated by an analysis of the number of ruptured aneurysms presenting at each of the collaborating hospitals per week before the rota is initiated. There is a possibility that hospitals without the collaboration may ask to transfer patients when their local vascular surgeons are not available. Some arrangement needs to be agreed between the vascular and ITU consultants as to their protocol when these requests arrive. Either all requests are accepted regardless or they are only accepted when appropriate facilities are available. It is much easier to deal with surges in demand where a *quid pro quo* arrangement exists and it may be that collaborating hospitals will agree to transfer ITU patients between each other to create space for the ruptured aneurysms at the on-call hospital. The creation of ITU networks has eased this problem.

Patients with vascular trauma may well have other injuries requiring expertise in other disciplines, such as Neurosurgery, Plastic Surgery and Orthopaedic Surgery. If these disciplines are only available at one site, if the patient is not fit for transfer or if the vascular injury has only come to light on the operating table then a patient transfer may not be appropriate and the vascular surgeon may need to travel instead. Strong liaison links are needed between the local general surgical team and the travelling vascular surgeon on-call in these circumstances to provide for immediate pre- and post-operative care when there is no local vascular surgical presence (A). In addition, the on-call vascular surgeon may need help from his general surgery colleagues to cover his home base emergency duties if he has to travel some distance to another hospital for a vascular emergency.

Mechanism of transfer

In the ideal world, every patient with a vascular emergency would be identified in the community and directed to the hospital on-call for vascular surgery. General practitioners need to be familiar with the emergency arrangements to facilitate this process. There is usually enthusiastic support from primary care for the idea of patients travelling if it means that they will get appropriate specialist treatment. Once the local medical communities become familiar with the rota arrangements, it is notable how many vascular emergency referrals are directed straight to the on-call hospital. It is essential for all the involved

hospital switchboards to have full rota and contact details to facilitate this process (A).

Not every vascular emergency is obvious though and not all patients present through their general practitioner. Some come through 999 calls to the ambulance service and some attend Accident and Emergency departments directly. Both of these services need to be involved in the protocol design.

The ambulance service is obliged to deliver an emergency patient to the nearest hospital unless specifically directed to pass its doors on the way to a more distant hospital on medical advice. Local GPs may not have details of which hospital is on-call for vascular emergencies, but the ambulance service can hold this information centrally and advise the GP accordingly. Robust arrangements need to be made with the ambulance service to keep them up to date with the on-call rota. Clear arrangements for leave are also needed to avoid last minute rota changes. All such administrative arrangements should be the responsibility of a designated manager from one of the participating hospitals (A).

There should also be established arrangements with the Accident and Emergency consultants regarding patient transfers. Transfers may need to be initiated by senior casualty medical staff if the general surgery on-call team are busy in theatre with another case. The ambulance service may prefer to respond to a 999 call from the A & E department to initiate a transfer when the patient is all set to go, rather than stand idle outside the door waiting for the patient to be resuscitated (A). Thought also needs to be given to who will accompany the patient, although this may vary from case to case and may best be left to the discretion of the referring hospital (B). There is little evidence that a doctor needs to accompany the patient. A paramedic ambulance is probably the best option.

Establishing the service

The first step in establishing an emergency vascular service involving more than one hospital is to ensure that all of the vascular surgeons and vascular radiologists enthusiastically endorse the principle and want to make the service work (A). All of these key participants should be involved in the service design and should feel ownership of it. The next step is to involve the local Health Authority(s), responsible for the provision of health care to the communities involved, and persuade them that the type of emergency service proposed is in the interests of the patients involved. A designated Public Health Consultant from the Health Authority can be a very useful facilitator when it comes to getting all the interested groups working together. The Chief Executives of the hospitals involved then need to agree the principles and direction from the Health Authority Chairman can smooth this process. A manager from each of the hospitals involved should then be designated to work with the clinicians in setting up the local arrangements. All of the clinical services affected by the arrangements need to be consulted and given the opportunity to provide advice **(A)**. These services include General Surgery, Interventional Radiology, Anaesthesia, Intensive Care, Accident and Emergency, Ambulance Services and local Primary Care Organisations.

There needs to be a strong commitment to audit of the service, especially the clinical outcomes **(A)**. The vascular surgeons should plan to hold regular meetings, not just to discuss audit outcomes, but also to iron out local problems as and when they arise **(A)**. Before instigating the service, a protocol which suits local arrangements needs to be written and agreed **(A)**. It should then be disseminated widely amongst the local medical staff.

An example of a local protocol is given below and is the one used in a collaborative network in Avon between the Bristol Royal Infirmary, Frenchay Hospital, Southmead Hospital and Weston General Hospital. Three of these hospitals lie within Bristol city and have local vascular units in close proximity, whereas Weston-super-Mare is some 25 miles distant and has no local vascular service. Weston General Hospital therefore sends all vascular emergency cases up to Bristol where Frenchay and Southmead share a week on-call, with the Bristol Royal Infirmary covering alternate weeks. This protocol therefore reflects these local arrangements and may not be suitable for collaborations between more geographically remote hospitals. The protocol is simply given as an example of the areas which need to be covered. The protocol is followed by a suggested clinical algorithm for the transfer of ruptured aortic aneurysm patients (Figure 1). Vascular surgeons interested in setting up an emergency service might

also read the recent Vascular Surgical Society of Great Britain and Ireland document describing mechanisms for the provision of vascular emergency services [22].

Avon emergency vascular rota - patient transfer protocol

◆ Vascular consultants will continue to provide 24 hour cover for their own patients unless they are out of town, in which case local arrangements to cover their patients should be clearly established and communicated to their junior staff.

◆ The emergency rota will be available for vascular patients who present acutely to hospital from outside with a condition requiring emergency treatment within 24 hours. These cases will predominantly be (a) ruptured aortic aneurysm, (b) acute limb ischaemia (c) vascular trauma.

◆ Vascular patients who present to the hospital with a condition that does not require emergency treatment within 24 hours (e.g. chronic limb ischaemia, symptomatic non-ruptured AAA) will be admitted to the surgical unit at the hospital where they present and will be handed over to the local vascular team the next morning. Until then they will be managed by the general surgical registrar at that hospital, who may take advice from the emergency on-call vascular consultant. If the local vascular team is not available within 24 hours (e.g. at weekends) then the patient may be transferred to the emergency on-call hospital at the discretion of the emergency on-call vascular consultant.

◆ Emergency cases which arise in house (e.g. graft thrombosis, post-operative haemorrhage, false femoral aneurysm or other interventional radiology complications), will normally be dealt with by the local vascular team regardless of whether they are on-call or not. If the local consultant is out of town then emergency assistance is given by the consultant designated to cover the local consultant's inpatients (see point 1 above). The emergency vascular rota is **NOT** a substitute for these arrangements.

◆ Emergencies which are identified by the GP as having a vascular cause will be diverted directly to the vascular on-call hospital by ambulance control. Cases referred on a 999 basis without GP input would be taken to the nearest A and E (i.e. ambulance staff are not expected to diagnose and divert vascular emergencies without medical staff input.) GPs may request admission of patients who are known to one hospital, back to that hospital even though it is not on-call, provided surgery is not required within 24 hours.

- Emergencies which are identified in an A and E Department as having a vascular cause **MUST** be assessed by the general surgical registrar on-call for that hospital. Patients who are haemodynamically stable and require treatment before the next day should be transferred promptly to the on-call hospital. If the General Surgery SpR is tied up with another case in theatre then a senior member of the A and E staff (i.e. Consultant or SpR) may initiate the transfer after discussion with the receiving SpR. The same would apply for consultants or SpRs in other specialties, to whom patients would be transferred back for further management and rehabilitation when their vascular surgical treatment has been completed.

  If there is doubt as to whether the patient needs emergency treatment before the next day, the registrar should discuss the case with the emergency on-call vascular consultant. Patients who are unstable (e.g. ruptured AAA with low BP, large vessel haemorrhage) should not be transferred but should be taken immediately to theatre by the registrar at the presenting hospital where they will be joined by the emergency on-call vascular consultant by request. Between 9 a.m. and 5 p.m. on Monday to Friday the local vascular team may be asked to help out under such circumstances if a consultant vascular surgeon is available to help.

- Where there is doubt about the diagnosis (e.g. abdominal pain but no obvious rupture) then investigation such as CT or ultrasound should be performed at the hospital of first presentation and a transfer to the on-call hospital initiated only **after** the diagnosis has been confirmed. The relevant CTs/ultrasound should be transferred with the patient.

- Patients should be ready to transfer before ambulance control is contacted. Ambulance control will then respond to a 999 call from the A and E department to transfer the patient and would not expect to be kept waiting on arrival at the referring A and E. The need for and number of escorts provided will be left to the discretion of the referring hospital. It is the referring hospital's responsibility to ensure that the ambulance is directed to the appropriate vascular on-call hospital according to the published rota.

- Emergency referrals from outside the Bristol and Weston catchment area should be dealt with as tertiary referrals on a consultant to consultant basis. Such cases should not be accepted by junior medical staff and cannot be accepted if they need ITU care unless ITU bed availability has been discussed beforehand with the ITU consultant. Emergencies within Bristol and Weston catchment area will be transferred regardless of ITU bed availability (subject to future review). Existing collaborative arrangements between the three Bristol ITUs would be invoked in cases where no ITU bed is available post-operatively, with the proviso that haemodynamically unstable patients would not be transferred between ITUs.

- At a junior staffing level, the emergency on-call general surgical team (PRHO, SHO, SpR) will continue to take clinical responsibility for all vascular emergency admissions at the on-call hospital. The general surgical SpR at a referring hospital must liaise with the SpR at the vascular on-call hospital before transferring a vascular patient.

- These protocols apply to Bristol hospitals only. Patients with vascular emergency conditions who present at Weston A and E department will all be referred up to Bristol according to current practice. Patients requiring emergency intervention the same day will be transferred to the vascular on-call hospital. Patients who do not require emergency surgery that day will be transferred, as now, to the Bristol Royal Infirmary. The vascular consultant on-call will be happy to advise in cases of doubt.

Figure 1 Clinical algorithm for transfer of ruptured AAA.

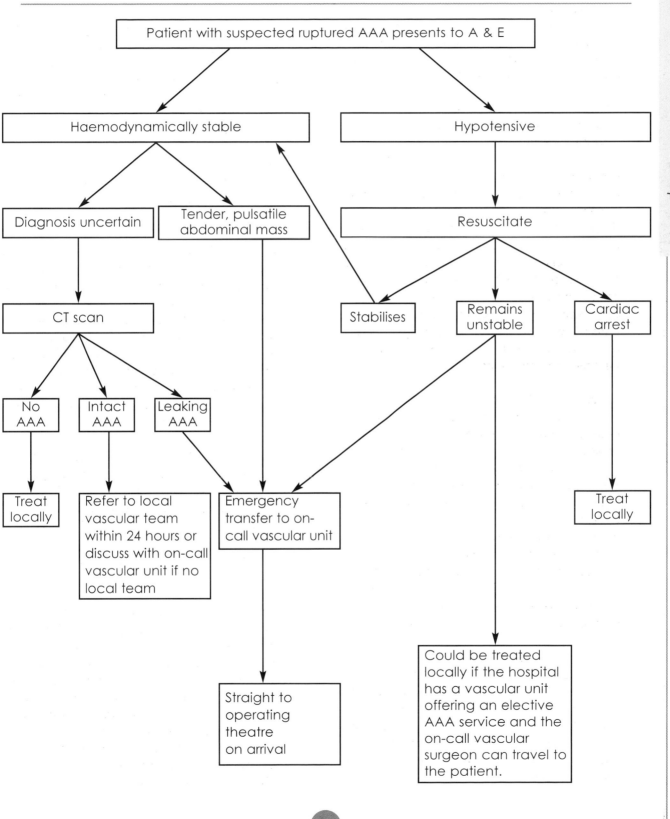

Chapter 38

Summary

♦ Patient transfers are an integral part of many different vascular emergency on-call collaborations.

♦ Patient transfers of up to one hour to adjacent vascular units are safe and any disadvantages are outweighed by access to a specialist vascular surgeon on-call **(II)**.

♦ The diagnosis should be established before initiating transfer **(A)**.

♦ The decision to transfer should be taken at SpR or Consultant level **(A)**.

♦ Patient transfers should follow locally agreed protocols, which have been designed with input from all involved parties **(A)**.

Further Reading

1   The Provision of Vascular Services, 1998 and The Provision of Vascular Emergency Services, 2001; both from the Vascular Surgical Society of Great Britain and Ireland.

References

1   Michaels JA, Rutter P, Collin J, Legg FM, Galland RB. Relation between rates of leg amputation and distal arterial reconstructive surgery. Oxford Regional Vascular Audit Group. *BMJ* 1994; 309: 1479-80.

2   Rutledge R, Oller DW, Meyer AA, Johnson GJ Jr. A statewide, population-based time-series analysis of the outcome of ruptured abdominal aortic aneurysm. *Ann Surg* 1996; 223: 492-502.

3   Kantonen I, Lepantalo M, Salenius JP, Matzke S, Luther M, Ylonen K. Mortality in abdominal aortic aneurysm surgery - the effect of hospital volume, patient mix and surgeon's case load. *Eur J Vasc Endovasc Surg* 1997; 14: 375-379.

4   Darke S. The provision of vascular services. The Vascular Surgical Society of Great Britain and Ireland 1998.

5   Woodcock SA, Hulton N. Provision of an emergency vascular service: a three-hospital model. *Br J Surg* 1999; 86: 703-704.

6   Cook SJ, Rocker MD, Jarvis MR, Whiteley MS. Patient outcome alone does not justify the centralisation of vascular services. *Ann R Coll Surg Engl* 2000; 82: 268-271.

7   Baird RN, Baker AR, Hine C, Lamont PM, Lear PA, Loveday E, Mitchell DM, Morse M, Munro EN, Murphy KP, Rees MR, Smith FCT, Thornton MJ. Interhospital provision of emergency vascular services for a large population: early outcomes and clinical results. *Br J Surg* 2001; 88: 598.

8   Wen SW, Simunovic M, Williams JI, Johnston KW, Naylor CD. Hospital volume, calendar age and short term outcomes in patients undergoing repair of abdominal aortic aneurysms: the Ontario experience, 1988-92. *J Epidemiol Community Health* 1996; 50: 207-213.

9   Tu JV, Austin PC, Johnston KW. The influence of surgical specialty training on the outcomes of elective abdominal aortic aneurysm surgery. *J Vasc Surg* 2001; 33: 654-656.

10   Lobo DN, Riddick AC, Iftikhar SY, Nash JR, Callum KG, Gudgeon AM. An audit of emergency abdominal aortic aneurysm repair to establish the necessity for an emergency vascular surgical rota. *Ann Roy Coll Surg Engl* 1999; 81: 156-160.

11   Basnyat PS, Biffin A, Moseley L, Hedges R, Lewis MH. Deaths from ruptured abdominal aortic aneurysm in Wales. *Br J Surg* 1999; 86: 693.

12   Adam DJ, Mohan IV, Stuart WP, Bain M, Bradbury AW. Community and hospital outcome from ruptured abdominal aortic aneurysm within the catchment area of a regional vascular surgical service. *J Vasc Surg* 1999; 30: 922-928.

13   Campbell WB, Collin J, Morris PJ. The mortality of abdominal aortic aneurysm. *Ann R Coll Surg Engl* 1986; 68: 275-278.

14   Vohra R, Abdool-Carrim AT, Groome J, Pollock JG. Evaluation of factors influencing survival in ruptured aortic aneurysms. *Ann Vasc Surg* 1988; 2: 340-344.

15   Cassar K, Godden DJ, Duncan JL. Community mortality after ruptured aortic aneurysm is unrelated to the distance from the surgical centre. *Br J Surg* 2001; 88: 1341-1343.

16   Barros D'Sa AAB. Optimal travel distance before ruptured aortic aneurysm repair. In: *The cause and management of aneurysms*. Greenhalgh RM, Mannick JA, Eds. WB Saunders, London 1990; 409-431.

17   Farooq MM, Freischlag JA, Seabrook GR, Moon MR, Aprahamian C, Towne JB. Effect of the duration of symptoms, transport time and length of emergency room stay on morbidity and mortality in patients with ruptured abdominal aortic aneurysms. *Surgery* 1996; 119: 9-14.

18   Akkersdijk GJ, van Bockel JH. Ruptured abdominal aortic aneurysm: initial misdiagnosis and the effect on treatment. *Eur J Surg* 1998; 164: 29-34.

19   Cohen JR, Birnbaum E, Kassan M, Wise L. Experience in managing 70 patients with ruptured abdominal aortic aneurysms. *N Y State J Med* 1991; 91: 97-100.

20   Adam DJ, Bradbury AW, Stuart WP, Woodburn KR, Murie JA, Jenkins AM, Ruckley CV. The value of computed tomography in the assessment of suspected ruptured abdominal aortic aneurysm. *J Vasc Surg* 1998; 27: 431-437.

21   Weinbaum FI, Dubner S, Turner JW, Pardes JG. The accuracy of computed tomography in the diagnosis of retroperitoneal blood in the presence of abdominal aortic aneurysm. *J Vasc Surg* 1987; 6: 11-16.

22   The provision of emergency vascular services. The Vascular Surgical Society of Great Britain and Ireland 2001.

Chapter 39

Developing Integrated Care Pathways

Sue Johnson Director, Venture Training & Consulting Ltd. [1]

Harvey Chant Specialist Registrar [2]

[1] MANOR FARM BARNS, DONNINGTON, CHICHESTER, UK
[2] DEPARTMENT OF SURGERY, DERRIFORD HOSPITAL, PLYMOUTH, UK

Introduction

The word "pathway" is being used with increasing frequency in healthcare language: Care Pathways, Pathways of Care, Patient Pathways, Anticipated Recovery Pathways, Service Pathways, Integrated Care Pathways, are all commonly used. However, the word "pathway" and the many jargon-terms that use "pathway" in their titles have a range of meanings to different people. This has created a great deal of confusion when discussing the merits of various health care pathways. This chapter will explain the Integrated Care Pathway (ICP) tool, and distinguish it from other interpretations and models that take on the term "pathway"; in particular the "Care Pathways" in the draft National Service Frameworks of the National Health Service (NHS).

What the ICP tool is NOT

National Service Frameworks (NSFs) are core guidance documents for targeted service provision and a central part of the NHS agenda. The New NHS [1] and A First Class Service [2] introduced a range of measures to raise quality and decrease variations in service including the NSFs. The NHS Plan [3] also emphasises the role of NSFs as drivers to ensure the delivery of the Modernisation Agenda [4]. NSFs are designed to ensure that "people in every part of the country can get the top quality and treatment of care they need, whether from their local doctors or community services, local district general hospitals or specialist regional centres" (National Service Framework - Coronary Heart Disease 1999) [5]. Each NSF that has been published sets out:

- national standards and defines service models for a defined service or care group;

- puts in place strategies to support implementation; and

- establishes performance milestones against which progress within an agreed time-scale will be measured.

The rolling programme of NSFs, launched in April 1998, takes forward the established frameworks already produced for cancer and paediatric intensive care and more recent published NSFs now include mental health, coronary heart disease (CHD), and

JVRG

older people. Diabetes is the next NSF to be published, and a draft version is available on the Internet for consultation. Information about all NSFs can be found on http://www.doh.gov.uk/nsf/

The relevance of the discussion of NSFs is that the recent drafts of NSFs have in their appendices flow charts or process maps that are called "Care Pathways". The labelled Care Pathways of the NSFs are not ICPs. Care Pathways in the draft NSFs are process flow charts that set out the desired service provision routes for care sectors, and not for individual patients. The draft Diabetes NSF has "Care Pathways" that describe broad, non-detailed steps that local services are required to interpret into actual service provision and practice at a local level. There is value in such system process flows, but they lack sufficient detail to inform local teams on how they should be delivering day to day care when face to face with actual patients.

It is unfortunate that the term "Care Pathway" has been employed by the NSF authors within the past year, when the term Integrated Care Pathway (ICP), which denotes something different, has been used in the UK for 10 years now. This has, and will continue to contribute to much confusion amongst health care professionals and service managers alike. An ICP is far more than a simple process map of service provision.

What the ICP tool is

An ICP ... "amalgamates all the anticipated elements of care and treatment of all members of the multi-disciplinary team, for a patient or client of a particular case-type or grouping within an agreed time frame, for the achievement of agreed outcomes. Any deviation from the plan is documented as a "variance"; the analysis of which provides information for the review of current practice" [6].

An ICP is a tool that enables teams to set out locally agreed multi-disciplinary/multi-agency best practice, based on evidence and national standards where available, as a record that is used as part or all of the patient's record of care. Variances to the anticipated pathway of care are documented as the

patient progresses along the ICP. Tracking and analysis of the variances for patient groups provides valuable information about standard and guideline adherence and about the outcomes of care, related to the processes of care delivery, thereby meeting the core requirements of true clinical governance.

The vital ingredient of an ICP is the facility to record, monitor, analyse and respond to the variances, and it is this function that is missing in other clinical record systems. Variance tracking is the only truly unique element of the ICP tool. Furthermore, a well-developed and effectively implemented ICP can deliver many of the requirements of clinical governance (B);

♦   Evidence-based practice at the point of care delivery.

♦   Risk management at the point of care delivery.

♦   Co-ordinated multi-disciplinary/multi-agency working.

♦   Improved documentation.

♦   Clinical audit.

♦   Outcome monitoring linked to processes of care.

♦   Development and education of staff.

♦   Standard and guideline implementation.

♦   Performance monitoring.

Developing and implementing ICPs properly has an impact on documentation, working processes and clinical practices, and demands that members of the patient care teams work in an integrated manner, thereby having an impact on multi-disciplinary and multi-agency team working.

Although there is confusion in the United Kingdom about the term "pathway", the ICP tool is distinct from other "pathways" in that an ICP sets out very specific best practice to be applied to individual patients, becomes the record of care, and vitally allows tracking of variances from planned care. If variances are not recorded, analysed and acted upon, the ICP is not working.

How to write an ICP

There are three stages in the development and implementation of ICPs:

♦ Writing the individual ICPs.

♦ Launching or implementing the written ICP.

♦ The contextual aspects of ICP development in terms of the infrastructure requirements and change management strategies that need to be employed for effective ICP development and ongoing maintenance at a directorate or organisational level.

There is not sufficient space in this chapter to give justice to all three stages - we will therefore concentrate on the first stage, of writing an ICP.

There are several key steps in the process of writing an ICP:

♦ Engage with multi-disciplinary/multi-agency team.

♦ Identify patient grouping.

♦ Identify episode.

♦ Map out best care/practice.

♦ Baseline audit.

♦ Set out as ICP record of care, ready for implementation

Engage with multi-disciplinary/ multi-agency team

Because ICPs by definition are "integrated", it is clear that to develop and implement this tool, all members of the health care team must be involved **(A)**. When an ICP is created, it attempts to describe locally agreed best multi-disciplinary care, based on evidence where it is available, in a document (paper or electronic) that will be an integral part of the patient's record of care. This requires a change in the way certain disciplines record their care. This change in practice is challenging and often threatening for many care professionals, and requires consultation and involvement of all stakeholders at the earliest opportunity so that the resulting ICP may be trusted and thus accepted by all health care professionals within that care setting.

The first practical step to gain involvement of all is to identify all the disciplines or members of the care team involved in the delivery of care. In vascular surgery, the team would involve as a minimum, the following staff:

Vascular surgeon

Vascular nurse (ward, theatre and angiography suite)

Vascular anaesthetist

Diabetologist

Vascular technologist

Interventional radiologist

Radiographer

Occupational Therapist

Physiotherapist

Wound care / tissue viability nurse

Limb fitter / prosthetist

Pharmacist

Clinical chemist

Haematologist

Ward Clerk

Porter

Involving all of these people need not mean many time-consuming meetings of 20 or more staff, which is both expensive and intimidating, often with little value. However, the process of drafting an ICP will require consultation with these people, and each team must find the most appropriate and effective manner of sharing the ICP writing process, so that opinions and expertise can be contributed from all levels and abilities. This could involve one-to-one sessions, or written drafts being distributed via internal mail or e-mail for consultation and edits to be gained from all in the team.

Gaining knowledge of patients' experiences is an important contribution to an ICP's development, so that patients' experiences can inform the order or timing or manner in which care processes are set out in the ICP and thus delivered.

Identify patient grouping

To write an ICP the patient group must be precisely defined **(A)**. Traditionally ICP groupings have been made by diagnosis (e.g. intermittent claudication or varicose veins) or by procedure (e.g. carotid endarterectomy). Certainly elective surgical procedures are reasonably predictable and are often the most simple ICPs to write.

However, diagnostic or procedural groupings are not the only methodology for determining an identifiable group of homogenous patients for whom you can set out an expected best practice process of care. An ICP can also be drafted for patients undergoing a common treatment, irrespective of their underlying diagnosis (e.g. electro-convulsive therapy, or smoking cessation classes). Generic ICPs are becoming more common, where the patient grouping is larger and less specific (e.g. pre-admission assessment, day surgery procedure, first consultant out-patient assessment).

Within vascular surgery, there are several patient groups that cover a majority of the caseload such as varicose veins, abdominal aortic aneurysms, carotid disease. But one point that makes ICPs so exciting for vascular surgeons is the fact that, in the main, they are dealing with a systemic disease (if atherosclerosis affects one site it is almost certain to affect another).

Identify episode

An episode of care can be as long or as short as required. For example, ICPs may be used in the treatment of varicose veins as day cases or be used for the conservative management of intermittent claudication over a long, supervised exercise programme. It is, however, important to accurately identify the target group (e.g. open aneurysm surgery as opposed to including open and endovascular approaches) and also to define the length of episode. Therefore there must be clear entry and exit, or start and end points for the ICP. Many ICPs within acute care start at admission and end at discharge from the inpatient setting. However, this is not the only episode that can be considered. An ICP could start in primary care, and go all the way through referral and treatment in secondary care, and back into primary care. However, a linear ICP of care that a patient is expected to follow over such a long period of care is unlikely to be appropriate, especially within vascular surgery, as even the most predictable arterial operations will have "variances from the expected pathway" if they are followed from primary care through hospital and out into primary care sometime later. This problem is a function of the often complex nature of vascular disease.

It may be more appropriate to consider each ICP as a smaller "bite-sized chunk" of the overall process, that then enables the clinicians to use each ICP chunk in turn, to build up the total care episode of the patient by bolting one ICP chunk onto the next. In this way the patient's progress can determine the type of ICP used, as their whole episode of care is built up from initial assessment in primary care through to final discharge from secondary care.

Figure 1 sets out some examples of such bite-sized ICPs that could be developed within a vascular surgery service. Once a patient enters the service, the appropriate ICPs would be selected and used as the patient progresses through the service, to build up a total record of care for the whole episode, made up of bite-sized ICPs bolted together (Figure 2). Using this system, one has the opportunity to apply guidelines, standards and best practice at every stage of care, with the facility to monitor what really occurs to patients at all times, related to their outcomes.

Map out best care/practice

Having engaged a multi-disciplinary/multi-agency team, chosen the patient grouping and selected the episode of care to be covered by the ICP, the framework is set so that the team can consider what

Figure 1 Potential bite-sized ICPs for vascular surgery.

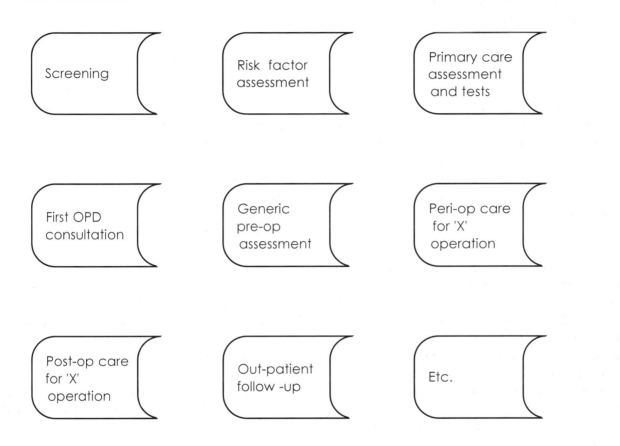

Figure 2 Bite-sized ICPs used for an individual patient.

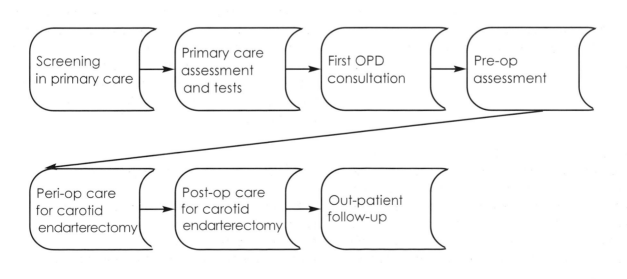

the best practice is for the chosen patient group, within the chosen episode of care. This requires the team to access and appraise the evidence of best practice, and to collate the standards and guidelines of practice for the topic area at hand.

This process can be simple if the team has the skills to access and appraise evidence. However, such skills are often lacking in clinical teams, as is the time to pursue such studies. Evidence-based practice is a core feature of clinical governance, so using this approach within the ICP tool system is no more than should be done already within existing professional duties. Although time is often a limiting factor here, library and internet resources, along with national guidance can be tapped into to reduce the time required to provide the evidence-base for the ICP.

Many teams find it useful to map out flowcharts of the care process, which often provokes healthy debate on what best practice should be for the patient population within the care episode you are considering. It is during this phase of writing the ICP that much consultation and involvement is needed from all members of the care team. It is important to reiterate that the involvement of all stakeholders at these early stages of development seem vital to avoid team members feeling left out and harbouring mistrust in the evolving ICP, which will hinder its effective implementation.

Baseline audit

In order to demonstrate the impact of the ICP on care, a baseline audit must be performed before the ICP is launched. The specific items to audit will depend on the particular ICP being developed. However, it is best to consider what aspects of care you most expect the ICP to have an impact on, or what areas are significant outcome measures for your patient group (e.g. graft patency, delay to discharge, length of stay, wound infection rates, patient being given information in writing, length of time on waiting list etc.) and to measure those in a baseline audit.

Baseline audit collection is important when developing an ICP. Once the ICP is written and implemented, and the ICP's variances have been analysed, the outcomes achieved with the ICP should be compared with the baseline audit, to show what impact the ICP has had.

Set out as ICP record of care

Determining the content of an ICP can be an exciting process that can build the team through wider understanding of each other's roles; however the difficult part of developing an ICP is to convert the care practices thus far mapped out into a record of patient care. It is the conversion of a detailed ICP process of care into a record of care that has often been the downfall of an otherwise good ICP care process.

Traditional records of care have been uni-disciplinary, and the Electronic Patient Record (EPR) developments in recent years have challenged this approach. ICPs challenge this too. The layout of an ICP is locally determined, as the ICP document (paper or electronic) must integrate carefully with the other documentation within a patient's record. Many Trusts in the United Kingdom have built their ICPs into the single multi-disciplinary record of care that replaces all other records. Some Trusts have used the ICP record to replace only part of the traditional notes employed by some disciplines.

The success of an ICP relies heavily on the quality of the data recording, and hence will depend on the style of the record of care (A). Producing records that do not integrate well, are time-consuming and complicated to complete, or constitute more paperwork for staff, will not encourage busy clinical professionals to use the ICP document. If the ICP record is not used, variances will not be recorded, thereby limiting the potential benefits of developing the ICP. No useful information is provided to the clinical team, to inform them of how to improve their care.

Discussion

The ICP tool offers many benefits for the vascular surgery multi-disciplinary team, including:

- Improved risk management.

- Improved team working.

- Identifying best, evidence-based multi-disciplinary practice.

- Implementing standards and guidelines into everyday practice.

- Monitoring of standards and guideline adherence.

- Equitable services for all patients.

However, are we not just re-inventing the wheel? One may argue that vascular surgery services have been providing evidence-based care to the best of its ability, using consistent records of care, in an equitable manner, for some time. Vascular surgeons have been at the forefront of monitoring and auditing their results and using the information to improve and upgrade their practices [7,8,9] (I).

In the 21st Century, all healthcare services in the UK are struggling under increasing bureaucracy, documentation, and cumbersome performance monitoring reporting systems that consume many precious hours of the clinical professional's time. Sadly, clinical governance seems to lead to more committees than effective quality improvement outcomes. One could thus argue that the ICP is simply compounding the scene by adding yet more to the full agenda of professionals.

Vascular surgeons and their teams must consider for themselves if they are really confident that they are providing the best care at all times, to all patients, consistently and equitably. If not, then what tools would you and your team consider to be the best to enable the team to provide care of a high standard at all times? The ICP is one such tool, that if implemented effectively, can meet the requirements of clinical governance and provide a means of not only identifying what best practice should be, but also monitoring whether or not it is being delivered at all times, and with what outcomes. In this way, the ICP can be considered as the glue that sticks all the responsibilities of risk management, evidence-based practice, etc., together for delivery through the one tool.

Summary

- The ICP offers a potential tool for improving the standard of care and providing a consistent and equitable service to vascular patients **(B)**.

- The development of high quality ICPs requires a multi-disciplinary/multi-agency approach **(A)**.

- Clarity is required about the patient population, procedure and/or diagnosis **(A)**.

- The combination of separate ICPs for smaller "bite-size chunks" of the care process may be advantageous **(B)**.

- ICPs must be developed on a foundation of agreed "best care" **(A)**.

- Special attention is required to the implementation, audit and documentation of ICPs **(A)**.

References (grade I evidence and grade A recommendations in bold)

1   The New NHS. Department of Health. 1997.

2   A First Class Service. NHS Executive. 1998.

3   NHS Plan. Department of Health. 2001.

4   The Modernisation Agenda, in the NHS Plan. Department of Health. 2001.

5   National Service Framework for Coronary Heart Disease. Department of Health. 1999.

6   Johnson S. *Pathways of Care*. Blackwell Science, Oxford, 1997.

7   **Ruckley CV, Stonebridge PA, Prescott RJ for the Joint Vascular Research Group. Skew flap versus long posterior flap in below knee amputations: Multicentre trial. *J Vasc Surg* 1991; 13: 423-427.**

8   **The UK Small Aneurysm Study Participants. Mortality results for the randomised controlled trial of early elective surgery or ultrasonographic surveillance for small abdominal aortic aneurysms. *Lancet* 1999; 352: 1649-1655.**

9   **European Carotid Surgery Trialists' Collaborative Group. Randomised trial of endarterectomy for recently symptomatic carotid stenosis: Final results of the MRC European Carotid Surgery Trial. *Lancet* 1998; 351: 1379-1387.**

Developing Integrated Care Pathways

Chapter 40

National Service Frameworks

Carolyn Nocton

Vascular Nurse Specialist & Cardiology Project Manager

Swindon and Marlborough NHS Trust, Swindon, UK

Introduction

This chapter provides an introduction to National Service Frameworks (NSFs) and identifies some of the key elements in the NSFs for coronary heart disease and older people and considers how these standards will influence the management of vascular patients or those at risk of vascular disease.

There are no immediate plans for a vascular NSF. An insight into current NSFs, in line with the evidence for vascular intervention and treatment outlined in this book, will enable the reader to consider the best evidence-based practice that should be implemented at a national level within the speciality and incorporated into care pathways.

National Service Frameworks

The Department of Health in 2000 introduced National Service Frameworks to facilitate "better, faster and fairer healthcare". These frameworks support the "Saving Lives: Our Healthier Nation" [1] National Priorities Guidelines for 2000-2003 document, whilst also reinforcing and facilitating the

NHS Plan [2] - a 10 year plan to modernise health and social care.

NSFs aim to:

- Specify interventions that are known to be effective.

- Identify, where possible, models of care that deliver those interventions reliably.

- Provide the means to implement systems of care.

- Develop audit tools and performance indicators to help ensure services are being delivered to an acceptable standard.

- Indicate the milestones and goals by which the NHS can monitor progress towards delivery.

- Identify gaps in knowledge or standards to inform research and other agencies.

- Institute a system for reviewing and updating the contents of the NSF in line with medical developments.

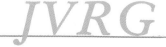

National Service Frameworks

The first priority areas for NSFs were identified as:

- Mental Health - 1999.

- National Cancer Plan - 2000.

- Coronary Heart Disease - 2000.

- Older People - 2001.

- Diabetes - strategy to be delivered 2002 and implemented from 2003.

These clinical areas represent the beginning of a series of NSFs to improve the quality and consistency of patient care. NSFs aim to stop the "post code lottery" of healthcare and provide recommendations for evidence-based quality treatment for everyone to prevent undesirable variations and inconsistencies in service delivery.

Each NSF reflects the principles of The NHS Plan [2], which states the NHS will:

- Provide a universal service for all based on clinical need, not the ability to pay.

- Provide a comprehensive range of services.

- Shape its services around the needs and preferences of individual patients.

- Respond to different needs of different populations.

- Work continuously to improve quality services and to minimise errors.

- Work together with others to ensure a seamless service for patients.

- Help to keep people healthy and work to reduce health inequalities.

- Respect the confidentiality of individual patients and provide open access to information about services, treatment and performance.

NSFs put in place strategies to support implementation of the standards including new money

and service redesign, recommending models of best practice. Beacon sites demonstrating best practice, high quality patient care and management are identified to share examples of service developments. These centres receive financial support to enable them to disseminate their learning to other organisations.

These NSFs are based on expert advice from External Reference Groups which reflect the wide range of expert professionals involved in each speciality. Management groups involved in care, organisations representing users and carers, service users, healthcare managers and partner agencies contribute to each NSF to cover primary prevention through primary, emergency and secondary care to rehabilitation.

An integrated approach to healthcare is required to implement NSFs and close working partnerships between primary and secondary care providers have evolved locally to provide a means of developing these standards. Collaboration and communication between Trusts and external agencies is essential to enable effective implementation of the NSFs. This work is intrinsically placed alongside collaborative working parties which focus on Health Improvement Plans and Local Modernisation Plans. The key principles of each underpin each other.

A First Class Service [3] identifies how clear quality standards would be set by the National Institute for Clinical Excellence (NICE) and National Service Frameworks to provide clear standards of service, delivered by local clinical governance networks and monitored by the Commission for Health Improvement (CHI), the NHS Performance Assessment Framework and The National Survey of NHS Patients. These systems provide a quality framework, which supports the implementation of NSFs.

Whilst recognising that there is not a specific NSF for Vascular Disease at this stage, there are some key elements of the Coronary Heart Disease and Older People NSFs that will undoubtedly have a direct impact on vascular patients and services. It can be expected that the Diabetes NSF will likewise influence the care of this well recognised high-risk group of patients with vascular disease.

National service framework - coronary heart disease

Coronary Heart Disease (CHD) remains amongst the biggest killers in the country. More than 110,000 die from heart disease in England each year, more than 1.4 million suffer from angina and 300,000 have heart attacks every year [4]. It is a Government priority to reduce incidence, suffering and death from CHD and it is recognised that this will have benefits for patients with other diseases. It is well recognised that over half of patients with peripheral arterial disease have coronary heart disease and therefore principles and recommendations of best practice within the CHD NSF could be applied to vascular patients. It is acknowledged within this framework that the standards will have a direct impact on the prevention and treatment of patients with peripheral arterial disease, transient ischaemic attacks and stroke. The summary of standards can be seen in Table 1.

Standards 1-4 include the benefit of health education programmes which could help reduce the incidence of peripheral arterial disease and stroke and specifically focus on those at high risk. Standard 2 is specific about reducing the prevalence of smoking in the local population and provides guidance on establishing specialist smoking cessation services for smokers who wish to quit. Vascular services should also have access to these specialist services.

The health education standards (3 & 4) include people with diagnosed CHD or other occlusive arterial disease and make the following recommendations:

♦ Advice about how to stop smoking including advice on the use of nicotine replacement.

♦ Information about other modifiable risk factors and personalised advice about how they can be reduced (including advice about physical activity, diet, alcohol consumption, weight and diabetes).

Table 1 NSF standards for coronary heart disease.

Standard 1&2	Reducing heart disease in the population
Standard 3&4	Preventing CHD in high risk patients
Standard 5,6&7	Heart attacks and other coronary syndromes
Standard 8	Stable angina
Standard 9&10	Revascularisation
Standard 11	Heart failure
Standard 12	Cardiac rehabilitation

Shaded areas: Standards for primary care with greatest impact on vascular patients.

Chapter 40

- Advice and treatment to maintain blood pressure below 140/85mmHg.

- Antiplatelet therapy advice - low dose aspirin 75mg daily.

- Statins and dietary advice to lower serum cholesterol concentrations EITHER to < 5mmol/l (LDL-C to < 3mmol/l) OR by 30% (whichever is greater).

- ACE inhibitors for people who have also had left ventricular dysfunction.

- Beta blockers for people over 60 years who have had a myocardial infarction.

- Warfarin or aspirin for people > 60 years who have atrial fibrillation.

- Meticulous control of blood pressure and glucose in diabetics.

The cardiac framework describes the treatment that patients with chest pain and heart attacks should receive to reduce their risk of disability and death and also provides clear direction on waiting times for investigation, intervention and treatment. It recommends development of local networks for cardiac care between tertiary centres, Primary Care Groups and Trusts, which agree common referral criteria, treatment protocols and quality improvement methods. Examples of protocols for assessment and treatment including effective medication are provided from Beacon Sites for other centres to adopt.

These themes could be similarly adopted by vascular centres to systematically review current practice and develop national standards to improve the quality of care for vascular patients. It should also be noted that the delivery of these standards could mean that the number of patients requiring vascular investigation and treatment increases through better management of CHD and a demand forecast by vascular services should be considered.

National service framework - older people

In England, census information suggests that between 1995 and 2025 the number of people over the age of 80 is set to increase by almost half and the number of people over 90 will double. It is well recognised that the majority of patients presenting with peripheral arterial disease are elderly and it could therefore be suggested that the demand for vascular services is likely to increase in the future. The summary of standards can be seen in Table 2.

Stroke

The NSF for Older People 2001 [5] considers major diseases and conditions that are common in older people and of most relevance to vascular services is stroke.

This standard identifies prevention as a main component for the development of integrated stroke services. It identifies cardiovascular disease as the main evidence-based risk factor and lists the following additional risk factors:

- Previous stroke or TIA.

- Hypertension.

- Atrial fibrillation.

- Other cardiovascular disease such as coronary heart disease and peripheral arterial disease.

- Carotid stenosis.

It recommends that patients with TIAs should be referred to a rapid response neurovascular clinic, managed by a clinician with expertise in stroke for investigation and treatment and recommends carotid endarterectomy for those with 70-99% stenosis.

Although the care pathway for stroke in this standard suggests referral to a neurovascular clinic in patients with a suspected TIA, it does not move beyond this step and consider the pathway of surgical treatment or produce recommended time frames for assessment and surgery.

Table 2 NSF standards for older people.

Standard 1	Age Discrimination
Standard 2	Person Centred Care
Standard 3	Intermediate Care
Standard 4	General Hospital Care
Standard 5	Stroke
Standard 6	Falls
Standard 7	Mental Health
Standard 8	The promotion of health and active life in older age

Shaded areas: Standards with greatest impact on vascular patients.

The standard on person centred care includes dignity in end-of-life care and provides a breakdown of key aspects of care that can be applied to any patient requiring palliative care. This aspect of care is perhaps not fully recognised in acute vascular settings where it could be suggested that the emphasis is often on surgical intervention more than the care and management required by patients with end stage vascular disease.

This NSF also identifies the need to establish additional intermediate care beds and services to promote rehabilitation that will of course be required for many vascular patients, most specifically amputees. This intermediate care service aims to prevent unnecessary acute hospital admissions, support timely discharge and maximise independent living.

Hospital care is a standard that sets out guidelines to ensure that older people receive the specialist help they need in hospital including access to specialist teams and ensuring quality of care.

Within the Older People NSF, the National Institute for Clinical Excellence (NICE) is referenced with particular mention of the clinical guidelines being completed on:

- Pressure ulcer risk assessment / prevention.

- Pre-operative investigation.

◆ Leg ulcers - clinical audit methodologies.

All these guidelines will require implementation for vascular patients for whom these clinical areas will feature highly. In addition to these areas it should be noted that there are also guidelines issued for wound debridement which are relevant to vascular patients.

National service framework - diabetes

These NSF standards [6] will be published in two stages with a delivery strategy in summer 2002 and implementation from April 2003. Details of this are available on the Department of Health website [7].

It recognises that diabetes is a common chronic disease, which can have serious complications including, if poorly managed, a reduction in life expectancy by between 10 and 20 years, particularly by raising the risk of coronary heart disease and stroke. Cardiovascular disease is between two and four times more common in people with diabetes and is the main cause of death. Stroke and peripheral arterial disease are identified as frequently occurring prevalent features in diabetic patients and within diabetes services and recommends that regular screening for cardiovascular risk factors should be mandatory.

Diabetes is the leading cause of non-traumatic amputation. Outcomes can be improved by early detection and management of cardiovascular risk factors, including blood pressure and lipids and early detection and management of long-term complications and lists foot complications as one of these. It is noted that less than a third of GP practices have routine access to a chiropodist.

The Scottish Intercollegiate Guidelines Network [8] illustrates an example protocol for the assessment and management of diabetic foot disease which includes vascular assessment and revascularisation and this is likely to be used as a model in the Diabetes NSF. Standard setting in diabetic services can be expected to increase the need of vascular teams for specialist advice.

Considerations for a NSF for vascular disease

Clearly there are standards of the CHD, Older People and Diabetes NSFs that can be applied to the risk management of vascular patients. Additionally, other common themes represented in these NSFs that should be considered for a NSF for vascular disease include:

◆ Recognition of immediate clinical priorities.

◆ Clear milestones and performance indicators to drive implementation.

◆ Rapid access to specialist services for high risk groups.

◆ Appropriateness of investigations and timescales for these.

◆ Action needed to reduce risk and complications.

◆ Nationally recognised audit standards and data collection requirements.

◆ A systematic approach to develop service models and local delivery plans.

◆ Collaborative working between acute and primary care and Health Authorities to agree protocols for referral, investigation, treatment and follow-up.

◆ Patient and user group involvement.

Summary

◆ There is an increasing level of expectation from patients and carers of healthcare services at a time of challenge and opportunity in the NHS.

◆ Care pathways incorporating the themes, appropriate common standards and the structure of the NSFs currently in place, will ensure the consistent delivery of quality vascular services demonstrating evidence-based care.

Chapter 40

◆ Vascular surgeons, nurse consultants, nurse specialists and other multi-disciplinary healthcare workers in acute and primary care have responsibilities to collaborate and develop working parties, adopting present NSF structures to address the needs of vascular patients and services as a preliminary measure to developing a NSF for vascular disease.

◆ A Vascular NSF will assist in raising the profile of the implications of peripheral arterial disease to the public.

Further reading

1   Department of Health. The New NHS: modern, dependable. The Stationary Office, London, 1997.

References

1   Department of Health. White Paper on Public Health, Saving Lives: Our Healthier Nation. DoH, London, 1999.

2   Department of Health. The NHS Plan. A plan for investment. A plan for reform. DoH, London, 2000.

3   Department of Health. A First Class Service: quality in the new NHS. DoH, London, 1998.

4   Department of Health. National Service Framework for Coronary Heart Disease. DoH, London, 2000.

5   Department of Health. National Service Framework for Older People. DoH, London, 2001.

6   Department of Health. National Service Framework for Diabetes: Standards. DoH, London, 2001.

7   www.doh.gov.uk

8   Scottish Intercollegiate Guidelines (SIGN) Network. Management of Diabetes. A national clinical guideline. SIGN Executive Royal College of Physicians, Edinburgh, 2001.

Websites

1   www.diabetes.nsf@doh.gsi.gov.uk
2   www.doh.gov.uk/chi
3   www.doh.gov.uk/nsf/coronary
4   www.doh.gov.uk/nsf/olderpeople
5   www.nice.org.uk
6   www.nhsbeacons.org.uk
7   www.kingsfund.org.uk

Chapter 40